Materials and Media in Art Therapy

The second edition of *Materials and Media in Art Therapy* provides an overview of material and media theory and practice in the field, with an emphasis on advances since the first edition.

This book takes an intersectional, anti-oppressive, social justice framework to theory and practice. The contributing authors represent multiple countries, write reflexively from their own intersecting identities, consider the use of materials from culturally aware and respectful positions, and reflect critically on the socio-cultural-political implications of materials and media in the context of therapy. Overall, the chapters provide a range of material and media applications in diverse settings, from conventional therapy practices to public practices focused on activism and well-being.

Thoroughly updated with the ongoing historical development of material and media use in the field and including extensive coverage of social and cultural issues faced by art therapy participants, this second edition is broad enough to be integrated into a course for a graduate program and specific enough to serve as a shelf reference for those in practice.

Catherine Hyland Moon is Professor Emerit in the Department of Art Therapy and Counseling at the School of the Art Institute of Chicago.

"This bold and brave book embraces the complexities found at the inter-sectionality of artist-therapist-activist-human. The contributing authors robustly identify the social, political, global, and ecological concerns of con-temporary art therapy, equipping practitioners with practical and theoretical foundations for addressing intersectional considerations the field seldom names. The book advocates for creatively disrupting, reconfiguring, building upon, or abandoning classical therapeutic approaches that no longer meet the diverse needs of clients, and holding space to meaningfully explore the impact of the current global climate on personal positionality. The text not only calls for collective transformation from therapist-activist perspectives but also shows clear and practical interventions whereby self-reflexive own-ing of accountability for harm in the face of working with difference, and clear actions toward reparations, are modelled and demystified."

Corrina Eastwood, co-editor and contributing author,
Intersectionality in the Arts Psychotherapies

"Through a collection of diverse storytellers, this book moves to decon-struct colonial and hetero-patriarchal perspectives within art-making by expanding, honoring, and uplifting the sacred, the magic, and the healing potential of art materials. These narratives center around the intersection-ality within the creative process, weaving together a beautiful constella-tion of potential between the self and community(ies). This book both challenges and celebrates art materials as vehicles for social change."

Megan Kanerahtenha: wi Whyte, art therapist and social
justice advocate from the Kanien'kehá:ka First Nation, and
author of *Walking on Two-Row: Reconciling First Nations*
Identity and Colonial Trauma Through Material
Interaction, Acculturation, and Art Therapy

"Completely revised to reflect the growing cultural diversity and critical con-sciousness of the field, this second edition of an already seminal text brings together a compendium of fresh voices to lead art therapy discourse into new, innovative directions. This wonderful text will inspire and provoke readers to rethink art therapy traditions and engage in a greatly more expansive view of how materials serve as active, relational partners in healing and care."

Lynn Kapitan, Mount Mary University, former
editor of *Art Therapy and past president, AATA*

Materials and Media in Art Therapy

Contemporary Theory and Practice

Second Edition

Edited by
Catherine Hyland Moon

Routledge
Taylor & Francis Group

NEW YORK AND LONDON

Designed cover image: Cover by Farah Salem titled POWER TO SEE BUT NOT BE SEEN, 2019

Second edition published 2026
by Routledge
605 Third Avenue, New York, NY 10158

and by Routledge
4 Park Square, Milton Park, Abingdon, Oxon, OX14 4RN

Routledge is an imprint of the Taylor & Francis Group, an informa business

For Product Safety Concerns and Information please contact our EU representative GPSR@taylorandfrancis.com. Taylor & Francis Verlag GmbH, Kaufingerstraße 24, 80331 München, Germany.

First edition published by Routledge 2015

ISBN: 9781032720173 (hbk)
ISBN: 9781032710181 (pbk)
ISBN: 9781032720166 (ebk)

DOI: 10.4324/9781032720166

Typeset in Caslon
by codeMantra

Contents

Acknowledgements   VIII

About the cover art   XI

About the authors   XIII

Introduction   XXII

SECTION I
History, theory, ethics, research   1

1   A contemporary history of art materials, media, and practices in art therapy   3
CATHERINE HYLAND MOON

2   Theories of materiality and making   29
CATHERINE HYLAND MOON

3   Ethical dimensions of materials, media, and practices in art therapy   49
CATHERINE HYLAND MOON

4   "Women's Work": women in the helping professions using crafts as self-care   70
GAL AMRAM AND EPHRAT HUSS

SECTION II
ART MATERIALS, MEDIA, AND PRACTICES IN CONTEMPORARY ART THERAPY 85

5 SIS, U BELONG HERE: BLACK WOMEN MAKING AND TAKING UP SPACE 87
VERONICA PRECIOUS BOHANAN

6 CLAWING OUR WAY OUT: ART THERAPY MANICURE RITUALS AND A FEMINIST ETHICS OF CARE 103
ROXIE ROSE EHLERT

7 HONORING OUR RELATIONSHIPS AND MATERIALS FROM OUR HOMELANDS 116
ZOË HARRIS (MASHPEE WAMPANOAG), ELLA MAHONEY (AQUINNAH WAMPANOAG), MICHELLE NAPOLI (FEDERATED INDIANS OF GRATON RANCHERIA), ASA PETERS (MASHPEE WAMPANOAG/ NARRAGANSETT), LEANA PILET (MASHPEE WAMPANOAG), BRITTNEY PEAUWE WUNNEPOG WALLEY (NIPMUC), AND RACHEL PARKS WINTERS, (CHEROKEE NATION OF OKLAHOMA/ᏣᏯᎠᎠᏋᏒ)

8 ART FROM INSIDE: PEER ART THERAPISTS REFLECTIONS ON MATERIALS AND MEDIA IN EXPLORING COMPLEX IDENTITY SYSTEMS 131
MAHLIE JEWELL AND CATHERINE CAMDEN-PRATT

9 PLASTIC MANDALA: ECO-ART AS COMPASSIONATE ACTION 147
EUNHAE JUNG

10 TRANSGENDER JOY AS COMMUNITY ART IN A "TRANS REFUGE STATE" 163
OWEN PAUL KARCHER AND G. NIC RIDER

11 SOCIO-POLITICAL STRESS AND ARTMAKING: CLOTHING, IDENTITY, AND SOCIAL CHANGE 178
MICHELLE KENDRICK HARTNEY

12 DRAWING CONNECTIONS: COMICS IN ART THERAPY
   PRACTICE   194
   RAKSHANDA KHAN

13 THE IMMERSIVE WORLDS OF THERAPEUTIC GAMING AND
   SCANOGRAPHY FOR ART THERAPY   211
   CHRISTINA MARRERO AND NATALIE RAE CARLTON

14 THE KITCHEN AS METAPHOR: SHAPING TOGETHERNESS
   AND THERAPEUTIC MAKERSPACES IN MARGINALIZED
   COMMUNITIES   225
   ROCHELE ROYSTER

15 THE NEOLIBERAL CO-OPTATION OF MINDFULNESS AND
   MANDALA PRACTICES   238
   KIRTHANA SELVARAJ

16 PLAYING IN THE DEEP: APPLYING IMPROVISATIONAL
   PRINCIPLES TO THERAPY   252
   VICTORIA TE YOU MOORE AND KATHARINE JOY HOUPT

17 A BOX OF FIRED CLAY BRICKS: BUILDING HOME ON THE
   COMMUNITY TABLE WITH PEOPLE ON THE MOVE   266
   MIRIAM USISKIN AND BOBBY LLOYD

18 FESTIVAL PEDAGOGY: ACROSS AND
   BETWEEN   281
   PAMELA WHITAKER

   INDEX   295

ACKNOWLEDGMENTS

The home where I edited this book and wrote three of its chapters sits on stolen land, the traditional territory of multiple Native Nations prior to their forced removal. I name this reality to acknowledge my identity as an invader/settler-colonizer; to grapple with the violence, displacement, dispossession, and erasure that occurred—quite literally—in my own backyard and continues to be enacted locally and throughout Turtle Island and other parts of the world; to unsettle my own and my White colleague's complicity with the invisibilizing of Indigenous struggles and survivance; and to go beyond apologies and contrition by making a commitment to material reparations.

Erasures and historical inaccuracies have made it difficult to identify the Indigenous groups that once flourished in McClean County in Illinois, Turtle Island/USA, where I currently live. The following statement was drafted by the local history museum in collaboration with the Kickapoo Tribe in Kansas, and Nichole Body, Director of the Native American House at the University of Illinois Urbana-Champaign: "McClean County is the ancestral land of many Native groups, beginning with the Paleoindians 12,000 years ago, and most recently Algonquin-speaking groups, including the Kickapoo, who were forced west from this area in the 1830s. Other groups in this area include (but are not limited to) the Peoria, Kaskaskia, Piankashaw, Wea, Miami, Mascouten, Odawa, Sauk,

Kickapoo, Mesquaki, Lenape, Potawatomi, Ojibwe, and Chickasaw Nations. These lands were and are the traditional territory of these Native Nations prior to their forced removal; and these lands continue to carry the stories of these Nations and their struggles for survival and identity" (https://mchistory.org/about).

As a small gesture of material reparations, I commit to donating a minimum of 15% of the proceeds of this book to the NDN Collective (https://ndncollective.org), an Indigenous-led organization whose mission is to "build the collective power of Indigenous Peoples, communities, and Nations to exercise [the] inherent right to self-determination, while fostering a world that is built on a foundation of justice and equity for all people and Mother Earth."

Not only did I undertake my writing and editing in a specific place, but also in a particular period of time characterized by significant worldwide upheaval and the erosion of democracy, equity, human rights, and the health of the planet. A part of me wanted to hide my head in the sand, not write a book about art therapy! And yet, write I did. I drew on my relationships with people past and present to find my inner courage and to be part of a collective commitment to justice. Among those people: my mom, always and forever, my mom. In the last years of her life, she planted seeds in the flower beds behind her house as she was preparing to move out—so that the unknown strangers buying her house would be greeted by flowers in the spring. How about that as a metaphor for responding to these troubled times! And then there is my principled daughter who stood up for trans kids even when it made her a pariah among the neighborhood social group. And my son, who doesn't have a macho bone in his body and frequently tells his friends and family members how much they mean to him. And my husband who writes and performs songs that challenge injustice and sometimes make people uncomfortable. I also have to mention my "accountabilibuddies," Lauren, Mary, and Carol. We decided to keep meeting after our anti-racism training ended—and have been meeting now for years. My ArtWorks community studio co-facilitator, Jackie, has brought tenderness and authenticity and laughter to pretty much every encounter I've ever had with her or witnessed her having with others. The world needs more people like you! My East African colleagues—Eunice, Sane, Nelly, Grace, Maeda, Christa, Mukasa, and

Isaac—and my travel companions—Linda, Sarah, Michelle, Naimah, and Emily Anne—are all incredibly fierce, compassionate, creative, and committed people who know how to face hardship without conceding joy. You inspire me! Finally, there are the former colleagues and students from Marywood University and the School of the Art Institute of Chicago whose voices, artistic visions, and perspectives live on within me and have continued to teach and challenge me. For all of those I have named—and many more who have gone unnamed—I am so grateful for you. You are partly responsible for this book, as you have helped me keep my head out of the sand, my eyes wide open, my curiosity sharp, and my commitment strong.

Of course, there are also people who more directly made this book possible. Amanda Savage and Sophie Dracott at Routledge patiently supported my writing process and, when necessary, nudged me along. Farah Salem gave permission for her beautiful and poignant artwork to grace the cover of this book. I am so honored by your generosity. To all the contributing authors, I am immensely grateful to you for your willingness to share your stories, perspectives, theories, artworks, insights, and passionate convictions. You do important, essential work in a world that needs all the help it can get.

ABOUT THE COVER ART

POWER TO SEE BUT NOT BE SEEN (2019) by Farah Salem, video and fabric cutwork installation, 23" × 38" fabric panels, 16' × 16' installation space.

The artwork draws on a quote by Fadwa ElGuindi, "Who has the power to see, but not be seen?" The metaphor of Mashrabiya, the wooden lattice work on oriel windows featured in Islamic architecture, is used to reflect on this question. In the installation, fabric is used to reinterpret Mashrabiya screens, creating portals that negotiate the boundaries between visibility and invisibility through its flexible yet structured form. Projected videos show desert landscapes with rock formations created by vulnerable exposure to weathering while veiled in snow. There is also footage of kaleidoscopic eyes and a shadow figure wandering in white sands, appearing and disappearing through the landscape, echoing the tension between visibility and invisibility. The same occurs for the installation viewers' bodies as they move through the installation.

Special thanks to Kialo Winters (Diné of the Ta'neeszhanii, Kinyaa'áanii, Táchii'nii, Honghanii clans) for guiding the artist through the traditional homelands of the Diné, Pueblo, and Jicarilla Apache, also known as the Bisti/De-Na-Zin Wilderness in northwest New Mexico where the majority of the video footage was filmed. And for sharing the importance of this land and its history with Indigenous people of the region. Winters reminds us as viewers and visitors that upon encountering this landscape, "Witnessing erosion change will be miniscule in our lifetime, but as visitors, we can always wonder what it will look like thousands of years from now."

ABOUT THE AUTHORS

Gal Amram is a social worker (MSW) who supports individuals and groups through the healing power of crafts. With experience in working with survivors of sexual abuse and the LGBTQ+ community, she guides clients on a journey of self-discovery and emotional well-being. Gal also facilitates creative workshops for helping professionals, emphasizing the transformative power of the creative process and the benefits of collective expression.

veronica precious bohanan is a womanist cultural worker and multidisciplinary healing arts practitioner. She grounds her work at the intersection of art therapy, healing justice, ancestral wisdom, liberatory and somatic practices, and meaning-making. She founded create.heal.share. to center Black women's wellness and cultural resonance through every season of being and becoming. Through its signature program, *Sis, U Belong Here*, veronica curates sista-circles that honor Black women's lived experiences and foster self-expression, belonging, and a deep recognition of inherent worth. As an instructor at the School of the Art Institute of Chicago, she teaches in the Art Therapy & Counseling Department. She is also a playwright and poet.

Catherine Camden-Pratt (I/we, she/they) lives on unceded Gund-ungurra Country, is a social ecologist, artist, peer art therapist, writer, and casual lecturer in the Master of Art Therapy at Western Sydney University. They are co-editor of the *Journal of Creative Arts Therapies*. Catherine is a nationally awarded university arts-based experiential educator. She works with children, families, and adults in her clinical practice, and for ten years facilitated groups for people living with cancer. An exhibited mixed-media artist focusing on social justice, artistic themes emerge from personal stories of sexual assault, domestic violence, and 'madness,' using mirrors to invite questions about viewers' implicit locations in social justice.

Natalie Rae Carlton has facilitated multisystemic art therapy and counseling experiences focused on the therapeutic use of diverse materials, including fabric crafts, clay, drawing and painting, digital photography and video, sound recording, and printmaking. Justice, systems, feminism, and queer theories have been grounding orientations for Carlton's therapy support, graduate teaching, and leadership. Carlton has authored scholarship regarding digital media use in art therapy and the therapeutic use of comics, zines, and graphic novels. Natalie is an Associate Clinical Professor in the MA and PhD Creative Arts Therapies (CAT) Department at Drexel University in Philadelphia, Pennsylvania.

Roxie Rose Ehlert (she/her) is a disabled, queer femme artist, art therapist, and educator. She is a faculty member at Southwestern College and at the Institute for the Development of Human Arts. Her teaching explores disability justice and collective healing through an abolitionist and transformative mental health framework. Her scholarship addresses the need for anti-oppression approaches to art therapy education and practice that dismantle sanism, racism, and heteronormativity in the field. Her personal art practice explores themes of home, grief, dreams, and queer belonging, using stitch work, printmaking, broken glass, alphabet stickers, nail polish, and a #2 pencil.

Zoë Harris is a public health practitioner living in Chicago, Illinois. She is a citizen of the Mashpee Wampanoag Tribe and has worked with her tribe as well as urban Native populations on topics related to indigenous wellness. Zoë is also a Jamaican citizen and has family roots in Selma, Alabama. Therefore, she strives to bring an intersectional lens to all her work. She has also worked on projects related to infection prevention, mental health, police violence, and racism as a public health issue. In her free time, she loves cultivating plants and practicing traditional finger weaving.

Michelle Kendrick Hartney is a Chicago-based artist, activist, and art therapist whose work engages with issues of reproductive justice, gender, and healthcare in the United States. Through mediums like fiber, ceramics, wood, and social practice, she creates projects that address obstetric abuse, postpartum PTSD, gender-affirming care, and the impacts of racism and misogyny on maternal health outcomes. Her art not only highlights these pressing issues but also invites public discourse and advocacy for change. Her work has been published in *The New York Times*, CNN, BBC Radio, *The Guardian*, *Ms. Magazine*, *Vice*, PBS, *Women's Health*, *Art in America*, Artnet News, and *Hyperallergic*.

Katharine Joy Houpt is an art therapist and artist in Chicago. She works in private practice with adults using arts-based, relational, psychodynamic, and somatic approaches. Katharine's artistic practice includes collage, fiber art, watercolor, comics, and improv. She is Assistant Professor, Adjunct at The School of the Art Institute of Chicago. Katharine has presented nationally at conferences including "Yes And" Mental Health Therapeutic Improv Conference, the Graphic Medicine Annual Conference, and several art therapy conferences. She co-authored an award-winning paper, "Anti-Memoir: Creating Alternate Nursing Home Narratives Through Zine Making," with people living in a skilled nursing facility. Katharine exhibits artwork nationally and maintains a regular studio practice.

Ephrat Huss is Professor of Social Work and Art Therapy at Ben-Gurion University of the Negev. She heads an innovative MA social work specialization that integrates arts in social practice and has 40 students doing social arts projects per year. She has a background in fine arts. Her areas of research are the interface between arts and social practice and arts-based research, using art to access the voices of marginalized populations. Specifically, she has received competitive grants and published much on arts-based research with Indigenous Bedouin women and youth in unrecognized villages in the south of Israel.

Catherine Hyland Moon (she/her) is Professor Emerit in the Department of Art Therapy and Counseling at the School of the Art Institute of Chicago. Editor of this text and author of *Studio Art Therapy: Cultivating the Artist Identity in the Art Therapist*, her scholarship is focused on the unique contributions of arts-based approaches to therapy, community-based art studios as public healthcare, the ethics of international collaboration and exchange, and intersectional care within art therapy praxis. Currently, she co-leads cross-cultural therapeutic arts paraprofessional training programs in East Africa and co-facilitates a free community art studio in the United States to cultivate collective care across social differences.

Mahlie Jewell (she/they/I/we/us) is a proud autistic queer disabled Wiradjuri woman living perpetually displaced due to the housing crisis and currently living on Dharug Country. She holds a Master of Art Therapy and certifications in Narrative Therapy, Dialectical Behavior Therapy and co-design. Mahlie works alongside other autistic people who share her experiences of complex trauma and identity systems, queerness, blakness, chronic illness, and disability. She is completing post-graduate research with Latrobe university connected to autistic people and art therapy. Her lived experiences of trauma and the internal systems that enable survival are embraced and vital to her ability to support others.

Eunhae Jung is an artist and art therapist who works in eco-art, art therapy, and community art. She studied art at Queen's University in Canada and art therapy at the School of the Art Institute of Chicago. Now living on Jeju Island in South Korea, she seeks to address the climate crisis and societal issues through art and art therapy. She has authored several books in Korean, including *Transformative Art Journaling*. She has received awards for her eco-art initiative, including the Minister of Culture Citation in 2023 and the Beautiful Earth Human award from Green Korea United NGO in 2022.

Owen Paul Karcher (he/they) is an art therapist, lecturer, author, and manager of the Comprehensive Gender Care Program at M Health Fairview. Through embodiment and creative expression, he works with the individual and collective healing of trauma and oppression. He has 15 years of experience working in mental health, violence prevention and intervention, HIV/AIDS, building healthy relationships, LGBTQ resiliency, and transgender liberation and healthcare access.

Rakshanda Khan is a Registered Canadian Art Therapist, Registered Psychotherapist, and the Research and Publications Chair of the Canadian Art Therapy Association. As a South Asian immigrant and settler in Tkaronto (Toronto, Canada), Rakshanda approaches art therapy from an anti-racist, anti-oppressive, trauma-informed framework. Her scholarly interests include graphic medicine, digital and online creative processes, as well as traditional arts practices to guide healing.

Bobby Lloyd is an artist, art therapist, supervisor, lecturer, and CEO of Art Refuge. Since the early 1990s, her work has taken place in both statutory and community settings in the UK and internationally in contexts of conflict and upheaval. As a lead practitioner for Art Refuge with people who are displaced, she also develops and delivers training on psychosocial, trauma-informed ways of working for frontline workers across contexts. Her interests lie in the roles of socially engaged art and adapted art therapy in relation to displacement, crisis support, community and social justice, and she writes about this work.

Ella Mahoney is a teacher and artist living in Brooklyn, New York. She is a citizen of the Aquinnah Wampanoag Tribe, and much of her artwork is inspired by legends from her tribe and her experiences of indigeneity in Aquinnah. Her artwork centers around storytelling as a form of cultural resilience, survival, and visioning for the future. She has illustrated children's books for the Wampanoag Language Reclamation Project, collaborated with the Long Island Children's Museum to create visual accompaniments for their land acknowledgment, and occasionally shows work in galleries.

Christina Marrero (she/they) is an art therapist in private practice and adjunct faculty. She is focused on helping sensitive and creative neurodivergent adults build and maintain meaningful lives. Her practice integrates Compassion-Focused Therapy and Acceptance and Commitment Therapy frameworks with focus on burnout recovery, anxiety/depression management, grief, and unmasking. She sees the flexibility of art therapy as one of its greatest strengths. It is her hope that art therapy will continue to defy binaries, break down barriers, and be a relief from the suffering inflicted by rigidity.

Michelle Napoli is an art therapist whose community-based work focuses on cultural continuity, authentic identity formation, and Native language revitalization as prevention and wellness. Kanni he ka'inniiko tuppe kaa peta luumaamu ke tookawmu ke 'eyye kochchaamu. My family and I are from Peta Luuma, Tookaw, and 'eyye Kochcha. Michelle is an assistant professor in the expressive therapies department at Lesley University. She is a citizen of the Federated Indians of Graton Rancheria and lives on her homelands.

Rachel Parks Winters is a higher education scholar-practitioner from Oklahoma now based in the Boston, Massachusetts area. She is a citizen of the Cherokee Nation of Oklahoma/ᏣᎳᎩ ᎠᏰᎵ and works with Native communities within and beyond UMass Boston. With a background in student affairs and community engagement at institutions of higher education, her research focuses on tribal community-university relationships and the process of shaping higher education to be a tool for self-determination and nation-building for Native communities. She is a dancer, a crafter, and enjoys growing traditional Cherokee foods.

Asa Peters is a member of the Mashpee Wampanoag Tribe and part of the Narragansett Tribal community. He is an educator, researcher, and musician currently working as a Land Steward at the Native Land Conservancy. Asa enjoys engaging in collaborative and creative projects with Tribal communities in the northeast in the realms of history, archive development, dance and music, and plant relationships. He is trained in fields of Botany, Music, and Technology (BA, Connecticut College), and Critical Ethnic and Community Studies (MS, UMass Boston).

Leana Pilet is a licensed mental health counselor specializing in expressive arts therapy and serves as the director of youth and young adult treatment services. A citizen of the Mashpee Wampanoag Tribe and of Haitian descent, Leana's work highlights the importance of exploring intersectionality, fostering community-based healing and wellness, and the transformative power of the arts. Her experience spans from clinical practice, education, and consultation that is deeply rooted in trauma-informed approaches. In her free time, Leana enjoys spending time in nature and engaging in the arts.

G. Nic Rider (they/them) is Associate Professor and licensed psychologist at the Institute for Sexual and Gender Health and the Director at the National Center for Gender Health, both of which are housed at the University of Minnesota Medical School. Their research broadly focuses on social and structural factors affecting the lives of marginalized communities, including trans and gender-diverse individuals, and resilience/strengths identified by these communities. They participate in committees advocating for trans individuals of all ages locally, nationally, and internationally.

Rochele Royster is an art therapist, community psychologist, and educator with over a decade of experience in clinical and community settings. Holding a Doctorate in Community Psychology from National Louis University and a Master's in Art Therapy from The School of the Art Institute of Chicago, Royster specializes in healing-centered approaches and care and the therapeutic use of creative expression. As the founder of the Dolls4Peace project, Royster has led community-based art interventions to address gun violence and promote understanding and healing through art. As a faculty member at Syracuse University, she integrates practical experience with academic rigor, inspiring students to explore the healing potential of art.

Farah Salem (b.1991, Kuwait) [Book cover artist] is an interdisciplinary artist and somatic art therapist. These two practices exist independently, yet are intertwined as her professional training informs her artistic inquiry of how trauma manifests in the body. Her visual arts practice is rooted in photography and expands through video, performance, and installation,

finding subtle affinities between geologic time, somatic movement, gendered trauma, and Arabian Peninsula ceremonial healing rituals. Through
relational merging and mapping of human and geologic bodies, she envi-
sions their liberation by examining themes of agency, making the invisible visible, and the potential erosion of socio-cultural conditioning. www.
farahsalem.com

Kirthana Selvaraj is an academic and practicing contemporary artist
currently teaching at Western Sydney University within Sociology and
Art Therapy. Her research centers on decolonial praxis, critical pedagogy,
and intersectionality in art therapy education and practice. Kirthana
graduated with distinction in both a Bachelor of Fine Arts from University New South Wales Art & Design and a Master of Art Therapy
from Western Sydney University. Currently completing her Doctor of
Philosophy at the University of Sydney, she is focused on reimagining art
therapy pedagogy. Her work has been published in the Journal of Creative Arts Therapies (JoCAT) and her art has been exhibited at the Art
Gallery of New South Wales and the Art Gallery of Western Australia,
as well as being held in national and international private collections.

Victoria Te You Moore is an artist and psychotherapist in private practice. She provides individual and group psychotherapy to adults. She also
offers training groups and bilingual clinical consultation to clinicians in
the United States and China. She serves on the faculty of the C. G. Jung
Institute of Chicago and the American Group Psychotherapy Society, as
well as the board of Clowns Without Borders-USA. She has been integrating improvisation and physical theater into psychotherapy and the
training of psychotherapists for over a decade. In addition to English, she
is fluent in Mandarin and French and speaks passable Spanish.

Miriam Usiskin is an art therapist, supervisor, and co-programme lead
for the MA Art Therapy at the University of Hertfordshire, UK, with a
background in National Health Service (NHS) acute settings. Since 2016
she has been a lead practitioner for Art Refuge, working with people
who are displaced in the UK and internationally, and developing and
delivering training on psychosocial, trauma-informed ways of working

for frontline workers across contexts. Her interests include adapting art therapy for contexts of conflict and upheaval, resilience, and the role of hope. She is completing a Doctorate on The Community Table model of practice developed in northern France.

Brittney Peauwe Wunnepog Walley, Nipmuc, is an interdisciplinary thinker, traditional weaver, and tribal activist. Brittney earned an MS in Critical Ethnic & Community Studies and a concentration in historical archaeology from the University of Massachusetts, Boston. She earned a BA in Sociology with minors in philosophy and business management from Rhode Island College. Brittney's work encompasses cultural continuity, wellness, and history. Her weaving work has been featured in various museums in the northeast and beyond. Weaving enables her to honor her ancestors while uplifting present and future generations. Brittney & her fiancé have two tabby cats and a shared interest in martial arts.

Pamela Whitaker is a lecturer in art psychotherapy at the Belfast School of Art, Ulster University. Her art therapy practice contributes ecologies of care within higher education and community contexts, which support hospitality as art. She has written about festival art therapy, the walking studio, the art of home, and environmental art therapy. Her professional ethos is dedicated to anti-oppressive practices within art therapy and curating studios within streetscapes, localities, and civic society that meet people in their daily experience. She supports people in these life studios, encouraging the creative use of materials from home and the affordances of lived-in surroundings.

INTRODUCTION

Catherine Hyland Moon

This book takes a critical approach to theorizing art materials, media, and processes, and an intersectional, social, and environmental justice framework to applying these ideas in practice. Unlike many second editions that contain revised and new chapters but retain the majority of content from the first edition, this is an entirely new book. Since the first edition was published, there has been a proliferation of literature about art therapy materials, media, and practices. There have also been dramatic changes in social, political, and environmental conditions at a global scale, and they have had a profound impact on the well-being of people and the planet. These factors together made the complete overhaul of this book necessary.

There are fundamental aspects of this book that have been carried over from the first edition. Art materials and media still have a central role in art therapy as constituents through which meaning is made. They provide a sensorial, tangible, nuanced, intelligible, diverse vocabulary through which to communicate thoughts, ideas, and experiences, some of which would be impossible to convey in any other way. The definition of art also remains almost without boundaries, as do the materials used in contemporary art. Despite the more central role of art materials and processes in art therapy research and practice, the art therapy literature still often holds unquestioned reliance on Western, modernist, middle- or upper-class constructions of art and on individualistic, medicalized Eurocentric orientations to practice. This limited perspective is, in part, a reflection of the field's failure to locate art therapy within the broad context of historical and contemporary art practices.

What has changed since the first edition was published is the much wider range of art materials, media, and practices being employed in the field. They have become the focus of research and practice, rather than ancillary subtopics of clinical practice. Materials are no longer taken for granted, but rather reflect applications that are often intentional, contextually relevant, and culturally attuned. While some art practices, such as those that engage or embellish the body, remain largely absent from the literature, there are other approaches, like fiber arts and social practice that now have a much more prominent place in the field.

An extensive discussion of materials, media, and practices within contemporary art is beyond the scope of this book. However, two general trends are worth noting. First, there are themes in contemporary art practice that are strikingly congruent with the practice of art therapy. Contemporary artists are interested in transformative art practices aimed at interconnectedness, justice, reciprocity (LeBaron & Sarra, 2018) and bringing disparate people together despite divisions (Elkin, 2023). Also, themes of care are common, whether in relation to care ethics (Millner & Coombs, 2022), interpersonal care practices (Lee, 2022), or ecological care (Neal, 2023; Weintraub, 2019). Second, while the diversity of art-making materials continues to be limitless, materials are no longer viewed as inert substances but are understood as having liveliness, vitality, and agency (Cabañas, 2021; Weintraub, 2019). This view of materials is consistent with how many art therapists have described the making process, as a partnership between makers and materials, with each partner affecting and being affected.

The increased alignment between contemporary art and art therapy in relation to transformative care practices and appreciation for material vitality is a sign of an intentional practice of hope in the face of a world where profit is prioritized at the expense of individual, collective, and environmental well-being, and individual responsibility is valorized while the potential for flourishing is undermined (Mundt, 2021; Skaife & Martyn, 2022). This book does not position art materials, media, and practices as separate and unrelated to care for the world. Instead, it examines how approaches to artmaking are either implicated in—or working to repair— the fracturing of the world. Questioning our complicity with society's dominant assumptions, norms, ideologies, and values, particularly in relation to the arts and well-being, is an ethical responsibility.

As a White, middle-class, currently nondisabled, cisgender, heterosexual, female-identified, settler art therapist with U.S. citizenship status, I hold responsibility for critically reflecting on my complicity with unjust systems and acting to redress harms, even when my harmful in/action is inadvertent. I consider this self-reflexive and reparative stance a necessary counterpart to critiquing my profession, with both being expressions of hope and commitment to professional justice, care, and ethics (Moon & Faulkner, 2024). From reflecting on the entanglements of our individual identities, families, and cultures, to considering how we are complicit in the field's individualistic, Eurocentric, White, cis-hetero-patriarchal, ableist conventions (Eastwood, 2022; Gipson, 2015), art therapists can contribute to collectively fashioning a more inclusive and equitable profession, one that is committed to socially just, culturally respectful, ethically responsible use of arts media, symbols, motifs, and practices.

Overview of book

The first section of this book addresses overarching themes concerning the history, theory, and ethics of materials and media use in art therapy, along with a chapter focused on research. The second section of this book concentrates on the application of art materials, media, and processes in art therapy practice. The contributing authors present a diverse range of perspectives and approaches, from using conventional to innovative materials, from focusing on a single material to a wide selection of media, from addressing individual distress to social harm, from working in private to community-based settings, and from positioning their work as therapy to activism. Overall, the authors' material practices are responsive to the social, cultural, political, geographical, and environmental contexts within which their practices take place.

In the first chapter, *A Contemporary History of Art Materials, Media, and Practices in Art Therapy*, I provide an overview of contemporary developments in material and media use, with an emphasis on the advances most widely represented in the literature: crafts, ecological approaches, digital media, cultural considerations, and research. I also provide an overview of materials and practices that are underexamined or largely absent from the literature and highlight potential future directions.

The second chapter, *Theories of Materiality and Making*, addresses current theory related to the significance of materials and media. I describe two art therapy theories, the Expressive Therapies Continuum and the Social Constructivist Theory, and discuss the strengths and shortcomings of each. I then present two additional theories, Critical Theory and New Materialism, and discuss their implications for deepening socio-cultural-ecological theorizing relative to the therapeutic use of artmaking practices.

The third chapter, *Ethical Dimensions of Materials, Media, and Practices in Art Therapy*, begins with an in-depth discussion of cultural appropriation, followed by consideration of ecological, socio-cultural, economic, accessibility, and safety aspects of using art materials and processes in therapy.

In Chapter 4, *'Women's work': Women in the Helping Professions Using Crafts as Self-Care*, Gal Amram and Ephrat Huss share the results of their research on how women in the helping professions in Israel understand the role of craft making in their lives and its relationship to professional practice.

Chapter 5, *Sis, U Belong Here: Black Women Making and Taking Up Space* by veronica precious bohanan, explores the materiality of space, rituals, and embodied practices in a community-based art program for Black women that integrates creativity, spirituality, and cultural traditions within a womanist framework.

In Chapter 6, *Clawing Our Way Out: Art Therapy Manicure Rituals and a Feminist Ethics of Care*, Roxie Rose Ehlert discusses the use of manicure rituals in a rape crisis center to address issues like fatphobia, racism, ableism, misogyny, transmisogyny, and gender dysphoria through the frameworks of queer femme identity, disability justice, and a feminist ethics of care.

In Chapter 7, *Honoring Our Relationships and Materials from Our Homelands*, Zoë Harris, Ella Mahoney, Michelle Napoli, Asa Peters, Leana Pilet, Brittney Peauwe Wunnepog Walley, and Rachel Parks Winters discuss and employ Indigenous methodology, storywork, and Indigenous futurism to reflect on art materials as situated within the larger context of relationality with land- and place-based practices, honoring one's ancestors, and contemporary continuity with community-based traditions.

In Chapter 8, *Art from Inside: Peer Art Therapists (PAThR) Reflections on Materials and Media in Exploring Complex Identity Systems*, Mahlie Jewell and Catherine Camden-Pratt discuss their integration of Lived Experience of mental distress, training in peer support, and education as art psychotherapists. They discuss how these educational and life experiences inform their work alongside people living complex trauma, with particular attention paid to diverse forms of communication through art materials and making processes.

In chapter 9, *Plastic Mandala: Eco Art as Compassionate Action*, Eunhae Jung weaves together scholarship from environmental artist-activists, her experiences as an art therapist, and her eco-art practice of collecting micro-plastics from the beaches of Jeju Island in South Korea to create subtly activist artworks. Altogether, this chapter presents a relational ethics of care that extends to nature as kin.

Chapter 10, *Transgender Joy as Community Art in a 'Trans Refuge State,'* by Owen Paul Karcher and G. Nic Rider describes a call-and-response art project between transgender patients at a medical facility and the general public at a Pride festival. The project's aims were to raise awareness about the experiences of transgender people seeking gender-affirming healthcare and to inspire communal support in return.

In Chapter 11, *Socio-Political Stress and Artmaking: Clothing, Identity, and Social Change*, Michelle Kendrick Hartney shares her use of fiber-based art practices in collaboration with the public to raise awareness about issues like racism in maternal healthcare and gender-affirming parenting, and to attend to the resulting emotional, psychological, and interpersonal effects of socio-political turmoil and structural inequity.

Chapter 12, *Drawing Connections: Comics in Art Therapy Practice*, by Rakshanda Khan, discusses and portrays through cartoons and narrative the versatility, therapeutic potentials, and practical strategies of applying traditional, textile, and digital comic arts in group and individual art therapy.

In Chapter 13, *The Immersive Worlds of Therapeutic Gaming and Scanography for Art Therapy*, Christina Marrero and Natalie Rae Carlton discuss the use of digital media in art therapy education and practice, comparing the therapeutic possibilities and practical challenges of a relatively accessible art form, scanography, with a resource-heavy technology, virtual reality.

In Chapter 14, *The Kitchen as Metaphor: Shaping Togetherness and Therapeutic Makerspaces in Marginalized Communities*, Rochelle Royster reflects on how the kitchens of her youth cultivated a sense of identity and belonging, and uses the metaphor of the kitchen to examine how makerspaces similarly employ tangible materials and intangible elements like togetherness and storytelling to support identity, community, and well-being in marginalized communities.

In Chapter 15, *The Neoliberal Co-Optation of Mindfulness and Mandala Practices*, Kirthana Selvaraj addresses the appropriation of mandalas and mindfulness within Western art therapy research and practice, characterized by a lack of concern for the cultural and spiritual significance of these practices, and advocates for a more ethical and culturally respectful approach.

In Chapter 16, *Playing in the Deep: Applying Improvisational Principles to Therapy*, Victoria Te You Moore and Katharine Joy Houpt introduce art therapists to theatrical improvisation (improv), providing examples from their personal and professional experiences, key principles from improv for supporting group therapy and teaching practices, and a discussion of improv as an unconventional art material.

Chapter 17, *A Box of Fired Clay Bricks: Building Home on the Community Table with People on the Move*, by Miriam Usiskin and Bobby Lloyd, focuses on a box of miniature fired clay bricks used within a psychosocial support group for people along the France-UK border who have been displaced and are seeking asylum. They address the use of culturally resonant materials and the intersectional and socio-political complexities of working within a context of pervasive loss.

In Chapter 18, *Festival Art Therapy Pedagogy: Across and Between*, Pamela Whitaker examines the significance of urban festivals in Belfast as contexts for art therapy practicums, considering ideas related to public practice art therapy, the materiality of place, the city as campus, and civic engagement as a means of addressing historical legacies of conflict and segregation. This chapter highlights student learning goals and provides *the walking studio* as an example of an art therapist-facilitated event.

Overall, this book takes up where the first edition left off, updating the diverse applications of art materials, media, and practices in art therapy, offering new perspectives on material theory, and encouraging ever more critical thinking about the historical, socio-cultural, political, economic, and environmental implications of making practices.

References

Cabañas, K. M. (2021). *Imminent vitalities: Meaning and materiality in contemporary art.* University of California Press.

Eastwood, C. (2022). Intersectional reflexivity: Art psychotherapy practice and self. In J. Collier & C. Eastwood (Eds.), *Intersectionality in the arts psychotherapies* (pp. 33–47). Jessica Kingsley Publishers.

Elkin, L. (2023). *Art monsters: Unruly bodies in feminist art.* Picador.

Gipson, L. R. (2015). Is cultural competence enough? Deepening social justice pedagogy in art therapy. *Art Therapy, 32*(3), 142–145. https://doi.org/10.1080/07421656.2015.1060835

LeBaron, M., & Sarra, J. (Eds.) (2018). *Changing our worlds: Art as transformative practice.* Sun Press.

Lee, K. (2022). Mattering bodies in a mattering world. In J. Millner & G. Coombs (Eds.), *Care ethics and art* (pp. 83–93). Routledge.

Millner, J., & Coombs, G. (Eds.) (2022). *Care ethics and art.* Routledge.

Moon, C. H., & Faulkner, K. (2024). Intersectional care ethics in art therapy organizations. *Arts in Psychotherapy, 89.* https://doi.org/10.1016/j.aip.2024.102165

Mundt, K. (2021). Touch as passage: Inhabiting the colonial wound. *The Arrow, 8*(1), 120–140. https://arrow-journal.org/touch-as-passage-inhabiting-the-colonial-

Neal, L. (2023). *Playing for time: Making art as if the world mattered* (2nd ed.). Triarchy Press.

Skaife, S., & Martyn, J. (Eds.) (2022). *Art psychotherapy groups in the hostile environment of neoliberalism: Collusion or resistance?* Routledge.

Weintraub, L. (2019). *What's next? Eco materialism & contemporary art.* Intellect.

SECTION I
HISTORY, THEORY, ETHICS, RESEARCH

A CONTEMPORARY HISTORY OF ART MATERIALS, MEDIA, AND PRACTICES IN ART THERAPY

Catherine Hyland Moon

This chapter begins with a brief synopsis of materials and media use in the early years of the field (see the first edition for a more detailed account), with the remainder of the chapter focused on contemporary art therapy practice.

Materials and media, 1940s–2010

In the early years of the field, publications rarely focused on specific art materials, media, or practices, with the exception of photography and video due to their novelty at the time. Establishing the legitimacy of art therapy as a psychotherapy practice may have resulted in largely taking art materials, media, and practices for granted, despite their significance. When art practices were mentioned or illustrated in the context of publications about clinical practice, they were mostly limited to painting, drawing, and clay sculpture (Moon, 2010).

In the 1990s and 2000s, though conventional fine arts materials continued to dominate, digital media applications beyond photography and video emerged, as did a broader array of art materials and practices like found objects, altered books, collage, fiber arts, and natural materials. A more sophisticated examination of the impact of material choices began to develop in relation to treatment contexts and participant groups, and research on the effects of materials began to emerge (Moon, 2010).

DOI: 10.4324/9781032720166-2

There have been themes that have remained significant to the field since its inception. They include practical matters like affordability, ease of transport, safety, and accessibility, as well as interest in how the qualities of art materials might affect participants' physical, psychological, and emotional states, and the importance of considering participants' aesthetic tastes and culturally significant materials/practices (Moon, 2010).

Contemporary art materials, media, and practices

The proliferation of literature on art therapy materials and practices since 2010 has made an in-depth discussion of each material or practice impossible. Therefore, I focus on the five most robust areas of development—crafts, ecological approaches, digital media, cultural considerations, and research—followed by a brief overview of materials and practices that have received insufficient attention or have remained largely absent in the literature.

Crafts

Art therapy was slow to adopt craft practices despite their connection to cultural traditions and their appeal to people who consider themselves art world outliers. More recently, however, art therapists have recognized that all creative making methods require conceptual, intellectual, and emotional processes and have potential benefits for well-being (Talwar, 2019). There is also greater awareness of the discriminatory nature of the art/craft binary. Crafts, particularly fiber crafts, were once viewed as antithetical to the art historical canon because of their association with gendered domestic labor practices (Talwar, 2020), queer culture (Roberts, 2011), and Indigenous cultural expression and heritage (Henderson, 2021).

Today crafting is more prevalent in the United States than fine arts practices, providing a compelling argument for art therapy to break away from its reliance on Western art conventions (Kaimal et al., 2017b). Crafts can be used for autobiographical documentation, activism, bonding and empowerment, encoded expression of cultural ideas and philosophies, connection with ancestors (Henderson, 2021), economic empowerment, and enhanced social capital (Talwar, 2020). Crafters often derive satisfaction from mastering new skills, find pleasure in crafts' sensory and kinesthetic processes, experience cultural resonance, gain enhanced cognition through embodied learning, and receive support and validation when crafting occurs within a community context (Leone, 2021).

Fiber arts

Among all craft practices used in therapy, fiber arts are most common. They include knitting, crocheting, sewing, embroidery, quilting, weaving, knotting, wrapping, and felting.

Knitting and crocheting have been credited with decreasing depression (Alamri & Dabes, 2023), aiding pain management (Corkhill, 2012), and providing a means of storying Black identity and ancestry (Taylor-Johnson, 2023).

Sewing is inherent to many textile-based practices and can be a neurodevelopmentally respectful approach to working with adults who have experienced trauma, because stitching is relational, developmentally relevant, repetitive, rewarding, and rhythmic (Homer, 2015). Narratives conveyed through sewn *story cloths* offer a means for divulging personal, social, and political events through the coded language of patterns, colors, and textures (Garlock, 2016). Stitching can also be a meaningful process for exploring the disruption and renewal associated with medical procedures (Flahavan, 2024, p. 174), and for shifting the narrative of disability from fixing to archiving, and recontextualizing care as collective and political (Yi, 2021). Likewise, sex-positive workshops featuring the creation of fiber-based vulvas have been a reparative response to sexual violence and the inadequacy of bodily knowledge (Ferranto, 2023; Napoli & Kirby, 2019).

Historically, embroidery has given women a voice when other avenues of expression have been denied (Gaspar da Silva, 2023). It has been used by adolescent girls to experiment with the interplay between tradition and free self-expression (Wolk & Bat Or, 2023) and by South African women to document the intersections between emancipations and continuing injustice and resistance (Segalo et al., 2015).

Quilting has provided a culturally relevant practice for women of color activists addressing gentrification (Leone, 2019), incarceration (Talwar & Wallis, 2021), and homelessness (Moxley et al., 2011). Anderson (2021) used quilts to express emancipation from heteronormativity and disrupt gender binaries. Thus, quilts are not only for individualized comfort and care, but also for addressing structural inequalities and reinforcing collective responsibility for social change.

Weaving's slow, sensorial process has been used for creating a personal grief ritual following pregnancy loss (van Zyl, 2023), and for crafting infant wrapping cloths to offer care and empathy to bereaved parents (Nordström & Groth, 2022). A traveling loom has provided opportunities for people in different neighborhoods to connect despite social divisions and mistrust (Glinzak & Dunkelberger, 2023). Knot (un)tying provides an apt metaphor for exploring connections, entanglements, disconnection, and loss (Thrall, 2017), while the simple process of wrapping sticks with textiles can be a daily grounding ritual (McAvoy, 2018).

Other craft practices

Dolls are made from yarn, fabric, paper, found objects, clay, and other materials to address therapeutic, spiritual, and activist agendas. Art therapist/elementary school teacher Royster (2021) developed a project in which students wrapped and embellished fabric dolls to memorialize people they knew who had been killed by gun violence. The project was replicated by teachers in 55 Chicago schools, and many of the dolls have been included in public exhibitions to provide a healing ritual, foreground community strengths, and resist the dismissal of communities beset by gun violence.

Books—including zines, scrapbooks, altered, and artists' books—contain, order, archive, reveal/conceal, enclose/expose, collect, and preserve. They have an inherent structure, can be worked on over time, and are accessible and easily transportable (Dean, 2016; Kapitan, 2021). Each book form has its unique qualities and metaphoric potentials. Altered books can address themes of self-repair, reclamation, and reframing (Jacobson-Levy & Miller, 2022). Scrapbooks offer a way to remember lost loved ones and document family history (Kohut, 2011), while zines often focus on unconventional subject matter or underrepresented groups of people (Mageary, 2021). An art therapist and residents of a nursing home took copies of the zine they co-created to conferences and zine festivals, presenting a counter-narrative to dominant stereotypes about aging (Houpt et al., 2016). Artists' books are works of art that extend the concept of what a book can be and often contain narratives that contest dominant stories and knowledges (Kapitan, 2021). For example, (Orbach, 2023) altered the Talmud—a sacred text that, as a woman, she was not permitted to formally study—by layering parchment paper over it and inscribing her ideas and associations on the paper. This was a way to both rebel and respectfully reclaim this "stream of religious men's knowledge" that was part of her heritage (p. 174).

Additional artisanal practices employed in art therapy include ceramics, glassblowing and glass fusion, leatherwork, origami, puppet making, and papermaking.

Ecological approaches

In a time of global warming, rising sea levels, extreme weather events, and other indicators of climate crisis, it is not surprising that literature on ecological approaches to art therapy has proliferated. The voices of Indigenous arts therapists are particularly important, as they hold deep knowledge about being grounded in reciprocal relationships with all the natural world (e.g., Archibald & Dewar, 2010; Napoli, 2021; O'Connor, 2018; Warson, 2013; Whyte, 2020).

The essence of ecological art therapy is not about using materials from nature or working in green spaces. Rather, it is the recognition that humans are *of* and *in* nature. Making processes *always* involve embodied materiality entangled within multispecies encounters, no matter where and with what/whom we are working.

Environmental settings, materials, and relationships

Environmentally focused art therapy takes place in settings like farms, nature preserves, hospital gardens, beaches, city parks, or alongside window flower boxes. It also takes place indoors where hydroponic gardens, plant walls, or eco-art are made (Alders Pike, 2021).

Natural materials can be touched, smelled, dug into, climbed, arranged, etc. (Nash, 2020a). In turn, these elements act upon the person interacting with them. For example, materials like clay or sand, due to their malleability and responsiveness, can elicit *me/not me* awareness (Boon, 2020). Natural environments and materials also offer rich metaphors that can be experienced in an embodied way, such as walking through brambles, gazing into a dark pool, or experiencing shaded protection (Nash, 2020a). Change processes can be normalized through exposure to migratory patterns, seasonal cycles, and birth, disease, and death (Wardle, 2023).

Nature is a dynamic entity with diverse intelligences, forms of agency, and means of communication (A'Court, 2017). The relationship between therapist, participants, artmaking, and nature can vary depending on whether nature is framed as background, co-therapist, active participant, container, teacher, or provider of materials (Nash, 2020b).

Challenges of natural environments

McNiff (2022) warned against focusing only on the bucolic qualities of nature, noting that imperfections and struggle are part of the creative ecosystem. Working in nature presents challenges related to terrain, weather, lack of privacy, mobility, security (Whitaker, 2016), restricted daylight hours, suitable clothing, and access to sites (Wardle, 2023). Participants may view outdoor environments as unpleasant, dirty, or boring (Whitaker, 2016) or engage in aggressive acts like destroying plants or killing small creatures.

For participants in marginalized communities, challenges can include limited access to greenspaces due to historical/ongoing colonization and discriminatory city planning and housing practices. Systemic barriers like lack of transportation or the danger associated with playing outside (e.g., police violence, deportation fears, etc.) can also limit use of public greenspaces (Velasquez, 2022). In particular, girls and young women may experience greenspaces as rife with misogyny and gender-based harassment or violence (Cole et al., 2024).

Response to climate crisis

Among many possible responses to the climate crisis, I offer three recommendations for art therapists. First, we can be ecologically conscientious about our material choices. Second, we can ground art therapy practice in a relational aesthetic aligned with care for the planet. Third, we can extend our attention to climate justice. Because I address ecologically minded use of materials in the Ethics chapter in this book, below I discuss the two remaining recommendations: a relational aesthetic and climate justice.

Relational aesthetic

A relational aesthetic challenges art therapy's tendency to focus on individual distress to the exclusion of social causes and effects. While attending to the individual certainly has its place, "pathological individualism" (Neal, 2018, p. 260) is at the root of social and planetary degradation. Therapists can facilitate engagement with the grief, complexity, and uncertainty of a declining world, while also encouraging social responsibility directed toward planetary care (Alders Pike, 2021; Timm-Bottos, 2011).

A relational aesthetic in the creative arts therapies challenges dominant, neoliberal ideas about wellness as an individual responsibility and focuses attention on the interdependent nature of all of life. It activates art processes to bring forth interpersonal, social, and planetary healing in material and relationally informed ways (Moon, 2002, 2016).

Levine (2022) uses the term *ecopoiesis* to highlight the role of artists as makers and shapers in nature-assisted expressive arts therapies. He calls for shaping the world with an eye toward beauty and the world's flourishing. However, he cautions that this cannot be done through the imposition of one's will, but rather through a humble, receptive attitude of collaboratively and co-operatively enabling possibilities to come forth.

During the COVID-19 pandemic, people intuitively engaged in creative acts, including land art projects that reinforced the relationship between humans and nature, such as creating rock balancing sculptures (Hu, 2021) and forming architectural dens from fallen branches (Whitaker, 2021). These random acts of creativity, begun by individuals, became collective care practices in public realms as multiple copycat sculptures and dens appeared. Perhaps these responses to disaster provide hints about art therapy's potential to support the world's flourishing through social art practices that are site specific, collaborative, and centered in an ethic of care for people and the planet.

Climate justice

Climate justice addresses the systemically linked material, psychological, socio-economic, and political patterns that have resulted in marginalized groups least responsible for climate change experiencing its most damaging impacts. Due to the exploitation of Indigenous peoples and lands, and the extractive policies and capitalist production of countries that prioritize profit over people and planet, places populated predominantly by Indigenous, immigrant, Brown, Black, and low-income people are most likely to contain hazardous waste sites, experience extreme weather events, and have contaminated air, water, and land. In turn, these conditions create issues like food insecurity, public health threats, and unsafe working conditions (Barnwell & Wood, 2022; Pellow & Vazin, 2019).

Psychology fields, including art therapy, have mostly engaged with the climate crisis by promoting individuals' pro-climate behaviors or by endorsing coping strategies to mitigate the effects of climate change on psychosocial well-being (Kalwak & Weihgold, 2022). Often framed around resilience narratives, these practices ignore the historical and political contexts that create structural inequalities (Ranganthan & Bratman, 2021).

Moving beyond a resilience narrative that expects marginalized groups to have limitless capacity to cope, art therapy could adopt an intersectional framework that highlights the historical and political realities making some communities particularly vulnerable to environmental degradation. In recognizing that the environment includes everywhere people live, work, and play, art therapy practice could encompass concerns related to fair housing practices, labor rights, toxin-free land, quality healthcare, access to clean water, and other social justice issues (Ranganthan & Bratman, 2021). Rather than addressing these concerns through ameliorative processes that help people adapt to circumstances and overcome distressing emotions, art therapy might be directed toward liberatory processes that foster understanding of the origins and value of emotions and their potentials as drivers of social action (González-Hidalgo et al., 2022).

Cultural considerations

Art therapists have become increasingly attuned to the links between cultural identity and art's role in health/healing. Yet, the field continues to adhere to two ideas—that art is a symbolic representation of its maker and that it can be used for individual self-expression—despite many non-Western art practices that contradict these assumptions (Gantt, 2013). To counteract this ethnocentric tendency, therapists from both dominant and minority cultures have addressed the need for culturally relevant and respectful practice.

Non-Eurocentric perspectives

Art therapists from non-Western countries and from minoritized cultural groups have provided important counter-narratives to the dominance of individualistic, medicalized, fine arts, self-expressive orientations to the field. These art therapists challenge ideas about what counts as art/craft, what the arts are for, and how the arts might contribute to well-being.

For people in collectivist societies, art is often focused on traditional forms or motifs that convey cultural, spiritual, or religious identity and norms. In some cultures, there are prohibited art practices, such as in Arab Muslim society where drawing images of people or any living creature is forbidden (Zaken & Walsh, 2021). Rather than using art for emotional expression, participants may be more inclined to create utilitarian objects that express ethnic cosmologies, reinforce collective identity and pride, or generate income (Salom, 2015).

Park et al. (2021) assert that unilaterally applying Western materials/practices to all participants constitutes cultural blindness and overlooks significant information conveyed through participants' relationships with materials. Locally sourced materials are most likely to be familiar and culturally relevant; however, even local materials have nuanced significations. For example, though rice is common in Asian cuisines, its use as an art material might be viewed as wasteful or disrespectful by older Asian adults, less so by younger generations (Divya, 2021).

When offering art materials or practices that are culture-specific, it is important to resist assumptions about participants' connections to those traditions (Hanania, 2020). Both conventional Western media and traditional crafts materials can be meaningful for some communities, such as refugees, internally displaced persons (Salom, 2015), or Indigenous people living in settler societies (Whyte, 2020). For example, Ansloos et al. (2022) wrote about the support of cultural resurgence and therapeutic healing that Indigenous beading practitioners found in connecting through social media platforms. Cross-cultural media practices can foster the integration of cultural heritage and emerging facets of identity, recognizing that "individuals can belong to multiple and transitional cultural contexts simultaneously, which they can embrace and resist in different ways" (Katoshevski & Huss, 2021, p. 145).

Many art therapists from non-Western countries return to their homelands after graduating from educational programs in Western countries, only to be confronted by the dissonance between their education and the cultural norms and arts and healing practices in their home countries. This same dissonance exists for Indigenous art therapists whose dominant culture education erases or silences their history, worldviews, and identity (Napoli, 2021).

Decentering the institutional conceptualization of art therapy is required for the development of localized, culturally relevant practices (Lee, 2022; Moon et al., 2024). In some contexts, culturally resonant art forms include spiritual practices, dance, music, poetry, and spoken word (Valldejuli & Belnavis Elliot, 2023). In non-Western contexts, consulting with traditional artisans and Indigenous artists can deepen understanding of native arts practices and help prevent the domination of imported materials and conventions (Gómez Carlier & Salom, 2012; Salom, 2015).

Cultural collaborator perspectives

Art therapists whose work involves international or intercultural border crossings encounter unique challenges. It is helpful for outsiders to approach the work through an ethnorelative lens (Kapitan, 2015), prioritizing collaboration, long-term relationships, reflexivity, and respect for community protocols (Moon, 2013; Vivien, 2018). Despite sincere efforts, art therapy might still be rejected in an effort to avoid colonial practices and unwanted interventions (Vivien, 2018).

Art therapists are often drawn into collaborations in response to humanitarian disasters. The work of Kalmanowitz and Lloyd in refugee settlement areas demonstrates carefully considered applications of media within culturally diverse, politically complex, emotionally fraught contexts. They consider materials' cultural and historical significance, metaphoric potential, economic and contextual accessibility, site specificity, portability, local availability, ephemerality, and relationship to participants' needs and inner resources. In Calais, France, they asked for Afghani men's help in sourcing materials from abandoned tents and advising on construction techniques for kite making and flying, which has a long history in Afghanistan. The kites served as a form of cultural and political resistance, a way to cross borders into forbidden lands and experience a sense of freedom (Kalmanowitz, 2018; Kalmanowitz & Lloyd, 2016).

Digital media

The breadth and depth of art therapy literature on digital technology confirms that digital media is now fully integrated into the field. Multiple factors have led to this shift, including art therapists' exposure to digital culture and skill-building over time, a pandemic-induced increase in technology use, tech-savvy art therapists entering the field, and new media that are increasingly portable and affordable (Carlton, 2014; Peterson, 2010).

The *material* of digital technology is data, an invisible yet pervasive aspect of the systems that order daily life, from scheduling a meeting, to doing laundry, to meeting a potential life partner. The malleability and adaptability of data make them ideal for artmaking, as they can provide the "foundation of many different outputs and experiences, such as graphic visualizations, artworks, animations, sound and music, narratives, tactile experiences, objects, scent, textiles," etc. (Freeman et al., 2018, p. 75).

Advantages and challenges of digital media

Digital media has many advantages. It provides an art studio available at one's fingertips, creations can be endlessly modified and mistakes deleted, both art process and product can be recorded, and multiple iterations of an artwork are possible (Carlton, 2014; Evans, 2012; Orr, 2015). New media use and storage are compact, and art products are easily shared. Options to integrate visual images, sound, photo editing, and storytelling provide the potential for a holistic sensory experience (Kim & Chung, 2023) while remote interactions available via voice, webcam, and virtual avatars make art therapy more democratically accessible, particularly for those who find face-to-face contact or the use of traditional art media intimidating (Diggs et al., 2015). Digital media also offers access alternatives for people with disabilities, and a clean art form for people who are immunocompromised, have aversions to messiness, or have heightened sensory reactivity (Kometiani, 2018; Zubala et al., 2021).

Challenges to digital media include connecting with participants who become absorbed by screen interactions, potentially creating distance from the therapist, the artmaking, and their own bodies (Diggs et al., 2015). There are also losses associated with technology as compared to working with conventional art materials—losses of smell, of varied tactile experiences, of the ability to work aggressively or messily, of the benefits that can be derived from working through mistakes and imperfections. Other challenges include technical glitches and content that is accidentally altered or deleted (Choe, 2014).

Digital art tools and technologies

Art apps enable the creation of digital drawings, paintings, collages, sculptures, comics, books, and videos. Choe (2014) identified three ideal qualities for art apps used in therapy: ease of use, powerful but uncomplicated features, and responsiveness to sensorial input like speed and pressure.

Artificial Intelligence (AI) technologies for human-AI co-creation in art therapy are under development at the time of this writing. Du et al. (2024) used a co-design approach to develop four core principles for human-AI co-creation in art therapy: low threshold for artmaking expertise; interactive balance between AI and human participants; multidimensional artmaking options with flexible switching between tools; and allowance for both synchronous and asynchronous artmaking.

Design collaborations among art therapists, human-computer interface designers and developers, and other professionals have focused on digital technology applications for specific participant groups. For example, Lazar et al. (2016) used an empathic design approach to develop a digital prototype for creating and sharing art among older adults with dementia, guided by consultations with art therapists who modeled a *third hand* approach in their work with older adults.

Photography can be used to explore identity and elicit personal and cultural history by making use of found images, family albums, documentary images, self-portraits, costumes, and props. Photos can be a means of making visible the complexity and contradictions of life stories and intersecting identities (Eastwood, 2022; Martin, 2020; Weiser, 2014).

In art therapy, photography techniques include camera-less photographic processes like cyanotypes; image transfer processes onto 2D or 3D surfaces; scans and photocopies modified with various media (Horovitz, 2015); and mobile devices and editing software for creating and altering images. Original and found photos are also used in art forms like photo-collage or digital stories, and they can be altered or embellished with embroidery, paint, or other media (Kopytin, 2018). Like most media, photography has been used with diverse groups of people for a range of therapeutic and research purposes.

Social media encompasses interactive technologies that enable users to connect with each other; create, edit, and share content; and participate in virtual communities. At minimum, participation requires creating an online persona, which can vary from a simple name and photo to the ongoing, dynamic curation of a self-system that is performed and revised over time (Ottiger & Ehemann, 2019, p. 247).

While art therapy literature often extols the virtues of social media for artmaking inspiration, resources, and supportive networks (e.g., Chilton et al., 2009; Miller, 2018, 2022), recognizing its more toxic features is crucial for guiding art therapy participants to use it productively. Through mining data and analyzing user behaviors, social media platforms manage what users are exposed to, thereby influencing what it means to be citizens and where to invest creative and material resources. Social media can pervert creativity into branding and commodification, feed a craving for external validation through "likes," and seduce makers into prioritizing trends over authenticity, social capital over integrity, and competition over collaboration.

Tele-art therapy became a common form of practice when the COVID-19 pandemic triggered a broad-scale move to conducting therapy online, which also forced the reconceptualization of art therapy materials. Material options were often determined by what was available in participants' homes, and extended beyond visual art to activities like music sharing, singing, dancing, and gardening (Walters, 2022).

The word *pivot* characterized abrupt changes in practice to meet the realities of lockdown and social distancing. Usiskin and Lloyd (2020) transitioned their in-person work with displaced people to two concurrent socially engaged art practices aimed at countering isolation and fostering creativity and resilience. They established an online version of their *community table* where refugees and frontline workers could meet to share artmaking experiences, and they hosted the *Coronaquilt*, a crowdsourced "quilt" of uploaded art images, made in responses to the theme of *daily rituals to help people cope*.

Video and animation are time-based and timeless, inherently collaborative, and can incorporate sound, music, visual arts, movement, text, photos, and narration to address diverse issues (Tuval-Mashiach et al., 2018). Green screen technology can be used for exploring identity through mirrored self-images (Ehinger, 2015), and 2D work can be transformed into videos to better express the fullness and dynamic nature of life experiences (Keaveny, 2018). Video productions that lead to public screenings can enable people from marginalized groups to participate in self-representation and activism. For example, a video project focused on domestic violence and sex trafficking that was initiated by adolescent boys led to film screenings and interactive workshops in which community members shouldered some of the burden of stories usually held alone and in silence by survivors (Rubin, 2016).

In animation, a series of still images viewed in rapid succession creates the illusion of movement. *The Animation Project* serves at-risk youth to address both workforce development and therapeutic goals through the collaborative creation of short computer animation videos. The youth develop career path skills by learning to use an industry-standard 3D modelling program and develop interpersonal skills by learning to collaborate, practice coping skills, and safely process story content (Kavitski & Austin, 2018).

Virtual reality and avatars are, at the time of this writing, in the early stages of use in art therapy. Virtual reality (VR) is a computer-generated environment that uses graphics, audio, and other sensory inputs to simulate a partial to fully immersive experience. Interactive devices, most commonly headsets and hand motion controllers, provide multisensory input and facilitate interactions with the virtual setting, objects, and scenarios. Users can experience *presence*, meaning that the immersive, sensorimotor effects of the virtual space feel like real life, even when users maintain an awareness of its computer-generated nature.

Strengths of VR (in additions to those generally associated with digital media) include its facilitation of presence; the enjoyable, playful nature of the experience; the opportunity to take a break from reality and explore facets of the self without real-world implications (Shamri Zeevi, 2021); the experience of moving around and even through what one has created (Carlton et al., 2018); and the ability to integrate virtual, 2D, and

3D work, for example, through documenting the VR experience with video, scanning an image or object and incorporating it into the virtual artwork, or translating virtual artwork into tangible objects by connecting to a 3D printer (Kaimal et al., 2019; Shamri Zeevi, 2021). Challenges include the sense of disconnect between therapists and participants; possible nausea and fatigue for participants (Hacmun et al., 2018); accessibility problems for people with balance, headache, or reality orientation issues (Kaimal et al., 2019); and cost, transport, and setup of technology equipment (Haeyen et al., 2021).

In VR, an avatar is a virtual representation of a user that enables interaction and communication within the virtual environment. Research on specific applications of avatars have included their use in creating life-review videos with cancer patients (Ryu & Price, 2022) and in gender exploration among participants diagnosed with either depression or personality disorders (Ottiger & Ehemann, 2019). In both of these studies, it seemed to be the playful, embodied nature of the VR avatars that allowed participants to become agents of themselves, whether to reconstruct self-narratives or try on alternate identities.

Digital futures

Art therapists have expressed interest in the promise of additional technologies, such as augmented reality, sensory absorbed experiences, and robotics (Miller, 2022). Other digital media, like video games, gesture-based technology, podcasts, live streaming, wearable technologies, 3D printing, code as a material for interactive installations, and even the most ubiquitous digital tool of all—smartphones—could be explored for the ongoing development of art therapy's creative engagement with technology.

Research

Research aimed at better understanding the therapeutic implications of artmaking materials, processes, and structures has greatly increased in recent years. This brief overview identifies key themes and a few examples.

Acknowledgment of the role materials play in art-based assessments has led to research examining the potential significance of participants' interactions with specific art materials (e.g., Pénzes et al., 2014). More commonly, research has focused on media comparisons, such as collage versus drawing, in relation to therapeutic outcomes (Raffaelli & Hartzell, 2016). The effects of art processes have also been explored, such as structured versus nonstructured art activities (Cross & Brown, 2019).

Participants' responses to the qualities and characteristics of different materials have been studied to better understand their therapeutic potentials and contraindications (e.g., Snir et al., 2017). Factors that impact the effect of art materials and processes have also inspired research, including investigations of using one material for differing purposes (e.g., Smolarski et al., 2015), and one theme executed through different art techniques (e.g., Becerra et al., 2021). Researchers have also examined how the therapeutic relationship affects participants' experience of working with art materials (e.g., Gazit et al., 2021).

Studies on specific materials and practices have focused on particular populations (e.g., Elkis-Abuhoff & Gaydos, 2018) and explicit techniques (e.g., Isis et al., 2023). Numerous studies have also been conducted on the effects of drawing or coloring mandalas, but the majority are highly problematic in that they do not consider the ethical issues associated with cultural appropriation.

An emerging theme in research is the use of physiological measures, alone or in tandem with qualitative methods, to gauge participants' responses to art materials and processes. Examples include the use of heart rate/variability measures (Rankanen et al., 2022), blood pressure readings (Keogh & Creaven, 2017), electroencephalogram (EEG) (Belkofer et al., 2014), and Functional near-infrared spectroscopy (fNIRS) (Kaimal et al., 2017a).

Finally, arts-based research (ABR), though identified as an approach ideally suited to understanding the nature and significance of art therapy practice (McNiff, 2013), has remained relatively rare in the field. ABR can be wide in scope, such as Hogan's (2019) Birth Project, which included birth professionals, fathers, obstetricians, and new mothers as research participants. It examined women's birthing experiences and transition to motherhood through studio art, performance, video documentation, and therapeutic art approaches. Alternatively, ABR can focus on the researcher's self-reflexive process, such as Wong's (2024) use of papermaking to explore the deconstruction and reintegration involved in her and her research participants' emigration processes.

Future research

Given the almost limitless range of art materials, media, and practices, the quest to better understand their applications in art therapy will likely be ongoing. While amassing empirical evidence about the effects and usefulness of various art materials and processes is needed (Hinz, 2015), evidence-based practice is also supported by the expertise of art therapy practitioners and participants. In the future, it will be essential to more conscientiously and consistently include art therapy participants in the design and implementation of research methods and the presentation of results (Springham & Xenophontes, 2021). In particular, centering the experiences of participants from marginalized groups through co-produced research will challenge therapist-researcher biases and lead to research that is socially, culturally, and politically situated, as well as results that are more relevant and useful for art therapy participants.

Other materials and practices—now and next

There is a wealth of information about the use of materials, media, and processes in art therapy. Yet, gaps remain, as do opportunities for ongoing expansion of the field's knowledge base.

Of the most frequently used and least theorized practices in the field, painting and drawing top the list (for exceptions, see Dean, 2016; Lorenzo de la Peña, 2015). There is a need for broad exploration of these two practices, as well as closer examinations of their applications using specific materials. Three-dimensional sculpture is also underexplored, despite its potential for fully embodied, dynamic approaches to artmaking (e.g., Bechtel et al., 2020). A third art form, collage, is widely applied in art therapy practice, but an exploration of contemporary art could enhance its potential. Collage can be so much more than magazine images glued onto paper!

There are some art materials, such as found objects, for which a solid research and practice base is developing (e.g., see Wong & Lay, 2021). Matott and Miller's (2024) book on papermaking is a strong start to exploring both the topic of paper arts and the marriage of therapeutic and social activist approaches to well-being. Comics is a slowly emerging but still underused art therapy practice, despite its widespread, interdisciplinary applications for addressing individual, social, and environmental health and well-being.

Finally, there are art forms and practices with much to offer art therapy that are seldom addressed in the literature. As discussed in Chapter 2 of this book, art practices that directly engage the body as ground or material have been largely overlooked. Place-based art forms such as architecture, installation, and built environments are almost completely absent from the field's literature. Fenner's (2019) research on the material effects of art therapy spaces offers an enticing invitation for expanding research and practice in this area.

These are just a few examples of the many possibilities for expanding art materials, media, and practice applications in art therapy. Our field would greatly benefit from more research, practice examples, viewpoints, and critical theorizing that addresses the *why, when, how, with whom,* and "how about this?" of diverse art materials, media, and practices.

References

A'Court, B. (2017). The art of mindful walking in earth-based art therapy. In A. Kopytin & M. Rugh (Eds.), *Environmental expressive therapies: Nature-assisted theory and practice* (pp. 123–160). Routledge.

Alamri, E., & Dabes, R. (2023). The effectiveness of a training program for providing the art of crochet skills as an adjunct for depression patients' therapy. *Journal of Architecture, Arts, and Humanistic Sciences, 8*(41), 705–720.

Alders Pike, A. (2021). *Eco-art therapy in practice.* Routledge.

Anderson, M. (2021). Queer ethos in art therapy. In L. Leone (Ed.), *Craft in art therapy: Diverse approaches to the transformative power of craft materials and methods* (pp. 218–236). Routledge.

Ansloos, J., Caranto Morford, A., Santos Dunn, N., DuPré, L., & Kucheran, R. (2022). Beading Native Twitter: Indigenous, arts-based approaches to healing and resurgence. *The Arts and Psychotherapy, 79*, 101914. https://doi.org/10.1016/j.aip.2022.101914

Archibald, L., & Dewar, J. (2010). Creative arts, culture, and healing: Building an evidence base. *Pimatisiwin: A Journal of Aboriginal and Indigenous Community Health, 8*(3), 1–25. https://journalindigenouswellbeing.co.nz/media/2018/12/1_Archibald.pdf

Barnwell, G., & Wood, N. (2022). Climate justice is central to addressing the climate emergency's psychological consequences in the Global South: A narrative review. *South African Journal of Psychology, 52*(4), 486–497. https://doi.org/10.1177/00812463211073384

Becerra, L. A., Hill, E. M., & Abraham, K. M. (2021). Self-portraits: Literal self-portraits, mandalas, and free drawings to reduce anxiety. *Art Therapy, 39*(1), 34–42. https://doi.org/10.1080/07421656.2021.1976024

Bechtel, A., Wood, L., & Teoli, L. (2020). Re-shaping body image: Tape sculptures as arts-based justice. *Arts in Psychotherapy, 68*, 101615. https://doi.org/10.1016/j.aip.2019.101615

Belkofer, C. M., Van Hecke, A. V., & Konopka, L. M. (2014). Effects of drawing on alpha activity: A quantitative EEG study with implications for art therapy. *Art Therapy, 31*(2), 61–68. https://doi.org/10.1080/07421656.2014.903821

Boon, L. (2020). The wild inside: Offering children natural materials and an ecopsychological understanding of self within art therapy. In I. Siddons Heginworth & G. Nash (Eds.), *Environmental arts therapy: The wild frontiers of the heart* (pp. 47–60). Routledge.

Carlton, N. R. (2014). Digital culture and art therapy. *The Arts in Psychotherapy, 41*, 41–45. https://doi.org/10.1016/j.aip.2013.11.006

Carlton, N. R., Sit, T., & Yu, D. R. (2018). Transcendent media: Tangible to digital and their mixed reality. In R. Carolan & A. Backos (Eds.), *Emerging perspectives in art therapy: Trends, movements, and developments* (pp. 74–90). Routledge.

Chilton, G., Gerity, L., LaVorgna-Smith, M., & MacMichael, H. (2009). An online art exchange group: 14 secrets for a happy artist's life. *Art Therapy, 26*(2), 66–72.

Choe, N. S. (2014). An exploration of the qualities and features of art apps for art therapy. *Arts in Psychotherapy, 41*(2), 145–154. https://doi.org/10.1016/j.aip.2014.01.002

Cole, S., Goodenough, J., Haniff, M., Hussain, N., Ibrahim, S., Jani, A., Jiggens, E., Khan, A., Langford, P., Montgomery, L., Moore, L., Rowe, R., & Skinner, S. (2024). Greenspace & us: Exploring co-design approaches to increase engagement with nature by girls and young women. *Gateways: International Journal of Community Research and Engagement, 17*(1), 1–17. https://doi.org/10.5130/ijcre.v17i1.8881

Corkhill, B. (2012). Knitting and pain. *Pain News, 10*(1), 44–46. https://www.britishpainsociety.org/static/uploads/resources/files/Pain_News_Mar2012.pdf

Cross, G., & Brown, P. M. (2019). A comparison of the positive effects of structured and nonstructured art activities. *Art Therapy, 36*(1), 22–29. https://doi.org/10.1080/07421656.2019.1564642

Dean, M. L. (2016). *Using art media in psychotherapy: Bringing the power of creativity to practice*. Routledge.

Diggs, L. A., Lubas, M., & De Leo, G. (2015). Use of technology and software applications for therapeutic collage making. *International Journal of Art Therapy, 20*(1), 2–13. https://doi.org/10.1080/17454832.2014.961493

Divya (2021). The use of non-traditional mediums in doll making with children who have experienced trauma. In D. Wong & R. P. M. H. Lay (Eds.), *Found objects in art therapy: Materials and process* (pp. 73–87). Jessica Kingsley Publishers.

Du, X., An, P., Leung, J., Li, A., Chapman, L. E., & Zhao, J. (2024). DeepThInk: Designing and probing human-AI co-creation in digital art therapy. *International Journal of Human-Computer Studies, 181*, 1–17. https://doi.org/10.1016/j.ijhcs.2023.103139

Eastwood, C. (2022). Intersectional reflexivity: Art psychotherapy practice and self. In J. Collier & C. Eastwood (Eds.), *Intersectionality in the arts psychotherapies* (pp. 33–47). Jessica Kingsley Publishers.

Ehinger, J. (2015). Filming the fantasy: Green screen technology from novelty to psychotherapy. In J. L. Cohen, J. L. Johnson, & P. P. Orr (Eds.), *Video and filmmaking as psychotherapy* (pp. 43–54). Routledge.

Elkis-Abuhoff, D. L., & Gaydos, M. (2018). Medical art therapy research moves forward: A review of clay manipulation with Parkinson's disease. *Art Therapy, 35*(2), 68–76. https://doi.org/10.1080/07421656.2018.1483162

Evans, S. (2012). Using computer technology in expressive arts therapy practice: A proposal for increased use. *Journal of Creativity in Mental Health, 7*, 49–63. https://doi.org/10.1080/15401383.2012.660127

Fenner, P. (2019). Material sensibility: A sense of place in art therapy practice and theory. In A. Gilroy, S. Linnell, T. McKenna, & J. Westwood (Eds.), *Art therapy in Australia: Taking a postcolonial, aesthetic turn*. Brill/Sense.

Ferranto, J. (2023). Vulva education through fiber arts: The +cunt Project. *Art Therapy, 40*(4), 220–224. https://doi.org/10.1080/07421656.2023.2206778

Flahavan, C. (2024). 'This space inside': An art-based autoethnographic exploration of the hysterectomy experience. *Journal of Applied Arts & Health, 15*(2), 171–187. https://doi.org/10.1386/jaah_00170_1

Freeman, J., Starks, G., & Sandler, M. (2018). A concise taxonomy for describing data as an art material. *Leonardo, 51*(1), 75–79. https://muse.jhu.edu/article/686140

Gantt, L. (2013). Stories without words: A cultural understanding of trauma and abuse. In P. Howie, S. Prasad, & J. Kristel (Eds.), *Using art therapy with diverse populations: Crossing cultures and abilities* (pp. 234–244). Jessica Kingsley Publishers.

Garlock, L. R. (2016). Stories in the cloth: Art therapy and narrative textiles. *Art Therapy, 33*(2), 58–66. https://doi.org/10.1080/07421656.2016.1164004

Gaspar da Silva, M. (2023). Storytelling embroidery art therapy group with Portuguese-speaking immigrant women in Canada. *Canadian Journal of Art Therapy, 36*(2), 86–104.

Gazit, I., Snir, S., Regev, D., & Bat Or, M. (2021). Relationships between the therapeutic alliance and reactions to artistic experience with art materials in an art therapy simulation. *Frontiers in Psychology, 12.* https://doi.org/10.3389/fpsyg.2021.560957

Glinzak, L., & Dunkelberger, L. (2023). The traveling loom: Example of community-based art therapy. *Art Therapy, 40*(3), 157–161. https://doi.org/10.1080/07421656.2023.2172948

Gómez Carlier, N., & Salom, A. (2012). When art therapy migrates: The acculturation challenge of sojourner art therapists. *Art Therapy, 29*(1), 4–10. https://doi.org/10.1080/07421656.2012.648083

González-Hidalgo, M., Del Bene, D., Iniesta-Arandia, I., & Piñeiro, C. (2022). Emotional healing as part of environmental and climate justice processes: Frameworks and community-based experiences in times of environmental suffering. *Political Geography, 98*, 1–11. https://doi.org/10.1016/j.polgeo.2022.102721

Hacmun, I., Regev, D., & Salomon, R. (2018). The principles of art therapy in virtual reality. *Frontiers in Psychology, 9.* https://doi.org/10.3389/fpsyg.2018.02082

Haeyen, S., Jans, N., & Heijman, J. (2021). The use of VR tilt brush in art and psychomotor therapy: An innovative perspective. *Arts in Psychotherapy, 76.* https://doi.org/10.1016/j.aip.2021.101855

Hanania, A. (2020). Embroidery (*tatriz*) and Syrian refugees: Exploring loss and hope through storytelling. *Canadian Journal of Art Therapy, 33*(2), 62–69. https://doi.org/10.1080/26907240.2020.1844416

Henderson, P. L. (2021). *Unravelling women's art*. Supernova Books.

Hinz, L. (2015). Media considerations in art therapy: Directions for future research. In D. E. Gussak & M. L. Rosal (Eds.), *The Wiley handbook of art therapy* (pp. 135–145). John Wiley & Sons.

Hogan, S. (2019). The birth project: Mothers and birth professional make art. In S. Hogan (Ed.), *Arts therapies and gender issues: International perspectives on research* (pp. 90–109). Routledge.

Homer, E. S. (2015). Piece 2work: Fabric collage as a neurodevelopmental approach to trauma treatment. *Art Therapy, 32*(1), 20–26. https://doi.org/10.1080/07421656.2015.992824

Horovitz, E. G. (2015). Photography as therapy: Through academic and clinical explorations. In D. E. Gussak & M. L. Rosal (Eds.), *The Wiley handbook of art therapy* (pp. 180–187). Wiley Blackwell.

Houpt, K., Balkin, L. A., Hunt Broom, R., Roth, A. G., & Selma (2016). Anti-memoir: Creating alternate nursing home narratives through zine making. *Art Therapy, 33*(3), 128–137. https://doi.org/10.1080/07421656.2016.1199243

Hu, J. (2021). Rock balancing land art: A more-than-human approach. *Creative Arts in Education and Therapy, 7*(1), 26–33. https://doi.org/10.15212/CAET/2021/7/9

Isis, P., Bokoch, R., Fowler, G., & Hass-Cohen, N. (2023). Efficacy of a single session mindfulness-based art therapy doodle intervention. *Art Therapy, 41*(1), 11–20. https://doi.org/10.1080/07421656.2023.2192168

Jacobson-Levy, M., & Miller, G. M. (2022). Creative destruction and transformation in art and therapy: Reframing, reforming, reclaiming. *Art Therapy, 39*(4), 194–202. https://doi.org/10.1080/07421656.2022.2090306

Kaimal, G., Ayaz, H., Herres, J., Dieterich-Hartwell, R., Makwana, B., Kaiser, D. H., & Nasser, J. A. (2017a). Functional near-infrared spectroscopy assessment of reward perception based on visual self-expression: Coloring, doodling, and free drawing. *Arts in Psychotherapy, 55*. https://doi.org/10.1016/j.aip.2017.05.004

Kaimal, G., Carroll-Haskins, K., Berberian, M., Dougherty, A., Carlton, N., & Ramakrishnan, A. (2019). Virtual reality in art therapy: A pilot qualitative study of the novel medium and implications for practice. *Art Therapy, 37*(1), 16–24. https://doi.org/10.1080/07421656.2019.1659662

Kaimal, G., Gonzaga, A. M. L., & Schwachter, V. (2017b). Crafting, health and wellbeing: Findings from the survey of public participation in the arts and considerations for art therapists. *Arts & Health, 9*(1), 81–90. https://doi.org/10.1080/17533015.2016.1185447

Kalmanowitz, D. (2018). Displacement, art and shelter: Art therapy in a temporary refugee camp. *Journal of Applied Arts & Health, 9*(2), 291–305. https://intellectdiscover.com/content/journals/10.1386/jaah.9.2.291_1

Kalmanowitz, D., & Lloyd, B. (2016). Art therapy at the border: Holding the line of the kite. *Journal of Applied Arts & Health, 7*(2), 143–158. https://doi.org/10.1386/jaah.7.2.143_1

Kalwak, W., & Weihgold, V. (2022). The relationality of ecological emotions: An interdisciplinary critique of individual resilience as psychology's response to the climate crisis. *Frontiers in Psychology, 13*, 1–10. https://doi.org/10.3389/fpsyg.2022.823620

Kapitan, L. (2015). Social action in practice: Shifting the ethnocentric lens in crosscultural art therapy encounters. *Art Therapy, 32*(3), 104–111. https://doi.org/10.1080/07421656.2015.1060403

Kapitan, L. (2021). Crafting the artist book as embodied, relational practice. In L. Leone (Ed.), *Craft in art therapy: Diverse approaches to the transformative power of craft materials and methods* (pp. 23–39). Routledge.

Katoshevski, M., & Huss, E. (2021). Using crafts in art therapy through an intersectional feminist empowerment lens: The case of Bedouin embroidery in Israel. In L. Leone (Ed.), *Craft in art therapy: Diverse approaches to the transformative power of craft materials and methods* (pp. 144–154). Routledge.

Kavitski, J., & Austin, B. (2018). The animation project. In C. Malchiodi (Ed.), *The handbook of art therapy and digital technology* (pp. 175–201). Jessica Kingsley Publishers.

Keaveny, R. (2018). Navigating grief: Using digital narrative as an intervention in art therapy. *Irish Association of Creative Arts Therapists Journal, 5*(1), 17–27. https://polyphony.iacat.me/uploads/ed/archive-journals/PDF_IACAT%20JOURNAL%20APRIL%202018_FINAL.pdf

Keogh, K., & Creaven, A. M. (2017). Evaluating the impact of a brief artistic intervention on cardiovascular recover from acute stress. *Art Therapy, 34*(4), 167–175. https://doi.org/10.1080/07421656.2017.1386038

Kim, J., & Chung, Y. J. (2023). A case study of group art therapy using digital media for adolescents with intellectual disabilities. *Frontiers in Psychiatry, 14*, 1–18. https://doi.org/10.3389/fpsyt.2023.1172079

Kohut, M. (2011). Making art from memories: Honoring deceased loved ones through a scrapbooking bereavement group. *Art Therapy, 28*(3), 123–131. https://doi.org/10.1080/07421656.2011.599731

Kometiani, M. K. (2018). Utilizing digital art therapy with hospitalized youth. In C. Malchiodi (Ed.), *The handbook of art therapy and digital technology* (pp. 247–264). Jessica Kingsley Publishers.

Kopytin, A. (2018). Photo-art therapy. In C. Malchiodi (Ed.), *The handbook of art therapy and digital technology* (pp. 106–126). Jessica Kingsley Publishers.

Lazar, A., Cornejo, R., Edasis, C., & Piper, A. M. (2016, June 4–8). Designing for the third hand: Empowering older adults with cognitive impairment through creating and sharing, *DIS '16: Proceedings of the 2016 ACM Conference on Designing Interactive Systems*, Brisbane, Australia, pp. 1047–1058. https://doi.org/10.1145/2901790.2901854

Lee, L. C. B. (2022). Shifting ethics of care in Hong Kong. *Arts in Psychotherapy, 79.* https://doi.org/10.1016/j.aip.2022.101916

Leone, L. (2019). Crafting change: Craft activism for community-based art therapy. In H. Mandell (Ed.), *Crafting dissent: Handicraft as protest from the American revolution to the pussyhats* (pp. 247–261). Rowman & Littlefield.

Leone, L. (2021). *Craft in art therapy: Diverse approaches to the transformative power of craft materials and methods.* Routledge.

Levine, S. K. (2022). Ecopoiesis: Towards a poietic ecology. In S. K. Levine & A. Kopytin (Eds.), *Ecopoiesis: A new perspective for the expressive and creative arts therapies in the 21st century* (pp. 59–69). Jessica Kingsley Publishers.

Lorenzo de la Peña, S. (2015). 2D expression is intrinsic. In D. E. Gussak & M. L. Rosal (Eds.), *The Wiley handbook of art therapy* (pp. 146–153). John Wiley & Sons.

Mageary, J. (2021). Zines, the DIY ethic, and empowering marginalized identities. In L. Leone (Ed.), *Craft in art therapy: Diverse approaches to the transformative power of craft materials and methods* (pp. 177–189). Routledge.

Martin, R. (2020). Look at me! Representing self, representing ageing: Older women represent their own narratives of ageing using re-enactment phototherapeutic techniques. In S. Hogan (Ed.), *Arts therapies and gender issues: International perspectives on research* (pp. 188–209). Routledge.

Matott, D. L., & Miller, G. M. (Eds.) (2024). *The art and art therapy of papermaking: Material, methods, and applications.* Routledge.

McAvoy, J. (2018). Yarn wrapping sticks – How my own arts practice informed my work with clients and students. *Creative Arts in Education and Therapy, 4*(2), 106–108. https://doi.org/10.15212/CAET/2018/4/17

McNiff, S. (2013). *Art as research: Opportunities and challenges.* Intellect.

McNiff, S. (2022). Foreward: Artistic expression as a force of nature. In S. K. Levine & Kopytin (Eds.), *Ecopoiesis: A new perspective for the expressive and creative arts therapies in the 21st century* (pp. 9–14). Jessica Kingsley Publishers.

Miller, G. (2018). *The art therapist's guide to social media: Connection, community & creativity.* Routledge.

Miller, G. (2022). Art therapists and digital community. In M. Winkel (Ed.), *Virtual art therapy: Research and practice* (pp. 208–219). Routledge.

Moon, C. H. (2002). *Studio art therapy: Cultivating the artist identity in the art therapist.* Jessica Kingsley Publishers.

Moon, C. H. (2010). *Materials and media in art therapy: Critical understandings of diverse artistic vocabularies.* Routledge.

Moon, C. H. (2013). Developing therapeutic arts programs in Kenya and Tanzania: A collaborative consultation approach. In P. Howie, S. Prasad, & J. Kristel (Eds.), *Using art therapy with diverse populations: Crossing cultures and abilities* (pp. 370–380). Jessica Kingsley.

Moon, C. H. (2016). Relational aesthetics and art therapy. In J. A. Rubin (Ed.), *Approaches to art therapy: Theory and technique*. Routledge.

Moon, C. H., Berman, H., Adhiambo, N., Kestone, L., Lema, I. S., Luzzatto, P., Mills, E., Osei, M., Pearce, J., & Reyes, P. (2024). Art therapy in the Global South: Now and next. *South African Journal of Arts Therapies, 2*(1). https://doi.org/10.36615/pk9fjt18

Moxley, D. P., Feen-Calligan, H. R., Washington, O. G. M., & Garriott, L. (2011). Quilting in self-efficacy group work with older African American women leaving homelessness. *Art Therapy, 28*(3), 113–122. https://doi.org/10.1080/07421656.2011.599729

Napoli, M. (2021). Ka Suwe: Culturally sustaining and responsive practices in expressive therapies education. *Arts in Psychotherapy, 76.* https://doi.org/10.1016/j.aip.2021.101854

Napoli, M., & Kirby, M. (2019). Crafting the vulva quilt: A community response to being silenced. In H. Mandell (Ed.), *Crafting dissent: Handicraft as protest from the American revolution to the pussyhats* (pp. 279–289). Rowman & Littlefield.

Nash, G. (2020a). Taking art therapy outdoors: A circle of trees. In I. Siddons Heginworth & G. Nash (Eds.), *Environmental arts therapy: The wild frontiers of the heart* (pp. 137–150). Routledge.

Nash, G. (2020b). Weaving the threads of theory and experience: A review of the literature. In I. Siddons Heginworth & G. Nash (Eds.), *Environmental arts therapy: The wild frontiers of the heart* (pp. 27–43). Routledge.

Neal, L. (2018). Finding stories in a form that can be acted: Creative states in response to climate change denial and biosphere destruction. In J. Adlam, T. Kluttig, & B. X. Lee (Eds.), *Violent states and creative states: From the global to the individual* (pp. 251–264). Jessica Kingsley Publishers.

Nordström, B., & Groth, C. (2022). The role of the weaver in the encounter with life and death. In T. Westerlund, C. Groth, & G. Almevik (Eds.), *Craft sciences* (pp. 292–314). Acta Universitatis Gothenburgensis.

O'Connor, N. (2018). Visual whakapapa: An arts therapy experiential. *Australian and New Zealand Journal of Art Therapy, 13*(1 & 2), 63–66. https://static1.squarespace.com/static/62cb6c4f3dd8c74a52efdb24/t/632175c71971a116a05ca4fd/1663137223936/12.ANZJAT-2018-NOC.pdf

Orbach, N. (2023). *The book of permission: Reflections on art, therapy, education, and being human.* Author.

Orr, P. (2015). Art therapy and digital media. In D. E. Gussak & M. L. Rosal (Eds.), *The Wiley handbook of art therapy* (pp. 188–197). Wiley Blackwell.

Ottiger, N., & Ehemann, R. (2019). Experimenting with gender roles in virtual reality. In S. Hogan (Ed.), *Arts therapies and gender issues: International perspectives on research* (pp. 247–259). Routledge.

Park, S., Lee, H., Kim, S., & Kim, Y. (2021). Traditional Korean art materials as therapeutic media: Multicultural expansion through materials in art therapy. *Art Therapy, 38*(2), 60–68. https://doi.org/10.1080/07421656.2020.1729077

Pellow, D., & Vazin, J. (2019). The intersection of race, immigration status, and environmental justice. *Sustainability, 11*(14), 1–17. https://doi.org/10.3390/su11143942

Pénzes, I., van Hooren, S., Dokter, D., & Hutschemaekers, G. (2014). Material interaction in art therapy assessment. *Arts in Psychotherapy, 41*, 484–492. https://doi.org/10.1016/j.aip.2014.08.003

Peterson, B. C. (2010). The media adoption stage model of technology for art therapy. *Art Therapy: Journal of the American Art Therapy Association, 27*, 26–31.

Raffaelli, T., & Hartzell, E. (2016). A comparison of adults' responses to collage versus drawing in an initial art-making session. *Art Therapy, 33*(1), 21–26. https://doi.org/10.1080/07421656.2016.1127115

Ranganthan, M., & Bratman, E. (2021). From urban resilience to abolitionist climate justice in Washington, DC. *Antipode, 53*(1), 115–137. https://doi.org/10.1111/anti.12555

Rankanen, M., Leinikka, M., Groth, C., Seitamaa-Hakkarainen, P., Makela, M., & Houtilainen, M. (2022). Physiological measurements and emotional experiences of drawing and clay forming. *Arts in Psychotherapy, 79*, 101899. https://doi.org/10.1016/j.aip.2022.101899

Roberts, L. J. (2011). Put your thing down, flip it up, and reverse it: Reimagining craft identities using tactics of queer theory. In M. E. Buszek (Ed.), *Extra/ordinary: Craft and contemporary art* (pp. 243–259). Duke University Press.

Royster, R. (2021). Dolls4Peace memorial: Liberatory community art action and praxis. *Voices: A World Forum for Music Therapy, 21*(1). https://doi.org/10.15845/voices.v21i1.3153

Rubin, R. (2016). The stuck in traffic film project: Engaging young me in community-bases expressive arts activism. *Journal of Applied Arts & Health, 7*(2), 2221–235. https://doi.org/10.1386/jaah.7.2.221_1

Ryu, S., & Price, S. K. (2022). Embodied storytelling and meaning-making at the end of life: VoicingHan avatar life-review for palliative care in cancer patients. *Arts & Health, 14*(3), 326–340. https://doi.org/10.1080/17533015.2021.1942939

Salom, A. (2015). Weaving potential space and acculturation: Art therapy at the museum. *Journal of Applied Arts & Health, 6*(1), 47–62. https://doi.org/10.1386/jaah.6.1.47_1

Segalo, P., Manoff, E., & Fine, M. (2015). Working with embroideries and counter-maps: Engaging memory and imagination within decolonizing frameworks. *Journal of Social and Political Psychology, 3*(1), 342–364. https://doi.org/10.5964/jspp.v3i1.145

Shamri Zeevi, L. (2021). Making art therapy virtual: Integrating virtual reality into art therapy with adolescents. *Frontiers in Psychology, 12*. https://doi.org/10.3389/fpsyg.2021.584943

Smolarski, K., Leone, K., & Robbins, S. J. (2015). Reducing negative mood through drawing: comparing venting, positive expression, and tracing. *Art Therapy, 32*(4), 197–201. https://doi.org/10.1080/07421656.2015.1092697

Snir, S., Regev, D., & Shaashua, Y. H. (2017). Relationships between attachment avoidance and anxiety and responses to art materials. *Art Therapy, 34*(1), 20–28. https://doi.org/10.1080/07421656.2016.1270139

Springham, N., & Xenophontes, I. (2021). Democratizing the discourse: Co-production in art therapy practice, research and publication. *International Journal of Art Therapy, 26*(1–2), 1–7. https://doi.org/10.1080/17454832.2021.1912939

Talwar, S. (2019). "The sweetness of money": The creatively empowered women (CEW) design studio, feminist pedagogy and art therapy. In S. Talwar (Ed.), *Art therapy for social justice* (pp. 178–193). Routledge.

Talwar, S. (2020). Feminism as practice: Crafting and the politics of art therapy. In S. Hogan (Ed.), *Gender and difference in the arts therapies: Inscribed on the body* (pp. 13–23). Routledge.

Talwar, S., & Wallis, R. (2021). Quilting across prison walls: Craftwork, social practice, and radical empathy. In L. Leone (Ed.), *Craft in art therapy: Diverse approaches to the transformative power of craft materials and methods* (pp. 237–252). Routledge.

Taylor-Johnson, H. (2023). Knitting as a way of honoring Black ancestry and creating storytelling through community, belonging, and the reframing of grief: A Womanist perspective. *Canadian Journal of Art Therapy, 36*(1), 12–19. https://doi.org/10.1080/26907240.2023.2199623

Thrall, J. (2017). Interpersonal knots: An art-based exploration of tying and untying. In B. MacWilliam (Ed.), *Complicated grief, attachment, and art therapy* (pp. 174–187). Jessica Kingsley Publishers.

Timm-Bottos, J. (2011). Endangered threads: Socially committed community art action. *Art Therapy, 28*(2), 57–63. https://doi.org/10.1080/07421656.2011.578234

Tuval-Mashiach, R., Patton, B. S., & Drebing, C. (2018). "When you make a movie, and you see your story there, you can hold it": Qualitative exploration of collaborative filmmaking as a therapeutic tool for veterans. *Frontiers in Psychology, 9*, 1–11. https://doi.org/10.3389/fpsyg.2018.01954

Usiskin, M., & Lloyd, B. (2020). Lifeline, frontline, online: Adapting art therapy for social engagement across borders. *International Journal of Art Therapy, 25*(4), 183–191. https://doi.org/10.1080/17454832.2020.1845219

Valldejuli, K., & Belnavis Elliott, L. A. (2023). Shifting the narrative: An intersectional exploration of art therapy in the Caribbean. *International Journal of Art Therapy, 28*(1–2), 58–64. https://doi.org/10.1080/17454832.2023.2174999

van Zyl, J. (2023). Re-storying pregnancy loss: Threading narrative, artmaking and textile-weaving into an embodied grief work ritual. *South African Journal of Arts Therapies, 1*(1), 203–225. https://doi.org/10.36615/sajat.v1i1.2571

Velasquez, M. (2022). Let's go outside: Nature-based play therapy through the lens of cultural humility. In J. A. Courtney, J. L. Langley, L. L. Wonders, R. Heiko, & R. Lapiere (Eds.), *Nature-based play and expressive therapies: Interventions for working with children, teens, and families* (pp. 45–56). Routledge.

Vivien, J. (2018). Reconciliation: A contemplation of the role of art therapy. *Canadian Art Therapy Association Journal, 31*(1), 43–48. https://doi.org/10.1080/08322473.2018.1453223

Walters, J. A. (2022). Online art therapy: Experiences of art therapists during the COVID-19 pandemic. In M. Winkel (Ed.), *Virtual art therapy: Research and practice* (pp. 26–35). Routledge.

Wardle, A. (2023). Landscape of loss: Art therapy outdoors and traumatic bereavement. *International Journal of Art Therapy, 29*, 1–7. https://doi.org/10.1080/17454832.2023.2267109

Warson, E. (2013). Healing pathways: American Indian medicine and art therapy. *Canadian Art Therapy Association Journal, 26*(2), 33–38. https://doi.org/10.1080/08322473.2013.11415584

Weiser, J. (2014). Establishing the framework for using photos in art therapy (and other therapies) practices. *Arteterapia: Papeles de Arteterapia y Educación Artística para la Inclusión Social, 9*, 159–190. https://revistas.ucm.es/index.php/ARTE/article/view/47490

Whitaker, P. (2016). A Review of 'Green Studio': Nature and the Arts in Therapy by A. Kopytin and M. Rugh. *Art Therapy, 33*(4), 220–221. https://doi.org/10.1080/07421656.2016.1230449

Whitaker, P. (2021). Habitats of composition: The nature of the commons. *Ecopoiesis: Eco-Human Theory and Practice, 2*(1), 26–32. https://en.ecopoiesis.ru/aktualnoe/news_post/habitats-of-composition-the-nature-of-the-commons

Whyte, M. K. (2020). Walking on two-row: Reconciling First Nations identity and colonial trauma through material interaction, acculturation, and art therapy. *Canadian Journal of Art Therapy, 33*(1), 36–45. https://doi.org/10.1080/08322473.2020.1724745

Wolk, N., & Bat Or, M. (2023). The therapeutic aspects of embroidery in art therapy from the perspective of adolescent girls in a post-hospitalization boarding school. *Children, 10*(6), 1–21. https://doi.org/10.3390/children10061084

Wong, D., & Lay, R. P. M. H. (2021). *Found objects in art therapy: Materials and process.* Jessica Kingsley Publishers.

Wong, T. Y. W. (2024). Emergent well-being: A qualitative study on cultural identity and belonging of emigrated Hong Kongers post-2019. *Art Therapy, 42*(2), 1–10. https://doi.org/10.1080/07421656.2024.2366576

Yi, C. S. (2021). Demystifying the individualistic approach to self-care: Sewing as a metaphorical process for documenting relational and communal care in disability culture. In L. Leone (Ed.), *Craft in art therapy: Diverse approaches to the transformative power of craft materials and methods* (pp. 72–89). Routledge.

Zaken, S. B., & Walsh, S. D. (2021). Bridging the cultural gap: Challenges and coping mechanisms employed by Arab art therapists in Israel. *Arts in Psychotherapy, 76.* https://doi.org/10.1016/j.aip.2021.101853

Zubala, A., Kennel, N., & Hackett, C. (2021). Art therapy in the digital world: An integrative review of current practice and future directions. *Frontiers in Psychology, 2,* 595536. https://doi.org/10.3389/ fpsyg.2021.600070

2

THEORIES OF MATERIALITY AND MAKING

Catherine Hyland Moon

Theory building is not just the prerogative of academics and researchers, but is a product of the everyday, ordinary experiences of observing, making, investigating, conversing, construing, trying something new, reflecting, writing, consulting, trying something else, etc. (Moon, 2014). Unfortunately, only those who have the social capital to speak and be heard have their ideas sanctioned as theory. When formally presented through academic norms and dominant cultural values and conventions, theories are reified as guiding truths, while creative practices of knowledge production by those on the cultural margins are often delegitimized, dismissed, co-opted, or erased (Norris et al., 2021).

Theory is often considered common sense not because of its objective truth, but because it preserves dominant values and practices. To develop anticolonial, anti-oppressive approaches to art therapy theory, we need to make visible how our theories and discourses are systemically entwined with power and take responsibility for how we support or resist them.

In this chapter I describe two art therapy theories, the Expressive Therapies Continuum and the constructivist theory of materiality, presenting the strengths and shortcomings of each. I then present two additional theoretical perspectives, critical theory and new materialism, and discuss their potential for centering art therapy materials/practices theory within a socio-ecological justice framework.

DOI: 10.4324/9781032720166-3

Expressive Therapies Continuum

The Expressive Therapies Continuum (ETC) theorizes art therapy participants' engagement with art materials and processes in relation to developmental levels and visual information processing. It was developed by Vija Lusebrink and Sandra Kagin, who published the first article about it in 1978. Initially, the theory was not well received, but interest in it has greatly increased since 2009 (Hinz, 2020; Lusebrink, 2016).

The ECT proposes a way to conceptualize artmaking along three continuums that, from bottom to top, represent increasingly complex developmental levels of information processing.

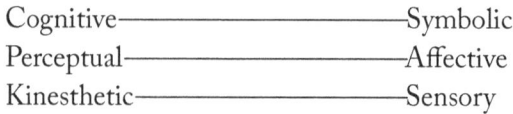

```
Cognitive————————————Symbolic
Perceptual————————————Affective
Kinesthetic————————————Sensory
```

The first level from the bottom, **Kinesthetic/Sensory,** is focused on bodily experiences. On the Kinesthetic end the emphasis is on motor expression, while on the other end sensory experiences are dominant. The second level, **Perceptual/Affective,** concerns the process by which materials become formed expressions. On the Perceptual end the formal elements of expression, such as figure/ground relationships, are pronounced. On the Affective end, attention to form recedes as emotional expression becomes dominant. The third level, **Cognitive/Symbolic,** is concerned with content and meaning. On the Cognitive end, concepts and problem solving are pronounced, while on the Symbolic end, intuition, metaphor, and personal insights are emphasized (Hinz, 2020).

A fourth part of the schema is the **Creative Dimension,** which can exist at any or all levels but is incorporated on the ETC diagram as a vertical line intersecting the three horizontal continuums. It represents the integrative function or self-actualizing effect elicited by artmaking, experienced as a flow state, a sense of well-being, and/or feelings of satisfaction and joy (Hinz et al., 2022a).

The other aspect of the ETC is the **Media Dimensions Variables** construct. These variables include the **structure** and **task complexity** involved in using a material or making a specific product, the **boundaries** of what's possible with a material given its quantity and capacity, the **mediators** (paintbrush, chisel, etc.) that come between the maker and direct sensory experiencing of materials, the **reflective distance** between making something and reflecting on it, and the effect of **novelty** related to introducing new media. Media **properties** have received the most attention in the field's literature, specifically in relation to *resistive* (dry, relatively nonmalleable, difficult to manipulate) and *fluid* (aqueous, malleable, relatively difficult to control) materials. It is theorized that resistive materials are more likely associated with cognitive processes, while fluid materials are more likely associated with affective processes. Altogether, these seven media variables can be used as change agents within the therapy process to shift or expand information-processing capabilities (Graves-Alcorn & Green, 2014; Hinz, 2020; VanMeter & Hinz, 2023).

Strengths

The strengths of the ETC include its applicability to diverse therapy approaches, using any media or material. The model is adaptable to participants' preferences and needs, and guides therapists' decision-making based on participants' responses to art materials and processes. Most significantly, it provides a uniquely art-based theory that considers the interactions of materials and embodied making practices. The ETC has wide appeal, as evidenced by research and practice publications.

The ETC's flexibility in relation to cultural relevance might be seen as a strength or shortcoming. Chapin Stephenson (2021) has adapted the model to the developmental stages of older adults and people with dementia, and Whyte (2023) has proposed alternative, culturally informed interpretations of behaviors and a revision of the model's diagram from hierarchical to circular. These modifications could be interpreted as evidence of the theory's flexibility or its lack of cultural relevance.

Shortcomings

While the ETC has made important contributions to art therapy theory, it also has deficiencies. First, since its inception the ETC has been theorized primarily in relation to conventional art materials and practices, and has not encompassed the much wider range of materials and methods currently employed in the field. Also, the resistive-to-fluid continuum provides insufficient consideration of the properties of art materials/media. Materials' textures, colors, weights, movements, durability/fragility, structures, temperatures, flexibility/stability, smells, sounds, interactions with light and space, etc. are not considered. It is hard to relate materials like an outdoor environment, the human body, or sound to simply a resistive/fluid continuum.

Second, authors with ETC expertise have acknowledged that a lack of training opportunities has led to misunderstanding and misuse of the theory (Hinz et al., 2022b). One of the most frequent misapplications, evident in the field's literature, is basing a material choice on the simplistic equation of fluid = emotive, resistive = cognitive. While inadequate training may be implicated in this misuse, so too is the ETC's limited consideration of material properties.

Third, through a reductionistic focus on biological systems and outdated developmental theories, the ETC ignores the role of socio-cultural factors and oversimplifies the complex nature of the art therapy process. For example, an Indigenous participant's engagement on the Kinesthetic/Sensory level might be mistakenly interpreted as their preferred means of information processing when it really reflects cultural connection to land and ceremony (Whyte, 2023). Or, in contradiction to the theory that fluid materials elicit spontaneity and emotional expression, a Chinese participant using paint is more likely to limit expression in favor of conveying nature-human harmony, making disciplined brush marks, and following a traditional landscape theme (Leung, 2020; Potash & Kalmanowitz, 2012).

Finally, the allure of neuroscientific knowledge can lead to broad, uncritical acceptance of even provisional theories like the ETC, without consideration of socio-cultural-environmental factors. At the same time, neuroscience's presumed authority and claims on normativity can lead to the "creation" of certain kinds of people by establishing classifications, interpretations, and practices. To judiciously integrate neuroscience developments into art therapy theory and practice, it is crucial for researchers, practitioners, and stakeholders to critically reflect on the ontological implications of the ETC and its resulting circulation of ideas and beliefs (Slaby, 2010).

Social Constructivist Theory of Materiality

In the first edition of this book (Moon, 2010), I presented the Social Constructivist Theory of Materiality (SCTM). As a postmodern theory, constructivism rejects essentialist "truths" and emphasizes that knowledge, meaning, and reality are socially created. The SCTM proposes that the import and meaning of materials are continually co-constructed within personal, social, cultural, historical, and political contexts.

A postmodern approach also deconstructs dominant beliefs to expose the underlying social forces that create and maintain them. For example, the common falsehood in art therapy that clay is a regressive material may have been derived from society's devaluing of manual labor as *dirty work*. The characterization of clay as regressive is particularly suspect given its attribution to psychiatrically hospitalized patients but not ceramic artists, suggesting the characterization is tied to the disparagement of Mad or mentally distressed people more than to the nature of clay. Such faulty beliefs come to be viewed as fact when they are repeated and maintained through sanctioned representations of expertise, such as academic institutions or journal publications, resulting in their unquestioned acceptance.

The SCTM proposes seven lenses through which to view materials. These lenses are not comprehensive, but merely representative of the multiplicity and potentially conflictual nature of material significations.

Aesthetic preference relates to assigned value or significance based on heightened awareness, feelings, or sense of beauty. Aesthetic preferences for art materials, practices, and products are informed by culturally bound tastes and values, which are influenced by factors, such as class, gender, race, geographic origins, religion, and educational opportunities.

Physical and sensual characteristics derived from the direct experiencing of materials evoke reactions from pleasure to aversion and conjure associations to particular times, places, and experiences. Materials provide embodied feedback and ground the maker in the physicality of the world. Visuality and tactility are most often ascribed to artmaking, but sounds, smells, and sometimes taste are also involved, as is engagement of the body's physiological systems.

Personal associations to materials and making practices are inevitable because there is no distinct separation between inner life and the outer environment. Recent literature in the field on the use of found objects attests to how even everyday materials/objects from the external environment can evoke inner thoughts, emotions, metaphors, experiences, losses, stories, and memories.

Associated language includes both descriptive words and idiomatic expressions. Exploring the nature of the words/expressions associated with art materials and processes can be enlightening. For example, cameras are used to *shoot*, *snap*, *take*, or *capture* images, suggesting that photography can be experienced as aggressive, intrusive, or controlling. Idiomatic expressions related to textiles—coming unraveled, patching things up, falling apart at the seams, being on the mend—suggest their connection to themes of rupture and repair.

Utilitarian function or purpose is significant for both single-use and multiuse or hybrid materials. For example, the sole purpose of a tube of watercolor paint is to add color to something, while a pair of scissors can be used for artmaking, office work, cooking, etc. Found objects used in artmaking often hold associations to their prior identities. For example, a wire clothes hanger holds garments for various purposes (organizing, protecting, displaying, selling, etc.). Hangers have also been used as tools to retrieve keys from accidentally locked cars, makeshift television antennae, and crude instruments for performing abortions. These visual and conceptual references to multiple functions and histories thicken an object's narrative.

Popular culture consists of beliefs, values, actions, or objects whose popularity is reinforced through mass media. It can include language, music, fashion, dance, television shows, lifestyles, social media, etc. For example, a Do It Yourself (DIY) ethos has been popular in recent years, as evidenced by interest in recycling and upcycling, television shows about renovating old houses, and communities that support sustainable lifestyles. Numerous "how to" videos provide instructions for creating from scratch, repairing rather than buying, or life-hacking. Art activities like visible mending, craftivism, found object art, and zines exemplify the DIY spirit, which can be associated with ecological concern, rejection of consumerism, anti-establishment stance, romantic idealism, mutual aid values, or adherence to trends.

Socio-cultural-historical relevance should be a primary consideration for using any art materials, media, and processes within therapy.

Art materials and practices are socially, culturally, and historically situated. Their valuation and meanings are constructed from social factors like their geographic origins, the intersectional identities of those who have historically employed them, and the ways (and by whom) they have been adopted, co-opted, and transformed over time.

Strengths

Like the ECT, strengths of the SCTM include its applicability to diverse therapy approaches using any media or material, and its adaptability to participants' preferences, needs, and responses to art materials and processes. Its most significant contribution to the field is that it considers the qualities and characteristics of materials and making practices in relation to their situatedness within historical, social, cultural, and political contexts. It offers a postmodern corrective to individualistic, positivist understandings of materials and media by asserting that multiple contextual factors are constitutive forces in the experiencing and semiotics of materiality.

Shortcomings

While the SCTM has made important contributions to art therapy theory, it also has deficiencies. First, the SCTM's basis in epistemological relativism means there are no irrefutable truths about the significance and meaning of art materials and practices, and thus its practical application is open to interpretation. Depending on the art therapist, this open-endedness could be experienced as invigorating (freedom to break through top-down, oppressive theories) or discouraging (unsure about what to do with this web of overlapping perspectives).

Second, to my knowledge, no research has examined the SCTM's validity, relevance, or practical implications. This is likely due to the challenge of researching an open-ended theory and the lack of broad endorsement of the SCTM.

Third, the theory's focus is anthropocentric. According to constructivism, the material world (both human and more-than-human) is viewed as simply the end result of humans' representational activities. Following this logic, matter only matters because of the meaning humans assign to it, and humans are the only beings who have agency. This theoretical position is no longer defensible given that anthropocentrism has been a significant driver of the worldwide climate crises.

Building art therapy theory

Despite their shortcomings, both the ETC and the SCTM have useful elements for theorizing art materials, media, and processes in art therapy. Two additional models, critical theory and new materialism, offer helpful perspectives for ongoing theory building. Critical theory is similar to the SCTM in its socio-cultural-historical-political perspective, but its focus is not limited to the meanings ascribed to materials. New materialism, as informed by Indigenous scholarship, provides a theoretical and philosophical approach to materiality that is inclusive of the human and more-than-human world.

Critical theory

Critical theory (CT) analyzes and exposes the effects of power relations and social inequities on theory and practice, examining the influences of relationships, ideologies, institutions, and systems. Nondominant discourses, such as queer, disability, feminist, and critical race theories, are all rooted in CT. A critical approach endeavors to create a more just world through rejecting fixed binaries and essentialist narratives, honoring diverse worldviews and sense-making frameworks, and promoting freedom from oppressive systems (Ki, 2025).

Art therapy materials, media, and processes can be considered through a critical lens by interrupting taken-for-granted assumptions and raising questions relevant to history, theory, research, and practice. For example: What is included in the canon of art history? Who is authorized to validate its inclusions and exclusions? Whose arts and cultural knowledges, perspectives, values, and traditions are privileged, and whose are overlooked, denied, exoticized, or appropriated? Whose artistic language is listened to and seen, and whose is ignored or devalued (lok, in Vellodi, 2020, p. 38)? What are art therapy students formally taught about visual arts and material culture, and informally taught through the materials made available and making practices introduced? Whose cultural capital does this curriculum reinforce and whose does it undermine? What dominant narratives about cultural art forms are reinforced through art therapy theory and practice? How does our use of visual arts reinforce or destabilize dominant gender, sexual, racial, class, and ability politics? How do art therapists contribute to the extraction, exploitation, and Westernization of art forms? (Hadley, 2013). I offer below a few examples of critical theory applied to art therapy theory and practice.

First, despite the incorporation of a more diverse repertoire of art materials/methods into art therapy in recent years, painting and drawing remain strikingly dominant. What is at issue is not simply the frequency with which these practices are employed, but that they are often employed unselfconsciously and uncritically. In particular, painting and drawing remain mostly untheorized beyond the fluid/resistive binary. The beneficial status of drawing/painting is simply assumed, or supported by weak rationales like familiarity or ease of transport. How and on whose authority have drawing and painting come to dominate the field? Whose culture-specific knowledges, perspectives, and values do they represent, and at whose expense?

Second, why has scholarship about the *art* of art therapy been underdeveloped relative to scholarship about the *therapy* of art therapy? The field's relationship to art history has been largely ignored. A recent exception to this trend (Dean, 2016) is focused almost exclusively on White, European, male artists, an unfortunate echo of the exclusion of art therapists of color from art therapy history. Positioning the field in relation to psychology rather than art has undoubtedly been motivated by access to power and status. While there are arguments about the practical implications of this alignment, such as employment opportunities and reimbursement for services, the question must be asked: At what cost? What asymmetrical relations of power have been reinforced by this hierarchy of clinical over arts-based skills? How has this hierarchy colluded with the privileging of White dominant cultural art forms and the silencing of art forms associated with racialized others?

Third, the art therapy field has been slow to adopt art practices that directly engage the body as ground or material. While art therapists have developed sophisticated theories about kinesthetic and sensorially based encounters with art materials (e.g., Elbrecht, 2021), there has been little scholarship on the use of the body as a creative ground for marking, modifying, or embellishing through art forms such as makeup, hairstyling/dyeing, fashion, costuming, jewelry, tattooing, piercing, or culture-specific practices like henna or scarification. Likewise, the body is seldom considered a material and engaged through art forms like cosplay, ritual, and performance art. There are many issues that could be sensitively addressed through direct body engagement, such as gender-based violence, chronic illness, and pregnancy loss. In particular, people from marginalized groups whose bodies are sites through which oppression is enacted could benefit from body-based approaches that transgress body norms and question how and why we read bodies through binary constructs. How might art therapy shift from viewing the body only as a noun that can be (re)presented through artworks to experiencing the body as a verb that *is* material, moves, processes, and performs actions (Johnson, 2021)? Whose cultural capital is reinforced and whose is undermined when we separate "a person's health and wellbeing from their bodies in the world" (Gipson, 2017, p. 115)?

Fourth, there are some glaring gaps in the literature that have implications for the field in relation to art materials and practices. To name just three, there is a dearth of literature on disability studies, social class, and the ethics of material use in relation to climate crisis. The overarching question is why these three topics have received inadequate attention, particularly given that they each hold relevance to a central aspect of our field. The first, disability studies, is obviously germane, given that its scholarship comes from people who self-identify as Disabled, Mad, Sick (chronically ill), Deaf, and Autistic (Yi & Moon, 2020), that is, from the very people who hold the primary identities around which our field constellates. Connecting with this literature not only provides important critiques of ableist, individualized, pathologizing approaches to art therapy (Ehlert, 2020; Yi, 2019), but also offers alternative models of collective care through the arts and exposes art therapists to disability arts and culture resources that could be of significant benefit to participants (Beck, 2020; Miller, 2020; Yi, 2010, 2021). The second and third topics—social class and the environmental ethics of materials—each raise timely concerns about material resource use in art therapy. Though art therapy literature often focuses on work within marginalized communities, the practical, ethical, and justice issues related to (un)sustainable access to art materials are seldom addressed (Moon & Faulkner, 2024). Likewise, though there is a plethora of literature on ecological approaches to art therapy, the field's complicity with the degradation of the environment through the use of toxic materials (paints, plastic beads, glitter, etc.) is rarely mentioned. What is behind these glaring absences? Are we collectively avoiding exposure of misaligned professional values and norms in relation to disability, economic, and environmental justice? How might we instead commit ourselves to "a justice of (re)distribution of land, resources, and opportunities, and also a justice of recognition in terms of dignity, identity, history, and collective biography" (Segalo et al., 2015)? How might we give ourselves permission to name our gaps in knowledge or awareness and our failures in practice so that we might better live out the social justice values to which we aspire?

New materialism

New materialism (NM) is a domain within posthumanism that has been taken up by the arts, social sciences, and humanities. It presents a broadly inclusive understanding of the nature of matter, contrasting with both modernism's positivist views (matter as inert, objective) and postmodernism's constructivist views (matter shaped by socially and culturally inscribed meanings). Below I outline key concepts of NM.

Matter is inclusive of all human and more-than-human entities. Objects, buildings, plants, animals, atmospheres, technologies, microbes, stars, gravity, time, imagination, and memory, as well as physical, biological, psychological, social, and cultural matter all co-constitute the continuous production of what is understood as reality.

Matter is dynamic, animate, has agency, exerts forces, and thus is constantly forming and re-forming in unpredictable ways, creating assemblages of evolving, emergent configurations, and co-producing knowledge among human and more-than-human, social, and material entities (Hickey-Moody et al., 2016). By collapsing the distinction between the physical world and social constructs, NM invites exploration of how each affects the other, as well as how nonhuman entities exert influence and shape what unfolds (Fox & Alldred, 2019). *Intra-action* refers to this mutual, dynamic exchange of actions and influences. It differs from *interaction* in that there are no pre-established, discrete entities involved, only phenomena that are constantly becoming (Barad, 2003).

Agential realism refers to the dynamic exchange among all human and nonhuman entities whereby "agency is not an attribute but the ongoing reconfigurings of the world" (Barad, 2003, p. 818). Agency is also not a unique capacity of humans, but is constantly enacted across the co-production of bodies and things. *Agential cuts* are the intentional but temporary pauses or stabilizations that simultaneously delineate boundaries and acknowledge ongoing entanglements (Barad, 2014, p. 168).

Rejection of binaries like mind/matter, culture/nature, subject/object, and living/nonliving is a consequence of conceptualizing matter as flexible and permeable. NM, therefore, also rejects "identity and difference defined through a colonizing logic whereby the 'self' maintains and stabilizes itself by eliminating or dominating what it takes to be the other" (Barad, 2014, p. 169).

Challenging anthropocentrism is a key precept of NM. Humans are not merely *in* the world as detached observers but are *of* the world, engaged in its ongoing intra-activity and co-creation (Barad, 2003). The universe is not divided into humans who are actively aware and making choices, and things and ideas that are inert and passive; everything is intertwined, vital, active, and constantly changing (Braidotti, 2020).

Ethical concerns are inherent to a worldview in which everything is interconnected. Not only does NM posit the intimacy and proximity of the universe, but it also asserts that, as a byproduct of our entanglements, we cannot extricate ourselves from ethical concerns. We are part of the world, and the world is part of us (Ringrose et al., 2019).

Indigenous knowledges

But is NM really new? The centering of nonhuman ethics, respect for the vitality and agency of both the biological and nonbiological conceptualizations of the body as an assemblage of interconnected life forms, and understanding that planetary life is foundational to political worldbuilding is not new. These perspectives have long been familiar to Indigenous peoples and to followers of other non-Western medical and spiritual practices (Wazana Tompkins, 2016).

NM, because of its Euro-American philosophical origins and the whiteness of its current scholarship (Strom et al., 2019), has been criticized for positioning materialism as *new* while ignoring the long-held understanding of materiality as a source of deep epistemological value within Indigenous ways of knowing (Todd, 2016). As a non-Indigenous scholar myself, and a citizen of a White supremacist settler society (Turtle Island/USA), I acknowledge the long-standing Indigenous scholarships and practices that predate NM. Eurocentric perspectives are neither the only nor the universal authority on this topic. Yet, I also do not have the competence to present Indigenous knowledges without the risk of misinterpreting, flattening, or distorting them (Sundberg, 2014). I lack deeply embodied and spiritually grounded understanding of Indigenous ontologies and epistemologies. For example, I deeply respect and am moved by Cameron's (2021) description of Country from an Australian Aboriginal perspective, but I *do not hold this knowledge in my bones.*

However, I can unsettle the racial/colonial biases that shaped my scholarly interests in NM and led me only secondarily to Indigenous scholarship. With the aim of disrupting, even in a small way, the oppressive historic and current knowledge practices of NM, I recognize below some of the aspects of Indigenous knowledge that are more developed than—and could enrich—new materialism and art therapy theorizing.

NM focuses on justifying nonhuman agency to a Eurocentric audience, while Indigenous knowledge holders presume the pervasive existence and influence of nonhuman agency, enabling them to concentrate their scholarship and practices on productive, reciprocal, ethical relationships with the more-than-human world (Rosiek et al., 2019).

NM posits that relational intra-actions occur among all human and nonhuman entities. However, unlike Indigenous studies, NM literature seldom refers to rocks, thunder, or lakes as relatives, ancestors, or persons. Indigenous scholars offer a more developed knowledge, language, and practice base from which to create a relationally democratic world where humans and inanimate objects like rocks are "cohabiting one another, or feeding one another, or making and re-making one another" (TallBear, 2011, para. 17).

NM tends to refer to intra-actions between humans and the more-than-human in general terms. The Eurocentric generalization and objectification of nature have led to its being mapped, used, owned, and destroyed. In contrast, Indigenous scholarship emphasizes the formation of relations with *particular* places and entities, as agency emerges from locally specific circumstances, cosmologies, and place-based knowledges. For example, Indigenous communities understand land/Country's role in the dissemination of life lessons for future generations (Rosiek et al., 2019).

NM literature sometimes misrepresents Indigenous origin stories as lore or legend rather than actual events, which is a colonizing act (intentional or not) that can undermine people's beliefs in themselves and their histories. It exposes Eurocentric perspectives that distinguish between place and thought, "where land is simply dirt and thought is only possessed by humans" (Watts, 2013, p. 32). TallBear (2011) points out that it is important to present Indigenous ontologies as *knowledge* rather than *beliefs*. Indigenous people are in relation to land that is alive, thinking, spiritual, and—for some communities—gendered. Thus, theorizing and place are intertwined.

Ideally, transdisciplinary exchange among Indigenous and NM scholars will grow. If undertaken with *ethical relationality*, which is not about assimilation, but about recognizing difference as ecologically necessary and seeking "deeper understanding of how our different histories, memories, and experiences position us in relation to one another" (Donald, 2016, p. 11), then such an exchange could support the futurity Indigenous, NM, and art therapy scholars hope for.

Implications of new materialism/Indigenous scholarship for art therapy

Below I describe a few ways that NM and Indigenous knowledges can support and deepen art therapy theory and practice.

Provides art-compatible theory

Art's capacity to hold complex, multilayered meanings is consistent with the concept of material forces continually composing and recomposing. In contemporary art, these forces engender affect, agitate and provoke, manifest ideas that flow and transform, are able to tolerate what is ill-defined, enable emergent knowledges, tell alternative narratives, and are concerned with ethical response-ability related to patterns of injustice (Strom et al., 2019).

Supports relational vitality and agency among makers and materials

Many accounts from artists, therapists, and practice-led arts researchers vividly convey intra-active relationships with materials, citing how
materials "behave, their feel, diversity, idiosyncrasies, and the rules they
inherently impose…, how materials exert themselves" (Fenner, 2019,
p. 410). Materials provide artists with feedback, affect their ideas, and
perhaps teach them how to make differently than they had planned
(Aktaş & Mäkelä, 2019; Hickey-Moody & Page, 2015). An artist's
belief that they are the sole producer, fully in charge of an emerging artwork, "may be betrayed by the unexpected dynamism of the materiality"
(Havsteen-Franklin et al., 2024, p. 10).

Supports development of trust

The idea of working *with* materials means the art process is one of
co-evolvement within a shared process of interchange. Initially, participants new to an art material or process might desire "rules" that enable
them to gain confidence or a sense of mastery. However, over time, if
participant-artists are able to develop trusting relationships with materials as creative partners, reliance on rules will recede and participants will
be able to allow the materials to co-lead (Aktaş, 2019). This way of working has relevance to the development of trusting relationships in other
areas of life—not only with other humans, but also with one's embodied
self and with the other-than-human world.

Encourages intra-active relational well-being

NM and Indigenous knowledges support an approach to artwork that is
not tied simply to its representational function, but rather to its potential
as a site for "the assemblage and intra-action of environment, materiality,
maker, and social context" (Havsteen-Franklin et al., 2024, p. 4). For art
therapists attuned to the social determinants of well-being and the role
injustice plays in degrading physical, mental, social, and planetary health,
this wider perspective is a necessity (Moon, 2023). It shifts the emphasis
in art therapy from an individualistic, human-centric practice to a relational aesthetic whereby artmaking leads to the deepening of relational
bonds and the expansion of care practices from the self to other people,

the socio-political context (Moon, 2002, 2016), and all that constitutes the more-than-human world.

Allows for reflection and meaning-making

Establishing an environment conducive to the development of collaborative, trusting, intra-active relationships with materials does not preclude setting goals with participants or co-creating structures to facilitate reaching those goals. What Barad (2014) calls *agential cuts* include all the ways art therapists create the space to pause, focus, reflect, and consider possibilities. Whether an art therapist offers participants a question, gesture, comment, empathic murmur, invitation to journal, mirrored movement, or any other such response, these types of actions can temporarily separate phenomena from the ongoing flow of intra-actions. If done sensitively, participants are then able to examine, ponder, and gain knowledge that helps them (re)build meaningful, livable lives (Hickey-Moody, 2018).

Disrupts binaries of normativity

Intersectionality is an inherent feature of NM, given that overlapping and interdependent systems of advantage/disadvantage are part of the "matter" of life that is actively and already unfolding and mixing together. This blurring of boundaries leads to questions such as: "What is 'natural' vs. 'unnatural, what is 'healthy' vs. 'sickness,' and what is 'compulsory' vs. 'deviant'?" (Bauman, 2015, p. 70). The same human/animal split that engenders violence is evident in harm directed toward human bodies that deviate from the norm (TallBear, 2011), bodies that are dark, disabled, queer, Indigenous, neurodivergent, immigrant, female, old, young, fat, or poor. If we look to biodiversity as crucial to a healthy planet and biomimicry as a guide to ethical care, we can radically alter norms around who/what is considered worthy of care and protection, who/what is viewed as threatening or disposable, and what it means to be an ally (Bauman, 2015; Clare, 2014; Crilley, 2016). For art therapy practice, such a vision could inspire spaces that intentionally welcome the *Other*, art materials and practices that disrupt high art norms for alternative aesthetic and material practices, and a *making* ethos that holds diversity (of thought, experience, identity, bodies, ideas, etc.) as crucial to health and well-being.

Supports an eco-relational ethic of care

Not only do NM and Indigenous studies challenge anthropocentrism, but they also dispute the very concept of a discrete, autonomous individual. However, they also acknowledge that agency is inequitably distributed among all humans and nonhumans. There are imbalances of power to which we humans must be accountable if we are to take seriously our ethical response-ability for co-shaping the world. For art therapists, NM theory demands both humility (abandoning anthropocentric notions) and responsibility (acknowledging our power). It challenges us to take the humble position of serving as conduits or scribes for materiality (Fairbairn, 2023) and collaborating with it in the telling of co-constitutive stories. It challenges us to reckon with what it means to be entangled with our nonhuman kin in a biosphere that is ailing.

References

Aktaş, B. M. (2019). Using wool's agency to design and make felted artefacts. *RUUKKU: Studies in Artistic Research, 10.* https://www.researchcatalogue.net/view/453632/453633

Aktaş, B. M., & Mäkelä, M. (2019). Negotiation between the maker and material: Observations on material interactions in felting studio. *International Journal of Design, 13*(2), 55–67. https://www.ijdesign.org/index.php/IJDesign/article/view/ 3267/857

Barad, K. (2003). Posthumanist performativity: Toward an understanding of how matter comes to matter. *Signs: Journal of Women in Culture and Society, 28*(3), 801–831. https://www.journals.uchicago.edu/doi/10.1086/345321

Barad, K. (2014). Diffracting diffraction: Cutting together-apart. *Parallax, 20*(3), 168–187. https://doi.org/10.1080/13534645.2014.927623

Bauman, W. A. (2015). Disability studies, queer theory, and the new materialism: Environmental metaphors for a planet on the move. *Worldviews, 19*(1), 69–73. https://www.jstor.org/stable/43809766

Beck, B. (2020). Embodied practice: Reflections of a physically disabled art therapist in social and medical disability spaces. *Art Therapy, 37*(2), 62–69. https://doi.org/10.1080/07421656.2020.1756137

Braidotti, R. (2020). "We" may be in *this* together, but we are not all human and we are not one and the same. *Ecocene, 1*(1), 26–31. https://doi.org/10.46863/ecocene.31

Cameron, L. (2021). Australian Indigenous sensory knowledge systems in creative practices. *Creative Arts in Education and Therapy, 7*(2), 114–127. https://caet.inspirees.com/caetojsjournals/index.php/caet/article/view/329

Chapin Stephenson, R. (2021). *Art therapy and creative aging: Reclaiming elderhood, health and wellbeing.* Routledge.

Clare, E. (2014). Meditations on natural worlds, disabled bodies, and a politics of cure. In S. Iovino & S. Oppermann (Eds.), *Material ecocriticism* (pp. 204–218). Indiana University Press.

Crilley, M. (2016). Material disability: Creating new paths for disability studies. *The College English Association Critic, 78*(3), 306–311. https://www.jstor.org/stable/10.2307/26574824

Dean, M. L. (2016). *Using art media in psychotherapy: Bringing the power of creativity to practice*. Routledge.

Donald, D. (2016). From what does ethical relationality flow? An "Indian" act in three artifacts. *Counterpoints, 478*, 10–16. https://www.jstor.org/stable/45157205?seq=1

Ehlert, R. (2020). A little less alone: Surviving sanism in art therapy. *Art Therapy, 37*(2), 99–101. https://doi.org/10.1080/07421656.2020.1756139

Elbrecht, C. (2021). *Healing trauma in children with clay field therapy*. North Atlantic Books.

Fairbairn, M. (2023). Spadix, stems and scar wounds: Finding inter/intra-sentient language through dialogue with material-other(s). *Journal of Creative Arts Therapies, 18*(2). https://www.jocat-online.org/a-23-fairbairn

Fenner, P. (2019). Material sensibility: A sense of place in art therapy practice and theory. In A. Gilroy, S. Linnell, T. McKenna, & J. Westwood (Eds.), *Art therapy in Australia: Taking a postcolonial turn* (pp. 383–417). Brill.

Fox, N. J., & Alldred, P. (2019). New materialism. In P. A. Atkinson, S. Delamont, A. Cernat, J. W. Sakshaug, & M. Williams (Eds.), *SAGE research methods foundations* (pp. 1–16). Sage.

Gipson, L. (2017). Challenging neoliberalism and multicultural love in art therapy. *Art Therapy: Journal of the American Art Therapy Association, 34*(3), 112–117. https://doi.org/10.1080/07421656.2017.1353326

Graves-Alcorn, S. L., & Green, E. J. (2014). The expressive arts therapy continuum: History and theory. In E. J. Green & A. A. Drewes (Eds.), *Integrating expressive arts and play therapy with children and adolescents* (pp. 1–16). Wiley.

Hadley, S. (2013). Dominant narratives: Complicity and the need for vigilance in the creative arts therapies. *Arts in Psychotherapy, 40*, 373–381. https://doi.org/10.1016/j.aip.2013.05.007

Havsteen-Franklin, D., Myles, A., Stolfi, D., & De La Cruz, L. M. (2024). A matter of dis/embodied non/relation in art/s psychotherapies practices. *Matter: Journal of New Materialist Research, 9*, 1–22. https://doi.org/10.1344/jnmr.v9.46749

Hickey-Moody, A. C. (2018). New materialism, ethnography, and socially engaged practice: Space-time folds and the agency of matter. *Qualitative Inquiry, 26*(7), 724–732. https://doi.org/10.1177/1077800418810728

Hickey-Moody, A., & Page, T. (2015). Introduction: Making, matter, and pedagogy. In A. Hickey-Moody & T. Page (Eds.), *Arts pedagogy & cultural resistance* (pp. 1–20). Rowman & Littlefield.

Hickey-Moody, A., Palmer, H., & Sayers, E. (2016). Diffractive pedagogies: Dancing across new materialist imaginaries. *Gender and Education, 28*(2), 213–229. https://doi.org/10.1080/09540253.2016.1140723

Hinz, L. D. (2020). *Expressive therapies continuum: A framework for using art in art therapy*. Routledge.

Hinz, L. D., Rim, S., & Lusebrink, V. B. (2022a). Clarifying the creative level of the Expressive Therapies Continuum: A different dimension. *Arts in Psychotherapy, 78*. https://doi.org/10.1016/j.aip.2022.101896

Hinz, L. D., VanMeter, M. L., & Lusebrink, V. B. (2022b). Development of the Expressive Therapies Continuum: The lifework of Vija B. Lusebrink, PhD, ATR-BC, HLM. *Art Therapy, 39*(4), 219–222. https://doi.org/10.1080/07421656.2022.2131951

Johnson, R. (2021, August 17). Queering/querying the body: Sensation and curiosity in disrupting body norms. *Embodied Philosophy*. https://www.embodiedphilosophy.com/queering-querying-the-body-sensation-and-curiosity-in-disrupting-body-norms/

Ki, P. (2025). Leak everywhere: A critical disability analysis of the conceptualizations of trauma. *Social Work & Policy Studies, 4*(1). https://openjournals.library.sydney.edu.au/SWPS/article/view/14924

Leung, W. (2020). Two sides of landscape in ink-wash painting: Chinese landscape painting in expressive arts practice. *Creative Arts in Education & Therapy, 6*(2), 209–220. https://doi.org/10.15212/CAET/2020/6/23

Lusebrink, V. B. (2016). Expressive therapies continuum. In D. E. Gussak & M. L. Rosal (Eds.), *The Wiley handbook of art therapy* (pp. 57–67). John Wiley & Sons.

Miller, S. M. (2020). Disability art: Potential intersections in studio practice with artists labeled/with intellectual and developmental disabilities. *Art Therapy, 37*(2), 93–96. https://doi.org/10.1080/07421656.2020.1756136

Moon, C. H. (2002). *Studio art therapy: Cultivating the artist identity in the art therapist.* Jessica Kingsley Publishers.

Moon, C. H. (2010). *Materials and media in art therapy: Critical understandings of diverse artistic vocabularies.* Routledge.

Moon, C. H. (2014). Theorizing from the margins. *Art Therapy OnLine, 5*(1), https://doi.org/10.25602/GOLD.atol.v5i1.339

Moon, C. H. (2016). Relational aesthetics and art therapy. In J. A. Rubin (Ed.), *Approaches to art therapy: Theory and technique* (pp. 50–68). Routledge.

Moon, C. H. (2023). The art studio as public health practice: Mitigating the negative impacts of social inequality through community care. In In E. Boss & E. Huss (Eds.), *Using art for social transformation: International perspective for social workers, community workers and art therapists* (pp. 156–166). Routledge.

Moon, C. H., & Faulkner, K. (2024). Intersectional care ethics in art therapy organizations. *Arts in Psychotherapy, 89*, 102165. https://doi.org/10.1016/j.aip.2024.102165

Norris, M., Williams, B., & Gipson, L. (2021). Black aesthetics: Upsetting, undoing, and uncanonizing the arts therapies. *Voices: A World Forum for Music Therapy, 21*(1). https://doi.org/10.15845/voices.v21i1.3287

Potash, J. S., & Kalmanowitz, D. (2012). Reflecting on materials and process in Sichuan, China. In D. Kalmanowitz, J. S. Potash, & S. M. Chan (Eds.), *Art therapy in Asia: To the bone or wrapped in silk* (pp. 196–208). Jessica Kingsley Publishers.

Ringrose, J., Warfield, K., & Zarabadi, S. (2019). Introducing feminist posthumanisms/new materialisms & educational research: Response-able theory-practice-methodology. In J. Ringrose, K. Warfield, & S. Zarabadi (Eds.), *Feminist posthumanisms, new materialisms and education* (pp. 1–15). Routledge.

Rosiek, J. L., Snyder, J., & Pratt, S. L. (2019). The new materialisms and Indigenous theories of non-human agency: Making the case for respectful anti-colonial engagement. *Qualitative Inquiry, 26*(3–4), 331–346. https://doi.org/10.1177/1077800419830135

Segalo, P., Manoff, E., & Fine, M. (2015). Working with embroideries and counter-maps: Engaging memory and imagination within decolonizing frameworks. *Journal of Social and Political Psychology, 3*(1), 342–364. https://doi.org/10.5964/jspp.v3i1.145

Slaby, J. (2010). Steps towards a critical neuroscience. *Phenomenology and the Cognitive Sciences, 9*(3), 397–416. https://doi.org/10.1007/s11097-010-9170-2

Strom, K., Ringrose, J., Osgood, J., & Renold, E. (2019). PhEmaterialism: Response-able research & pedagogy. *Reconceptualizing Educational Research Methodology, 2–3*(2). https://journals.oslomet.no/index.php/rerm/article/view/3649/3404

Sundberg, J. (2014). Decolonizing posthumanist geographies. *Cultural Geographies, 21*(1), 33–47. https://doi.org/10.1177/1474474013486067

TallBear, K. (2011, November 18). Why interspecies thinking needs Indigenous standpoints. *Fieldsights.* November 18. https://culanth.org/fieldsights/why-interspecies-thinking-needs-indigenous-standpoints

Todd, Z. (2016). An Indigenous feminist's take on the ontological turn: 'Ontology' is just another word for colonialism. *Journal of Historical Sociology, 29*(1), 4–22. https://doi.org/10.1111/johs.12124

VanMeter, M. L., & Hinz, L. D. (2023). A deeper dive into the Expressive Therapies Continuum: Structure, function, and the creative dimension. *Art Therapy*, *41*(2), 107–110. https://doi.org/10.1080/07421656.2023.2240682

Vellodi, K. (2020). *Decolonizing art history*. Wiley-Blackwell.

Watts, V. (2013). Indigenous place-thought & agency amongst humans and non-humans (First Woman and Sky Woman go on a European world tour!). *Decolonization: Indigeneity, Education & Society*, *2*(1), 20–34. https://jps.library.utoronto.ca/index.php/des/article/view/19145

Wazana Tompkins, K. (2016). On the limits and promise of new materialist philosophy. *Lateral*, *5*(1). https://www.jstor.org/stable/48671431

Whyte, M. K. (2023). Stepping into the circle: Inviting Spirit through medicine wheel teachings in the Expressive Therapies. *Canadian Journal of Art Therapy*, *36*(1), 20–30. https://doi.org/10.1080/26907240.2023.2210984

Yi, C. S. (2010). From imperfect to I'm perfect: Reclaiming the disabled body through making body adornments in art therapy. In C. H. Moon (Ed.), *Materials and media in art therapy* (pp. 103–117). Routledge.

Yi, C. S. (2019). Res(crip)ting art therapy: Disability culture and art as a social justice intervention. In S. K. Talwar (Ed.), *Art therapy for social justice: Radical intersections* (pp. 161–177). Routledge.

Yi, C. S. (2021). Demystifying the individualistic approach to self-care: Sewing as a metaphorical process for documenting relational and communal care in disability culture. In L. Leone (Ed.), *Craft in art therapy: Diverse approaches to the transformative power of craft materials and methods* (pp. 72–89). Routledge.

Yi, C. S., & Moon, C. H. (2020). Art therapy and disability studies. *Art Therapy*, *37*(2), 59–61. https://doi.org/10.1080/07421656.2020.1764798

ETHICAL DIMENSIONS OF MATERIALS, MEDIA, AND PRACTICES IN ART THERAPY

Catherine Hyland Moon

This chapter addresses the ethics of working with art materials, media, and practices in art therapy. First, cultural appropriation is addressed in depth due to its concerning prevalence in the field. This is followed by a broader discussion of ethical dimensions of material and media use for ensuring the well-being of art therapy participants within the context of just, inclusive, and equitable care practices.

Cultural appropriation

If the art therapy field is to center care practices that respectfully accommodate diverse ways of being and knowing, then cultural appropriation in art therapy provides a key "opportunity to reset, unlearn, and relearn" (Ki, 2022, p. 100). While it is natural for art therapists to be interested in ancestral healing traditions that incorporate the arts, it is essential to discern when appreciation becomes appropriation.

Cultural appropriation defined

In its broadest sense, appropriation refers to taking possession of something without consent. Cultural appropriation occurs when a dominant group exercises sovereignty over the resources of a minority group, and expects the minority group to capitulate to their authority (Sheikhai, 2021). It reinforces the historically violent relationships of imperialism,

DOI: 10.4324/9781032720166-4

racism, and genocide, enabling the White dominant culture to simultaneously exploit people of color and deny their self-representations, knowledges, and worldviews.

In art therapy, appropriation is a form of cultural bypassing that denies structural oppression and feigns innocence around the unexamined incorporation of ideas and practices from other cultures (Franklin, 2016). By positioning culture-specific healing arts and healers as transcultural, art therapists uncritically adopt practices without being historically informed or relationally accountable (Kapitan & Kapitan, 2023). Knowledges are taken out of context, deprived of their "original rhythms, languages, practices, or stories," and then (re)presented as universal knowledge or historic artifacts (Napoli, 2019b, p. 78). Because art's role in some cultures is the generational transfer of stories to keep the culture alive, appropriation is a form of cultural genocide (Napoli, 2019a). Appropriating cultural arts practices constitutes the theft of Indigenous knowledges, undermines livelihoods, and dismisses established traditions (Ansloos et al., 2022).

Cultural appropriation in art therapy

Discussions about cultural appropriation have recently emerged in art therapy. Selvaraj (2021) recounted experiences in graduate school of having Eastern practices from her culture co-opted without context or history, and then being invalidated and gaslighted for speaking up about how "this 'sharing' has very real material consequences… where whiteness is positioned as standing separate from culture and is the collective archetype of human" (p. 71). Brandoff and Thompson (2019) characterized appropriation not only as potentially "disrespectful or marginalizing," but also possibly "appropriate, respectful, and relevant" if undertaken respectfully, with clear intentions, and with historical understanding (pp. 16–17). Yet, in describing directives for art forms such as Puerto Rican Vejigante masks, Tibetan prayer flags, and Guatemalan worry dolls, they provided only brief historical contexts, and failed to state their intentions or steps undertaken for respectful inclusion of these art forms in their book.

The most striking example of cultural appropriation in art therapy is the widespread use of the mandala "for commodified recipes and oversimplified use without context, reference, or credit to the true origin and ancient philosophy embodied in the art form" (Jhaveri, 2021, p. 126). Most authors writing about the use of mandalas fail to indicate their own cultural identity or their efforts to sensitively and ethically integrate mandalas into their practice or research.

Cultural symbols like mandalas and dreamcatchers, body adornments like bindis and kimonos, practices like henna tattooing and cornrow braiding, traditions like sweat lodge ceremonies and Cinco de Mayo, and disciplines like yoga and prayer are just a few examples of cultural objects and activities that have been appropriated by cultural outsiders. As art therapists, rather than plundering and commodifying these art forms, we could learn about their complex histories and meanings, empathize with the struggle to maintain cultural practices despite the threats of capitalism and colonization, and engage with them in ways that honor and uplift marginalized communities.

Responding to the potential harm of cultural appropriation

Globalization, migration, and colonization have led to transformations and adaptations of cultural art forms over time, often obscuring their origins. Meanwhile, the internet has catalyzed widespread exposure to cultural art forms stripped of their context and meaning, resulting in cultural practices that lack clearly defined boundaries. While some aspects of cultural traditions are common to many healing practices, each culture has particular stories, histories, rituals, and places through which they engage these common elements. Cultural specifics are what make healing practices "historically dense" (Mundt, 2021, p. 125). I learned this lesson when some of my graduate art therapy students critiqued an assignment in which I asked them to create talismans in preparation for brave conversations about racial justice.

Talismans are handcrafted or found objects imbued with magical properties that offer protection and empowerment. They have existed for millions of years and have been used by followers of faiths and traditions around the world to serve as mediators between humans and the more-than-human world, spiritual realm, or cosmos (Varner, 2008). Arslanbek et al. (2022) distinguished between *Indigenous* art forms, which are directly tied to a particular community, history, and region, and *traditional* art forms, which have existed across time but not in relation to a specific community. Because talismans have been a part of cultures around the world and across time, I considered them traditional art forms. It did not occur to me that some students might perceive my use of talismans as cultural appropriation.

I learned about a few students' discomfort with the talisman assignment through anonymous course evaluations, which meant I did not have the opportunity to speak with them about their perspectives. However, I surmised that some students experienced the making of talismans as culturally appropriative because they had specific, historically dense relationships with talismans. With the intention of repairing the harm I may have caused, I took three steps. First, I wrote to the whole class to let everyone know this concern had been raised and that I was taking it seriously. In that message I acknowledged steps I should have taken in presenting the assignment, which included providing information about the history and integration of talismans into the spiritual practices of multiple cultures, disclosing my own relationship to talismans (through the artifacts of my Catholic upbringing), and engaging the students in a discussion about the potential cultural significance of talismans in their lives and cultures. Second, I identified steps I had taken and would take as reparations. To make amends for the teaching opportunity I had missed, I created and attached a handout, along with a list of resources, on what cultural appropriation is and how to avoid it. I also made a commitment to them to carry this lesson into my future teaching and writing (the evidence of which you are now reading). The third step I took was to send an apology to the one student who had mentioned something in class about talismans and cultural appropriation, and to whom my response was woefully inadequate. I expressed my respect for their perspective, my appreciation for their bravery, and my regret for not having been better prepared to respond.

How to avoid cultural appropriation

To avoid appropriation, there are two core concepts to keep in mind. First, cultural appropriation is not about borrowing, experiencing, sharing, or appreciating; it is about power. It is the ahistorical denial by people from the White dominant culture of the roles colonialism, slavery, and genocide have played in the theft of cultural practices and the refusal to examine how this dynamic continues to contribute to the systematic oppression of minority cultures (Kuo, 2016).

Second, there is no simplistic, one-answer-fits-all approach to the ethics of cultural appropriation in art therapy. Renouncing the use of any and all art materials, symbols, and forms existing outside one's own culture may not be possible. Nor would this stance be advisable for anyone whose cultural identity differs from that of their participants, with the understanding that identity is inclusive of ethnicity, geographic affiliation, class, religion, race, gender identity, sexual orientation, disability, citizenship status, and other markers of difference.

Like many ethical questions, the challenge of avoiding cultural appropriation is not solved by rules and regulations alone, but must be engaged politically, affectively, relationally, and morally. Therefore, I offer the following list of questions as a framework for thinking through this complex aspect of the art therapy profession that has not yet received adequate attention.

In relation to using a culturally associated art form (material, symbol, motif, or practice) in art therapy that is not part of your cultural lineage:

- Are you knowledgeable about its history and cultural significance? Is it specific to one culture, or used in multiple cultures?
- Were you invited—or have you received permission—to use this art form by a member of the culture where it originated? Have you been educated by cultural leaders on its appropriate and sensitive use? What is your plan for remaining accountable to the culture's members?
- Have you made assumptions based on stereotypes to determine the art form's relevance to participants? Or have you also considered participants' circumstances and intersectional identities?
- Do you possess racial, ethnic, or religious privileges that make it easy for you to engage in using this art form with negligible repercussions?
- What are your motivations for using this art form? Are you enticed by its popularity, "exotic" nature, healing potential, difference from Eurocentric art forms, or potential cultural cachet?

- What are your intentions for using this art form? Are they consistent with the intentions of its originators?
- Have you explored why your own culturally rooted arts and healing practices do not seem as compelling or useful as those belonging to another culture? If you have been cut off from your own cultural lineages and traditions, what work have you done to reclaim them?
- Does the art form have religious or spiritual significance? Is it used in healing ceremonies or practices? If the answer is yes to either question and you believe participants would benefit from this healing art form, have you reached out to elders or traditional healers for their guidance and potential collaboration?
- Who has the power and financial resources to access this art form? Are the people who originated it able to access it in their own communities? Will you profit (economically, socially, or politically) from using this art form? Have you paid those who taught you the history, meaning, and techniques of the art form? If yes, did you pay them a fair wage that is commensurate with what you charge for your services?
- If you are a cultural outsider, do you understand the physical, mental, emotional, and spiritual implications and contraindications of the cultural form you plan to adapt and apply to your practice? How will you ensure your approach is culturally respectful? What harm reduction steps will you implement?
- How do you plan to appropriately credit the specific cultural origins and practitioners you are borrowing from? What is your plan for sensitively and respectfully introducing the context, history, and background of this art form when using it in your therapy, teaching, or research? Are you prepared to model cultural humility by being transparent about who you are and what you do and do not know?
- Have you considered the potential of generational trauma associated with using the ancestral art forms and healing traditions of marginalized groups?
- Given your class, citizenship, and other social privileges, what considerations are necessary for you to ethically use the art forms and healing practices of other cultures?

- Given the current heightened sensitivity to cultural appropriation, especially in countries experiencing the ongoing effects of imperialism, settler colonialism, and slavery, are you prepared to receive critique thoughtfully, with an open mind and heart, to learn from it and then do better?

(Carter et al., 2013; Jhaveri, 2021; Sheikhai, 2021;
Weinberg, 2018)

Ethical guidelines for material and media use in art therapy

Ethical dimensions in art therapy are complex, given the plethora of art materials and processes available, and the varied responses they evoke, including sensory experiences, emotional reactions, physical and neurological activations, socio-cultural connections, and ecological concerns. How people understand and respond to materials is a dynamic process affected by factors such as developmental level, emotional state, psychological makeup, cognitive strengths and challenges, prior experiences with artmaking, physical abilities/constraints, sensory sensitivity, worldview, social context, cultural traditions, and exposure to the arts.

In discussing the ethical use of art materials, media, and practices, I consider the interplay of personal, social, cultural, political, and environmental factors. Rather than quoting codes of ethics already readily available online, my aim is to include factors not often discussed in ethical guidelines, such as the impact of relational power dynamics, our potential as therapists for complicity with oppression, non-Western knowledges and practices, and our responsibility to respect participants' expertise about their needs (Ki, 2022). As a basis for ethical, socio-culturally aware art therapy, Awais and Keselman (2019) recommend structural competence (recognition of the social, political, and economic conditions that contribute to health disparities), cultural humility (ongoing self-reflexivity related to implicit bias and openness to participants' expertise about their worldviews, values, and cultural practices), and intersectionality (framework for understanding and challenging the interlocking systems of social oppression and advantage). On the basis of these overarching frameworks, I offer below some considerations for the ethical use of art materials, media, and methods in art therapy.

Therapist familiarity with art materials, media, and processes

A common assertion is that art therapists should not use art materials or processes with which they are unfamiliar. However, failing to offer materials that are potentially beneficial to participants could be ethically problematic if it impedes the progress of therapy (Scarborough, 2022). What is an art therapist to do?

No one can know everything about all art materials and processes, but personal artmaking enables us to better understand participants' potential experiences of inspiration, creative block, flow, frustration, satisfaction, etc. Through challenging our biases, assumptions, and preferences related to art practices, we can gain insight into how they limit us. We can also commit to ongoing learning of new skills, which refreshes our empathy for participants who find artmaking unfamiliar and intimidating. Finally, we can be transparent with participants about what we do not know, and willing to learn from them about their interests, skills, and knowledges.

Participants' familiarity with material, media, and processes

Exploring with participants their personal art histories can provide helpful information about their lifetime exposure to arts/crafts and related creative practices, and the influences that have shaped their ideas about the arts and about themselves as makers. This history can be reconstructed through dialogue, a fillable form, or an art-based project.

Provision of materials

The range, quality, and quantity of materials offered to participants can vary greatly. Aside from practical considerations like budgetary constraints, the quality of materials should correspond with their potential for successful outcomes. Poor quality materials and tools can be infantilizing, suggest participants are unworthy of quality care, or cause unnecessary frustration during artmaking. They can also lead to disappointing results, which participants might assume they caused. However, materials should not be so precious that they inhibit use. Fine arts materials, in particular, can have an intimidating effect because they are often associated with preconceived aesthetic standards.

The range and quantity of materials can evoke either abundance or scarcity. While most art therapists probably prefer a sumptuous buffet of materials to entice exploration and experimentation, there may be economic, environmental, therapeutic, or other reasons for a more restrained offering of materials.

Sometimes limiting material use is necessary, such as when a child becomes fixated on squeezing paint bottles to disgorge their contents. Limits can be based on budgetary, educational, environmental, relational, or therapeutic considerations. Honestly and sensitively communicating the reasons for limits is important, especially when they are not strictly related to therapeutic goals (Orbach, 2023).

Ecological responsibility

The ecological impact of art materials is one of the most urgent concerns for art therapists, and one of the most challenging. It may be the very materials we or our participants desire and find meaningful that are environmental hazards. For example, glitter, which can symbolize beauty, joy, seduction, or celebration, is also an ecological menace impacting water, air, and marine life. Its overuse might be indicative of emotional hunger, covering over emotions, or "an industrial and capitalist world wanting limitlessness" (Orbach, 2023, p. 57). Havard (2022) proposed *glitter grief*, a queer disabled approach to holding pleasure and ache in tension while identifying alternative materials that evoke glitter's magical, transformative qualities.

Given that nearly all media and processes have environmental impacts, we are responsible for taking actions to mitigate harm, ration use, find nontoxic alternatives, or eliminate some materials/processes altogether. Responsible use of resources also includes researching how materials are produced to avoid products made with child or forced labor, in unsafe work environments, or through using an excessive quantity of natural resources (Timm-Bottos & Chainey, 2015). Ecologically responsible practices also include mindful participation in a circular economy (reuse, repair, refurbish, remanufacture, and recycle) and purchasing products made available through fair trade principles. At the local level, we can reduce the waste that goes into landfills by using recycled art supplies, furnishings, and consumer waste (Brandoff & Thompson, 2019; Carpendale, 2010).

When harvesting natural materials for artmaking, an ethical approach includes modeling environmental respect and sustainability, which includes respect for biodiversity and avoiding the depletion of natural resources (see Alders Pike, 2021, for specific recommendations). It is also important to consider the intersecting impact of ecological issues and economic, racial, cultural, and therapeutic factors. For example, Matott and Miller (2024) suggested harnessing waste from cannabis and textile industries for use in papermaking, thereby preventing the fibers from ending up in landfills and providing a source of income for local communities.

Socio-cultural considerations

Socio-cultural-economic aspects of material and media applications require art therapists to challenge "Eurocentric values that prioritize individual psychological change, independence, and freedom of expression" (Gipson, 2019, p. 103), and consider artmaking as a potential means for mutual aid, social change, and collective transformation. Socially responsible practice begins with learning about a community's creative making practices. What creative practices are thriving, and how can those be supported? (Moon, 2023). Who does the making? What purposes do the arts serve? What materials are affordable? What art forms or other creative activities are participants interested in?

If we are community outsiders, we have to be humble about the limits of our knowledge and consult local experts. They can enlighten us about gendered, religious, or ritual norms associated with certain arts practices or materials, as well as taboo topics or practices. Even a mainstay of art therapy like encouraging self-expression can pose a threat to participants if it goes against cultural norms (Gopalakrishna, 2022).

When working in traditional therapy settings where the focus is on individual change, we must still challenge our ethnocentric assumptions about art media and practices (Sochanik, 2023). Offering a range of materials conveys a welcoming, inclusive message about participants and their diverse interests, needs, and art practices (Manthe & Carolan, 2018). Siano (2021) suggested that metaphors associated with materials enable participants to engage in dialogue without being forced to speak in a foreign language. Yet, for some participants their artmaking *mother tongue* is not metaphors, but rather social and cultural capital

(Talwar, 2020), cultural symbolism (Huss, 2010), cultural survival (Arslanbek et al., 2022), or direct spiritual connection (Napoli, 2019a).

It is also crucial to critically evaluate the gendered nature of art materials and practices and how these perspectives are reinforced through cis-heteronormative, ageist, and other stereotypes and assumptions (Partridge, 2020; Van Den Berg, 2024). Conscious awareness of associations between materials or colors and specific gendered identities enables us to question their potentially useful or harmful implications (Hetherington, 2020). We can explore culturally respectful ways to disrupt gender binaries and create more fluid use of materials.

Socio-economic considerations

Given that art therapy is situated within economic and material contexts, access may be enhanced by providing not only art materials, but also food or drink, assistance with childcare, and/or compensation for transportation (Gopalakrishna, 2022; Martyn, 2022).

For participants who have faced economic deprivation, lack of exposure to fine arts materials can evoke discomfort and inadvertently position the participants as unrefined (Lazar et al., 2018), whereas crafts materials might be experienced as culturally familiar and affirming. Awareness of abundant or limited materials in the art therapy studio can elicit varying responses in participants, from being overwhelmed to being inspired. Sometimes, these varied responses are pathologized as theft, hoarding, acting out, low self-esteem, or selfishness, rather than recognized as expressions of lived experience (Partridge, 2016) or "justified political protest" against systemic failures (Lambert, 2022, p. 94).

To address the needs of low-income individuals or communities, we can prioritize artmaking processes that are locally and financially accessible in the short term and sustainable in the long term. The use of found objects and recycled art supplies is not only environmentally responsible, but also economically just if we aim to inspire artistic interest and desires that can't be supported over the long term and avoid creating dependence on the art therapist (Bonz et al., 2020; Potash et al., 2017).

When providing online art therapy, it is important to determine participants' current and ongoing material needs and to co-develop a realistic plan for sustainable access to art materials. In the case of digital artmaking, sustainable practice requires ongoing access to reliable internet, technology literacy, and updated digital tools and equipment.

Access needs

Addressing access needs, which can range from the need for quiet during artmaking to the need for braille signage, helps ensure that everyone is able to fully participate in art therapy sessions. Beginning each session with an access check-in that includes the therapist disrupts the body-mind ideal and destigmatizes the need for care (Reinholz & Ridgway, 2021).

Accessible spaces and alternative or adapted tools and materials demonstrate commitment to accessibility. Needs may be based on physical constraints such as limited hand strength, visual impairment, exaggerated sensory responses, or restricted ambulation. Examples of adaptations include thickening a tool handle to make it easier to grasp, warming clay to make it more malleable, offering tactile and aromatic materials when vision is impaired, providing gloves to reduce sensory stimulation (Chapin Stephenson, 2021), supplying edible materials for people who confuse art materials with food (Pedersen, 2023), or offering unconventional material applications like painting with a rolling wheelchair to enhance autonomy and a sense of control (Awais & Keselman, 2019).

The concept of accommodations is commonly thought to include factors like wheelchair access or ASL interpretation, but it also can include access to gender neutral bathrooms, freedom from microaggressions in group dialogues, respect for prayer times, mask wearing on behalf of immunocompromised group members, or adequate childcare support (Reinholz & Ridgway, 2021). Just as trauma-informed care assumes that trauma is a barrier to care in multiple settings and systems, a critical social model of disability assumes that ableism is a barrier to care in multiple settings and systems. Though adaptations and accommodations are important, we have a collective responsibility to go further by aiming for the elimination of barriers and the creation of arts-based practices that center inclusive, liberatory, interdependent care (Mingus, 2017; Yi, 2021).

Creating safer spaces

Ethical practice includes addressing multiple aspects of safety: physiological, physical, psychological, emotional, cultural/intersectional, and relational (Kalmanowitz, 2022).

Physiological safety begins by asking new participants about allergies as well as sensitivities to smells, sounds, textures, messy materials, and image content (Schorr, 2022). When conducting art therapy in outdoor settings, inquiries about seasonal, insect, and plant/sap allergies should be included (Alders Pike, 2021). Remaining attuned to participants' needs, sensitivities, and responses is key because materials can have destabilizing or dysregulating effects (Hetherington & Gentile, 2022) or otherwise cause harm.

Physical safety is most straightforwardly addressed by considering the potential of materials, tools, and processes to cause corporeal harm. Comprehensive information about the safe use of commercial art materials is available online. Use of eco-materials requires research to determine safety related to skin, respiratory, and ingestion exposure (Alders Pike, 2021). Every material's potential toxicity, flammability, or other hazards, and each material or tool's procedures for safe use and storage should be evaluated (Horovitz, 2018; Moon & Nolan, 2020) in relation to participants' developmental levels, cognitive and physical abilities, allergies, sensory aversions, skin sensitivities, and psychological states.

The physical safety of participants may be addressed through mandated practices in some institutional settings. For example, in medical sites art therapists typically follow infection control guidelines, using only new or disinfected materials and performing required hand washing procedures (Elkis-Abuhoff & Gaydos, 2019). In the carceral system, limitations on materials and tools can vary from setting to setting or even over time within a given institution (Gussak, 2015).

In all settings, providing proper training for the safe use of tools, along with safety equipment like masks, gloves, protective eyewear, and fire extinguishers is essential (Timm-Bottos & Chainey, 2015). Adequate lighting, water access, proper ventilation (Moon & Nolan, 2020), first aid supplies, and a space that is free of obstructions or hazards are also priorities.

Online art therapy poses unique issues related to the safe use of art supplies because participants often provide their own materials and tools, and because the therapist is unable to closely observe participants' artmaking processes. These limitations need to be addressed in dialogue with participants or their legal guardians and through informed consents.

For art therapists working in natural environments, site accessibility can be a concern in relation to both reaching the site and navigating the environment once there (Nash, 2020). In addition, the therapist should warn of potential threats to physical safety, like inclement weather and poisonous plants and animals (Whitaker et al., 2022).

Psychological/emotional safety is often enhanced when a consistent, organized selection of well-maintained tools and materials is provided, reinforcing the sense that the environment is safe and the therapist trustworthy (Moon & Nolan, 2020). As a way to become acclimated to art therapy, new participants can be encouraged to walk around the therapy space, touch and look through the materials, and briefly test out unfamiliar media, thereby exploring their qualities and the embodied responses they elicit (Wilkinson & Chilton, 2018).

In collaborative artmaking that involves working in close proximity or physically touching one another, the therapist should clearly explain the process and engage participants in conversation about feelings proximity might provoke. In addition, the therapist should ensure that each participant has granted permission to be touched, provide the option of pausing or ending active involvement at any point, check in with participants periodically, and provide options for how to manage feelings that arise (Bechtel et al., 2020).

When working in outdoor settings, participants should be informed of limits to confidentiality and privacy. For participants who find open space unsettling or overstimulating, Whitaker et al. (2022) suggested ways to create containment and limits, such as providing blankets to sit on, drawing boundaries with sand or flour, or using cameras to encourage focus and framing.

Psychological/emotional safety is also enhanced when participants feel seen and acknowledged. Along with inclusive language and forms (Kapitan & Kapitan, 2023) and land/Country acknowledgments for practices located in settler societies, the space and materials are important aspects of conveying that participants' diverse experiences and identities are welcomed and valued. For example, when working with people with chronic pain, priorities include comfortable furniture, different types and levels of work surfaces, options for warming painful bodies, and opportunities to sit, stand, move, or lie down. In addition, the option of virtual therapy conveys sensitivity to the potential of travel to aggravate pain responses (Woodford, 2024).

Ideally, art therapy spaces convey that diverse ethnicities, religions, racial identities, abilities/disabilities, sexual orientations, gender identities, ages, body sizes, and other social identities and practices are affirmed and welcomed. Who is represented by the posters or artwork hanging on the walls or by the furniture? Whose perspectives and identities are associated with the books, pamphlets, and other resources available in the space? What do the artmaking aids convey? Metzl (2017) encouraged the provision of collage images, words, and magazines that normalize a variety of sexual, romantic, physical, mental, and emotional connections, fantasies, roles, and expressions. Ideally, these same approaches to materials and resources are extended to encompass a full range of ages, bodies, identities, lifestyles, abilities, and worldviews.

The use of digital media in art therapy requires additional psychological safety measures related to privacy, confidentiality, and emotional safety. Because digital creations can easily be uploaded to the internet, where security can never be guaranteed and uploaded materials never completely deleted, art therapists must ensure that participants (and their legal guardians) are fully aware of the risks. The potential ramifications of public exposure currently or in the future, ranging from embarrassment to appropriation to cyber violence, should be explicitly discussed with participants and outlined in writing. Measures to protect private information to the degree possible should be taken, such as using hardware that's under the therapist's or agency's control, employing password-protected computer filing systems, using locked storage cabinets, and creating encrypted backups of information in case digital equipment like a camera or computer is lost, damaged, or stolen (Alders et al., 2011; Choe & Carlton, 2019; Johnson & Cohen, 2015; Thayer, 2022).

When participants choose to share their digital artwork publicly due to the therapeutic significance and benefit of being seen and heard, ethical challenges can arise. Particularly in relation to producing videos that will be viewed publicly, participants should be engaged in ongoing conversations about their responsibility to protect not only their own rights, but also the rights of people discussed or appearing in their videos (Johnson & Cohen, 2015). As with exhibiting any artworks created in the context of therapy, the potential implications of public exposure should be discussed with participants. In relation to online sharing and discussion of one's artwork, therapists can also help participants understand the potential positive and negative connections between social media, power dynamics, and personal and collective well-being, as well as how to best cultivate online communities that provide positive support and civil engagement (Hunt et al., 2018).

Cultural/intersectional safety is demonstrated through awareness of participants' art traditions and values, as well as their generational traumas, and the sensitive, nonexoticizing, nonexploitative, nonappropriative provision of culturally relevant materials, symbols, and practices. However, care should be taken to avoid assuming that all participants from a cultural group will be familiar with and interested in employing traditional materials and practices (Gaspar da Silva, 2023).

Participants from marginalized communities who have frequently been misrepresented, stigmatized, and degraded in media produced by the dominant culture may be reluctant to create art that has the potential to reach a public audience. Art therapists cannot ensure that videos or other digitally created art will engender a uniformly supportive response. Participants' reticence, resistance, and refusal to engage in digital art processes may be justified forms of healthy limit-setting and should be honored (Mosinski, 2015).

Many settings frame restrictions on art materials, practices, or content as protective of participants, staff, or both. It is the ethical responsibility of art therapists to critically engage with such restrictions, questioning whether they are genuinely aimed at safety or are evidence of culturally targeted discrimination, punishment, censorship, or other forms of injustice. In some circumstances, challenging or resisting institutional restrictions might be the most ethical choice for an art therapist.

Relational safety concerns how people and their art materials, processes, and products are treated, as well as the general ethos of the milieu. The art therapist is responsible for establishing an environment that is conducive to artmaking and supportive of respectful, health-promoting relationships. This ethos can be cultivated in multiple ways, such as the sensitive use of materials for facilitating connections among participants, demonstrating care for art materials and tools, and humbly recognizing everyone's expertise as co-makers. Mims (2022) recommends educating colleagues about when, if, and how to respond to participants' artworks, and demonstrating respect for art products by providing safe storage, respectful finishes (frames, protective coatings, etc.), and secure means of transport. Altogether, these types of actions create relationally safer spaces through mutual care practices.

From the perspective of a relational aesthetic, it is the fostering and deepening of relationships that is of primary concern in art therapy (Moon, 2002, 2016). These relationships can be with our embodied selves, intersecting identities, art objects, beloved others, community, ancestral lands or Country, spirituality, ancestors, living and nonliving world, sense of justice, life purpose, cosmos, etc. The beauty of art is that it can give voice and substance to any and all of these relational endeavors, allowing for their development and deepening.

References

Alders, A., Beck, L., Allen, P. B., & Mosinski, B. (2011). Technology in art therapy: Ethical challenges. *Art Therapy, 28*(4), 165–170. https://doi.org/10.1080/07421656.2011.622683

Alders Pike, A. (2021). *Eco-art therapy in practice*. Routledge.

Ansloos, J., Morford, A. C., Dunn, N. S., DuPr´e, L., & Kucheran, R. (2022). Beading Native Twitter: Indigenous arts-based approaches to healing and resurgence. *Arts in Psychotherapy, 79*, 1–11. https://doi.org/10.1016/j.aip.2022.101914

Arslanbek, A., Malhotra, B., & Kaimal, G. (2022). Indigenous and traditional arts in art therapy: Value, meaning, and clinical implications. *The Arts in Psychotherapy, 77*, 101879. https://doi.org/10.1016/j.aip.2021.101879

Awais, Y. J., & Keselman, M. (2019). Culturally responsive care for art therapists in medical settings. In D. Elkis-Abuhoff & M. Gaydos (Eds.), *Art and expressive therapies within the medical model: Clinical applications* (pp. 224–234). Routledge.

Bechtel, A., Wood, L. L., & Teoli, L. (2020). Re-shaping body image: Tape sculptures as arts-based social justice. *Art in Psychotherapy, 68*, 101615. https://doi.org/10.1016/j.aip.2019.101615

Bonz, A. G., Del Carmen Casas, S., & Arslanbek, A. (2020). Conflict and displacement: Finding the space for creativity. In M. Berberian & B. Davis (Eds.), *Art therapy practices for resilient youth: A strengths-based approach to at-promise children and adolescents* (pp. 337–358). Routledge.

Brandoff, R., & Thompson, A. (2019). *Quick and creative art projects for creative therapists with (very) limited budgets*. Jessica Kingsley Publishers.

Carpendale, M. (2010). Ecological identity and art therapy. *Canadian Art Therapy Association Journal, 23*(2), 53–57. https://doi.org/10.1080/08322473.2010.11432338

Carter, T., Chenyek, R. K., M'kali-Hashiki, Montalvo, M. F. G., Piepzna-Samarasinha, L. L., & Daniel, J. A. (2013). A babe-ilicious healing justice statement from the BadAss Visionary Healers (BAVH). *Nineteen Sixty Nine, 2*(1). https://escholarship.org/uc/item/1z61z54j

Chapin Stephenson, R. (2021). *Art therapy and creative aging: Reclaiming elderhood, health, and wellbeing.* Routledge.

Choe, N. S., & Carlton, N. R. (2019). Behind the screens: Informed consent and digital literacy in art therapy. *Art Therapy, 36*(1), 15–21. https://doi.org/10.1080/07421656.2019.1565060

Elkis-Abuhoff, D., & Gaydos, M. (2019). *Art and expressive therapies within the medical model: Clinical applications.* Routledge.

Franklin, M. A. (2016). *Art as contemplative practice: Expressive pathways to the self.* SUNY Press.

Gaspar da Silva, M. (2023). Storytelling embroidery art therapy group with Portuguese-speaking immigrant women in Canada. *Canadian Journal of Art Therapy, 36*(2), 86–104. https://doi.org/10.1080/26907240.2022.2160546

Gipson, L. (2019). Envisioning Black women's consciousness in art therapy. In S. Talwar (Ed.), *Art therapy for social justice: Radical intersections* (pp. 96–120). Routledge.

Gopalakrishna, M. (2022). Practicing in an expanded paradigm: Case examples and ethical anchors for creative arts therapists working in community-based social justice contexts. *Arts in Psychotherapy, 80.* https://doi.org/10.1016/j.aip.2022.101921

Gussak, D. E. (2015). Art therapy in the prison milieu. In D. E. Gussak & M. L. Rosal (Eds.), *The Wiley handbook of art therapy* (pp. 478–486). John Wiley & Sons.

Havard, J. (2022). Glitter grief: Eco-crip affect for mourning and re-building. *Periskop, 28,* 16–33. https://tidsskrift.dk/periskop/article/view/134573/179440

Hetherington, R. (2020). Invisible complicity in LGBTQI art therapy: A series of case studies in response to Hadley's call for the need for vigilance. *Arts in Psychotherapy, 70.* https://doi.org/10.1016/j.aip.2020.101667

Hetherington, R., & Gentile, F. (2022). Healing boundaries: A teenager's experience of art therapy integrated with Somatic Experiencing. *International Journal of Art Therapy, 27*(4), 190–197. https://doi.org/10.1080/17454832.2022.2080239

Horovitz, E. G. (2018). *A guide to art therapy materials, methods, and applications: A practical step-by-step approach.* Routledge.

Hunt, D., Robertson, D., & Pow, A. (2018). The counselor's role in the age of social media and fake news. *Journal of Creativity in Mental Health, 13*(4), 405–417. https://doi.org/10.1080/15401383.2018.1462748

Huss, E. (2010). Bedouin women's embroidery as female empowerment: Crafts as culturally embedded expression within art therapy. In C. H. Moon (Ed.), *Materials & Media in Art Therapy: Critical understandings of diverse artistic vocabularies* (pp. 215–229). Routledge.

Jhaveri, K. (2021). Healing roots of Indigenous crafts adapting traditions of India for art therapy practice. In L. Leone (Ed.), *Craft in art therapy: Diverse approaches to the transformative power of craft materials and methods* (pp. 118–130). Routledge.

Johnson, J. L., & Cohen, J. L. (2015). A challenge to readers: Ethical considerations in film- and video-based therapies. In J. L. Cohen, J. L. Johnson, & P. P. Orr (Eds.), *Video and filmmaking as psychotherapy* (pp. 13–26). Routledge.

Kalmanowitz, D. (2022). Reinforcing a home in the mind: An art therapy and mindfulness-oriented approach to working with refugees, trauma and resilience. In H. Jury & A. Coles (Eds.), *Art psychotherapy and innovation: New territories, techniques, and technologies* (pp. 165–186). Jessica Kingsley Publishers.

Kapitan, A., & Kapitan, L. (2023). Language is power: Anti-oppressive, conscious language in art therapy practice. *International Journal of Art Therapy, 28*(1–2), 65–73. https://doi.org/10.1080/17454832.2022.2112721

Ki, P. (2022). Proceeding from our roots in the dust: An unfolding ethics of care through the arts. *Canadian Journal of Art Therapy, 35*(2), 95–102. https://doi.org/10.1080/26907240.2022.2139057

Kuo, R. (2016, September 6). How cultural appropriation becomes trendy - and the real cost of our consumerism. *Everyday Feminism.* https://everydayfeminism.com/2016/09/cultural-appropriation-trends/

Lambert, B. (2022). 'This is our group:' Art therapy with adolescents in the shadow of Grenfell. In S. Skaife & J. Martyn (Eds.), *Art psychotherapy groups in the hostile environment of neoliberalism: Collusion or resistance?* (pp. 80–95). Routledge.

Lazar, A., Feuston, J. L., Edasis, C., & Piper, A. M. (2018). Making as expression: Informing design with people with complex communication needs through art therapy. *CHI,* Canada. https://doi.org/10.1145/3173574.3173925

Manth, L., & Carolan, R. (2018). Ethics in art therapy. In R. Carolan & A. Backos (Eds.), *Emerging perspectives in art therapy: Trends, movements, and developments* (pp. 93–104). Routledge.

Martyn, J. (2022). Exploring experiences of exhibiting artwork from a therapeutic art studio for refugees and asylum seekers. In C. Brown & H. Omand (Eds.), *Contemporary practice in studio art therapy* (pp. 184–193). XXX.

Matott, D. L., & Miller, G. M. (Eds.) (2024). *The art and art therapy of papermaking: Material, methods, and applications.* Routledge.

Metzl, E. S. (2017). *When art therapy meets sex therapy: Creative explorations of sex, gender, and relationships.* Routledge.

Mims, R. (2022). *Art therapy with veterans.* Jessica Kingsley Publishers.

Mingus, M. (2017, April 12). Access intimacy, interdependence and disability justice. *Leaving Evidence.* https://leavingevidence.wordpress.com/2017/04/12/access-intimacy-interdependence-and-disability-justice/

Moon, B. L., & Nolan, E. G. (2020). *Ethical issues in art therapy* (4th ed.). Charles C Thomas Publisher.

Moon, C. H. (2002). *Studio art therapy: Cultivating the artist identity in the art therapist.* Jessica Kingsley Publishers.

Moon, C. H. (2016). Relational aesthetics and art therapy. In J. A. Rubin (Ed.), *Approaches to art therapy: Theory and technique* (pp. 50–68). Routledge.

Moon, C. H. (2023). The art studio as public health practice: Mitigating the negative impacts of social inequality through community care. In E. Bos & E. Huss (Eds.), *Using art for social transformation: International perspective for social workers, community workers, and art therapists* (pp. 156–166). Routledge.

Mosinski, B. (2015). Video art and activism: Applications in art therapy. In J. Cohen & J. L. Johnson (Eds.), *Video and filmmaking as psychotherapy: Research and practice* (pp. 135–145). Routledge.

Mundt, K. (2021). Touch as passage: Inhabiting the colonial wound. *The Arrow, 8*(1), 120–140. https://arrow-journal.org/touch-as-passage-inhabiting-the-colonial-wound/

Napoli, M. (2019a). Ethical contemporary art therapy: Honoring an American Indian perspective. *Art Therapy, 36*(4), 175–182. https://doi.org/10.1080/07421656.2019.1648916

Napoli, M. (2019b). Indigenous methodology: An ethical systems approach to arts based work with Native communities in the U. S. *Arts in Psychotherapy, 64,* 77–83. https://doi.org/10.1016/j.aip.2019.05.006

Nash, G. (2020). Weaving the threads of theory and experience. In I. Siddons Heginworth & G. Nash (Eds.), *Environmental arts therapy: The wild frontiers of the heart* (pp. 27–43). Routledge.

Orbach, N. (2023). *The book of permission: Reflections on art, therapy, education, and being human.* Author.

Partridge, E. E. (2016). Access to art and materials: Considerations for art therapists. *Canadian Art Therapy Association Journal, 29*(2), 100–104. https://doi.org/10.1080/08322473.2016.1252996

Partridge, E. (2020). Dismantling the gender binary in elder care: Creativity instead of craft. In S. Hogan (Ed.), *Gender and difference in the arts therapies: Inscribed on the body* (pp. 196–206). Routledge.

Pedersen, H. (2023). Adaptive art making: Materials and methods. In T. Weinberg & M. Carpendale (Eds.), *Walking with: An emerging dialogue with art therapists in the cultural commons* (pp.187–195). Essence.

Potash, J. S., Bardot, H., Moon, C. H., Napoli, M., Lyonsmith, A., & Hamilton, M. (2017). Ethical implications of cross-cultural international art therapy. *Arts in Psychotherapy, 56,* 74–82. https://doi.org/10.1016/j.aip.2017.08.005

Reinholz, D. L., & Ridgway, S. W. (2021). Access needs: Centering students and disrupting ableist norms in STEM. *CBE—Life Sciences Education, 20*(3), 1–8. https://doi.org/10.1187/cbe.21-01-0017

Scarborough, V. (2022). The ethics of art materials. In T. J. Ling & J. M. Hauk (Eds.), *Navigating ethical dilemmas in creative arts therapies: A case-based approach* (pp. 45–60). Routledge.

Schorr, M. (2022). *DBT and art for youth suicide prevention: When art saves lives.* Jessica Kingsley Publishers.

Selvaraj, K. (2021). Being Queer and Brown: A Queer, decolonial, arts-based, autoethnographic enquiry into art therapy pedagogical institutions and spaces. *Journal of Creative Arts Therapies, 16*(1), 66–76. https://www.jocat-online.org/a-21-selvaraj

Sheikhai, S. (2021). Returning to the sacred circle, immigrant and Indigenous allies: A heuristic perspective. In M. Kitazawa (Ed.), *Asian art therapists: Navigating art, diversity, and culture* (pp. 41–54). Routledge.

Siano, J. (2021). The magic of holy junk. In D. Wong & R. P. M. H. Lay (Eds.), *Found objects in art therapy: Materials and process* (pp. 105–122). Jessica Kingsley Publishers.

Sochanik, J. (2023). How does skin color affect the therapeutic relationship in art psychotherapy? *International Journal of Art Therapy, 28*(1–2), 84–91. https://doi.org/10.1080/17454832.2023.2185787

Talwar, S. (2020). Feminism as practice: Crafting and the politics of art therapy. In S. Hogan (Ed.), *Gender and difference in the arts therapies: Inscribed on the body* (pp. 13–23). Routledge.

Thayer, F. (2022). Technology and art therapy: Navigating the use of digital art and/or telehealth in the art therapy process. In T. J. Ling & J. M. Hauk (Eds.), *Navigating ethical dilemmas in creative arts therapies: A case-based approach* (pp. 139–152). Routledge.

Timm-Bottos, J., & Chainey, R. (2015). *Art hives how-to guide.* https://arthives.org/resources/art-hives-how-guide

Van Den Berg, Z. D. (2024). Addressing traumatic experiences of cis-heterosexism with LGBTQUIA+ clients in art therapy. *International Journal of Art Therapy, 29*(1), 57–66. https://doi.org/10.1080/17454832.2023.2261542

Varner, G. R. (2008). *The history & use of amulets, charms, and talismans.* Lulu Press.

Weinberg, T. (2018). Gaining cultural competence through alliances in art therapy with Indigenous clients. *Canadian Art Therapy Association Journal, 31*(1), 14–22. https://doi.org/10.1080/08322473.2018.1453214

Whitaker, P., Shaw, N., & Winkel, M. (2022). Integrating art therapy with nature-based practices. In M. Winkel (Ed.), *Virtual art therapy: Research and practice* (pp.150–166). Routledge.

Wilkinson, R. A., & Chilton, G. (2018). *Positive art therapy theory and practice.* Routledge.

Woodford, A. E. (2024). The creative arts therapies and bodies living with/in ongoing pain. *Journal of Creative Arts Therapies, 19*(2). https://www.jocat-online.org/e-24-woodford

Yi, C. S. (2021). Demystifying the individualistic approach to self-care: Sewing as a metaphorical process for documenting relational and communal care in disability culture. In L. Leone (Ed.), *Craft in art therapy: Diverse approaches to thea transformative power of craft materials and methods* (pp. 72–89). Routledge.

4

"WOMEN'S WORK"

WOMEN IN THE HELPING PROFESSIONS USING CRAFTS AS SELF-CARE

Gal Amram and Ephrat Huss

Social practice in the arts, including Photovoice, arts as communal expression, creative placemaking, and craftivism, is a rapidly growing phenomenon, with a literature base that includes arts-based methodologies for research and for both therapeutic and activist projects. However, there is scant literature on how women in the helping professions (aside from art therapists), such as social workers, nurses, and educators, use crafts for their own self-care and quality of life. Interestingly, art therapy is increasingly focused on social applications of the arts and on empowerment, and thus an understanding of how crafts enable self-care and give voice to women is relevant for their practices as well.

Practitioners of both helping professions and crafts are predominantly female, inherently practical, and interested in creating positive change on micro and macro levels, whether through new products or new realities. Craft practices focus not only on skills, but also on relationality, as through crafts circles or products made for others. Both helping professionals and crafters aim to enhance agency and creativity.

Helping professions that are predominantly female, such as nursing, education, and social work, are often low-paying and high-stress professions with accompanying dangers of burnout and compassion fatigue. Does the engagement in crafts help to regulate this stress? The aim of this

DOI: 10.4324/9781032720166-5

chapter is to explore how female social service practitioners who employ crafts practices as leisure activities connect their professional experience and work-related stress with their involvement in crafting. Using semi-structured interviews with social workers who engage in crafts, this study seeks to co-produce knowledge with them about how they connect their craft practices and their helping profession.

Literature review

What is handicraft?

Historians and researchers still struggle to define *craft* due to its complex, evolving history and the inferior status attached to it (Greenhalgh, 1997; Zehavi, 2015). A key characteristic of craft has to do with creating an aesthetic product that is functional and has potential benefit, either real or metaphoric (Zehavi, 2015). In addition, handwork is one of the most obvious features of handicraft, and the skills required for it are linked to the sensory and experiential use of materials (Shiner, 2012).

Compared to the craftsperson, the artist's intellectual claims have been given more weight than their technical skills (Lucie-Smith, 1981; Yam, 2002). The Industrial Revolution brought with it a distinction between practical artifacts, which underwent industrialization and were therefore seen as objects, and *fine art* works created solely by independent artists (Lucie-Smith, 1981; Yam, 2002).

The Industrial Revolution pushed traditional handicrafts out of daily economic and cultural life, though women held on to crafts like sewing, knitting, or lacework as part of their domestic duties (Adamson, 2007; Yam, 2002). One expression of gender and class divides in relation to the arts was the recurring association of specific crafts with women. Brown (1970) argued that some lines of work were designated *feminine* based on how closely they related to child-rearing, including activities that could straightforwardly be resumed after interruptions, didn't require high levels of concentration, and could easily be done at home. Throughout art history, decorative work and domestic handicrafts were seen as women's work, and as such were never deemed fine art (Lippard, 1978; Parker & Pollock, 2013).

Crafts and female empowerment

The history of art created by women reveals an intimate bond between the content of their art and women's lived reality, with personal experiences and history reflected and embodied in the artwork (Anderson & Gold, 1998). Women created using available materials and incorporated aspects of aesthetics and functionality into their work (Kapitan, 2011).

Crafts, in general, and textiles in particular played diverse roles in many women's lives, including helping them express the hardships and challenges they could not express in words. Crafting was used to cope with loss and anxiety, provide a source of pride and empowerment, cultivate a sense of community, foster a sense of control, enact mutual support, and stimulate social and political change (Anderson & Gold, 1998; Parker, 1996). Furthermore, forms of traditional art made by women had a subversive purpose in that they challenged patriarchal expectations of women. For example, in the 18th and 19th centuries, under the guise of embroidery women learned to read and write and to study what were then unacceptable subjects for women, such as geography. In addition, crafts offered women a socially acceptable context for gathering in groups, sharing their experiences, gaining support and validation, and penetrating the isolation of traditional domestic life (Anderson & Gold, 1998; Mainardi, 1982; Parker, 1996).

Another example of the subversive use of crafts occurred during the regime of Chilean dictator Augusto Pinochet from 1973 to 1990. Women in Chile sewed and quilted *arpilleras*, fabric pictures that portrayed the hardships and brutality they were experiencing. Their products were sold and exported, contributing both to the financial empowerment of the women and to exposing the harsh reality in Chile to the rest of the world, which helped generate international pressure toward regime change (Garlock, 2016; Youngson, 2019).

Handicraft today – reclaiming craft

The 1960s and 1970s heralded the conscious use of so-called *feminine crafts* as valid and relevant art forms, pointing to their subversive political value and their equivalence to fine art. Since then, an interest in crafts has grown. Over the past two decades, handicrafts have been given a more prominent position in both the domestic and public spheres and in Western popular culture (Adamson, 2009). Handcrafting has also become more widely accepted and popular, due in part to the emergence of social media that allows users to share their creations and DIY projects (Kaimal et al., 2017; Leenerts et al., 2016).

However, handicrafts are still used for financial purposes, as "tangible benefits are gained from the end products of the crafter's labor" (Pollanen, 2013, p. 217). Also, crafts continue to be an empowering and even subversive act by women who use them to celebrate gender, engage in political action, expand agency, and be creative and proactive. The use of craft circles by women creates natural spaces for shared reality, enhanced empowerment, and the exchange of knowledge and experience (Chansky, 2010).

With their rising popularity, crafts that were once considered women's work are now accepted and given prominent places in the contemporary art world (Kikuchi, 2015; Yam, 2002). Nowadays women are not limited to textile work and may opt for other craft forms such as carpentry or welding. Many artists in the current craft culture seek to challenge the domestic, gendered nature of handicrafts, especially textile works, and redefine them as a form of activism (Chansky, 2010).

Crafts as a therapeutic medium

Crafts have been shown to positively influence emotional and physical health (Reynolds, 2000, 2004) and to improve subjective well-being (Kaimal et al., 2017; Pollanen, 2013, 2015b; Riley et al., 2013). Crafts can also affect mood and help relieve depression (Collier et al., 2016; Collier & von Károlyi, 2014), be a way of coping with negative feelings and anxiety (Pollanen, 2015a; Reynolds, 2000), and stimulate empowerment (Tubbs & Drake, 2017). Crafts can enable people to access a state of flow that is simultaneously alert, calm, and creative, and to feel a sense of agency and achievement (Pollanen, 2015b). On a neurological level, crafts can help in dealing with trauma as it activates the hands and both sides of the brain and thus is a neurologically integrative activity (Garlock, 2016).

Crafts as an embodied sensory experience

An embodiment approach to the arts therapies views sensory experience as influencing cognition, perception, action, and emotion. Likewise, cognition, perception, action, and emotion influence sensory experience (Koch & Fuchs, 2011). Embodied sensory experiences can activate *past* autobiographical memories such as recalling the crafting activities of one's mother, *present* sensations through physical engagement with materials, and *future* visions inspired by perceptual innovations (Goshen et al., 2019).

Crafts as empowerment

While art therapy literature focuses primarily on the rehabilitative and calming or self-regulating effects of crafts, handiwork can also be experienced as empowering. Textile crafts and other craft work can provide a voice for women who are excluded from dominant verbal narratives (Parker, 1996). The use of crafts bolsters self-esteem, fosters a sense of agency, enables self-expression, provides *me time*, and stimulates physical and cognitive development associated with learning new skills (Parker, 1996; Pollanen, 2013).

Crafts can also be a source of cultural pride, a way to connect with one's ethnicity, origins, and family, and thus to develop a stronger sense of identity (Huss, 2010; Kaimal et al., 2017; Moon, 2010). They also can make elements of everyday life special by creating meaning, outcomes, and attachments to place (Tubbs & Drake, 2007).

A feminist perspective on stress in the helping professions

Feminist theories focus on patriarchal social constructions as sources of oppression for women (Carroll et al., 1999; Saulnier, 1996). Not only the clients who receive services, but also social service practitioners are predominantly female. Practitioners are often underpaid and dealing with overburdening workloads and very little support. Thus, they are marginalized in a process parallel to that of their clients (Krumer-Nevo, 2002). The caring nature of these jobs leads to their being considered extensions of the *natural* female role of looking after others, with the accompanying implication that fair financial compensation is unnecessary (Peled & Krumer-Nevo, 2012).

High levels of stress and burnout in social work, nursing, and education, all predominantly female professions, are endemic (Carpenter & Webb, 2012). Constant exposure to traumatic stories may be experienced as intrapersonal and invasive, and secondary trauma may include symptoms parallel with those of traumatized clients. A common stress reaction known as compassion fatigue results from the combination of listening and empathizing over time. Another related concept is that of burnout, manifesting in symptoms such as a lack of interest in the work, numbing of feelings, and clinical depression. Burnout may give rise to a sense of detachment and to avoidance behaviors employed for self-protection (Adams et al., 2008; Figley, 2002).

What actions do women take in their day-to-day lives to relieve stress and engage in self-care? Research shows that while social practitioners are encouraged to engage in self-care, they seldom do so. In addition, there is little research about the forms of self-care they do engage in (Lee & Miller, 2013; Miller et al., 2018).

In summary, we can make a connection between crafts and helping professions as predominantly female and thus marginalized activities. However, many women engage in crafts, and the question emerges as to whether this practice serves as a coping mechanism for them (Anderson & Gold, 1998). If it does, then crafts may also be relevant resources for female marginalized clients who are experiencing considerable stress. This chapter aims to explore these theoretical connections through accessing female social practitioners' lived experiences of engaging in crafts practices.

Research methods and participants

This study employed qualitative phenomenological methods to understand how female-identified social workers who engage in craft practices experience and understand their use of crafts. For the purpose of this research, craft practices were defined as the creation of products, both decorative and functional, that require skills to produce.

The research participants were gathered by snowball sampling. They received explanations about the research and signed consents to participate. Semi-structured interviews were conducted with seven cisgender female social work practitioners who engaged in decorative crafts such as knitting, ceramics, and embroidery.

The interviews included three types of questions. First, participants were asked general questions about themselves, their social service work, and their crafts practices. Second, they were asked follow-up questions to clarify and gain additional details about their responses. Third, they were asked conceptual questions including how they understood the role of crafts in their lives and what their views were on the connection between engaging in crafting and being a social worker.

Interviews were analyzed thematically according to a grounded theory approach, using the constructive perspective of Charmaz (2000). The objective of this method is to form a theoretical explanation for the phenomenon explored. Thus, the area of crafts is explored within the social context of being female social practitioners.

The researchers, both social work practitioners who engage in crafts practices, have personal experience with the topic explored through this research. The interviews were peer reviewed by the researchers and a group of women who engaged in similar crafts and were members of a group the first researcher belonged to (Shimoni, 2016). There were no dual relationships or overt imbalances in power between the researchers and participants. The research data was anonymized and shown to the participants before being used. This research received ethics approval from the university's Human Subjects Research Committee.

Findings

The themes that emerged from the data are divided into those that relate to the intimate, personal practice of crafting, and those that relate to the relational and interactive experience of crafting.

Crafts as intimate, personal experience

Crafts were described by the women as pleasurable because of the sensory experience of touch, color, smell, and movement activated when making crafts.

> For me touching the material is already therapeutic…just putting my hands on the clay is already significant.

In addition, the pleasure in creating something beautiful, the pleasure in aesthetics, was mentioned:

> I love to see beautiful things, and even more to create beautiful things – it is as if you are making the world better.

The pleasure in gaining new skills and achieving mastery was also stressed.

> I love to learn. It's true. It's a challenge. The challenge of learning
> something, to overcome it….

A sense of pride and mastery was also emphasized.

> I see that women who come to learn crafts with me gain compe-
> tence, confidence in their own abilities, their skill, creativity, deci-
> sion making, their ability to create something beautiful. These skills
> grow over time, and more complex challenges can be met. I sud-
> denly saw that I can. If I can do this, then I can also do other things.

> There's something very pleasant in seeing something finished,
> whole, that's yours… that you created.

Self-expression was another theme.

> It's a space of personal expression… it reflects me, my personality. In
> jewelry making I know that I think a bit differently, I need it to be
> unique, like it won't be the same. I give myself some creative space….

Other participants described crafts in therapeutic terms, as enabling regulation of stress and fostering a sense of emotional safety.

> I really experience it like therapy, it can be compared to therapy
> for the whole body.

> I allow the creation to look like something supportive, as a hobby,
> like some sort of refuge for the spirit.

The experience of entering a state of flow and mindfulness was also
mentioned:

> I feel that this really leads to relaxation, something that's more
> pleasant, that concentrates me more. It [knitting] creates a feel-
> ing over time that maybe things won't shake me up as much. Like
> it releases my head from dealing with certain subjects.

For some participants, crafting enabled a playful space where they allowed themselves to shed their duties and commitments and return to feeling like children and having fun with varied art materials.

> It is a sort of letting go and losing control, it's a bit like being a little girl.

Some viewed crafting as an experience in which mistakes are permissible.

> I say there aren't mistakes - everything is cool in art and crafting. Everything, it's yours, the opposite when you make a mistake—that's your fingerprint on the work.

> You can make mistakes but also correct things, always....

Other participants viewed crafting as an opportunity to create culturally sanctioned personal space.

> I do not sit down to paint and 'waste' my time, but create something useful for my needs or the needs of the home.

> When you do crafting, or functional art, or handiwork... it has a use, it's like, justified.... It seems like I have justification in clearing time for this.

Relational and interactive experience of crafting

Some participants discussed the pleasure of producing something beautiful for other people.

> So, to the one that creates them, it's like you donate something to the world. Something to the home, something to the world, something to the children, something real, something grounded in reality.

For some participants, their sense of giving extended to making the world a better place.

I also think that maybe part of the fun is that you create something, and you feel like you don't waste, like you guard the earth, like this is how you're one who protects it. It's something to be proud of.

Some participants discussed crafting in groups as a support system and a way to develop social connections outside of professional networks.

Interestingly, the fact that the women were not social workers enabled a new type of closeness and connection.

All day long I meet with women that overwhelm me with stories of sexual assault and post trauma, and stories that are very complex, and that's what I do all day, so I really appreciate the three hours that are, like, neutral time to talk to people about other things, to see people, to create.

Discussion

The data revealed that crafts practices have a broad range of benefits for the participants' well-being. These benefits included sensory and aesthetic pleasure, a sense of personal challenge and achievement, and experiences of playfulness and relaxation. According to the participants, crafting enables creation of personal space as well as relational space. Beneficial elements helped them manage the stress of social work through creating an alternative inner and outer world, and through enhancing creativity, decision-making, achievement, connectivity, and self-regulation in a safe, culturally sanctioned, gendered space. Thus, doing crafts expanded well-being on multiple levels. It enabled participants to experience a sense of agency and experiential and creative stimulation, to set aside a personal time, to engage in playfulness, and to learn new skills. In addition, they noted that creating crafts is a way to give to oneself and to others. Paradoxically, crafting can both provide a respite from cultural and gendered roles and a means to find a comfortable fit in relation to those roles.

In terms of skills, the ability while crafting to make decisions, solve problems, and see new possibilities, as well as to experience a sense of achievement and of making the world a better place have the potential to be transferred to social work practice. Additionally, participants addressed the potential of using crafts to foster these same experiences in service users. They also identified engaging in craft practices to connect with service users' cultural identities and strengths, as an alternative to problem-oriented encounters.

From a feminist perspective, crafts employed in the context of a female-dominated, underpaid, low-status profession enabled a space of privacy, agency, and playfulness, as well as a space for unstructured social interaction, productivity, and sense of achievement. These elements have the potential to be empowering for both women in so-called *female* professions and for clients who are marginalized based on their identity as women. At the same time, crafting is a culturally contextualized and accepted form of self-expression that enables multiply marginalized women to experience agency within overall patriarchal systems, in ways that do not create a conflict between the women and their social and cultural environments.

Culturally sanctioned, embodied, sensory opportunities for self-expression connect to third-world feminist principles of creating personal and relational spaces where skills and abilities can be enhanced in culturally acceptable ways. Craft practices can help to bring gender, culture, and embodiment into social work practice, making it more relational and holistic, and less clinically detached. It can help the field move away from de-contextualized practice, for the benefit of both practitioners and clients. The concept of making special through decorating, beautifying, engaging in personized gifting, and self-expression becomes a means of empowerment that is practiced in day-to-day life rather than in encapsulated therapeutic spaces. Making special through crafting enables the creation of place attachment and pride in one's body, home, or community, regardless of financial status. These aims are consistent with social work practice. The benefits of crafting could reach not only social workers, but also other social service providers and their clients.

References

Adams, R. E., Figley, C., & Boscarino, J. (2008). The compassion fatigue scale: Its use with social workers following urban disaster. *Research on Social Work Practice, 18*, 238–250. https://doi.org/10.1177/1049731507310190

Adamson, G. (2007). *Thinking through craft.* Berg Publishers.
Adamson, G. (2009). Directions and displacements in modern craft. *Australian and New Zealand Journal of Art, 10*(1), 18–33. https://doi.org/10.1080/14434318.2009.11432600
Anderson, L., & Gold, K. (1998). Creative connections: The healing power of women's art and craft work. *Women & Therapy, 21*(4), 15–36. https://doi.org/10.1300/J015v21n04_02
Brown, J. K. (1970). Notes on the division of labor by sex. *American Anthropologist, 72*(5), 1073–1078. https://doi.org/10.1525/aa.1970.72.5.02a00070
Carpenter, J., & Webb, C. (2012). What can be done to promote the retention of social workers? A systematic review of interventions. *British Journal of Social Work, 42,* 1235–1255. https://doi.org/10.1093/bjsw/bcr144
Carroll, L., Gilroy, P. J., & Murra, J. (1999). The moral imperative. *Women & Therapy, 22*(2), 133–143. https://doi.org/10.1300/J015v22n02_10
Chansky, R. A. (2010). A stitch in time: Third-wave feminist reclamation of needled imagery. *Journal of Popular Culture, 43*(4), 681–700. https://doi.org/10.1111/j.1540-5931.2010.00765.x
Charmaz, K. (2000). Grounded theory: Objectivist and constructivist. In N. K. Denzin & Y. S. Lincoln (Eds.), *Handbook of qualitative research* (2nd ed.) (pp. 509–536). Sage Publications.
Collier, A. F., & von Károlyi, C. (2014). Rejuvenation in the "making": Lingering mood repair in textile handcrafters. *Psychology of Aesthetics, Creativity, and the Arts, 8*(4), 475–485. https://doi.org/10.1037/a0037080
Collier, A. F., Wayment, H. A., & Birkett, M. (2016). Impact of making textile handcrafts on mood enhancement and inflammatory immune changes. *Art Therapy, 33*(4), 178–185. https://doi.org/10.1080/07421656.2016.1226647
Figley, C. R. (2002). Compassion fatigue: Psychotherapists' chronic lack of self-care. *Journal of Clinical Psychology: Psychotherapy in Practice, 58*(11), 1433–1441. https://doi.org/10.1002/jclp.10090
Garlock, L. R. (2016). Stories in the cloth: Art therapy and narrative textiles. *Art Therapy, 33*(2), 58–66. https://doi.org/10.1080/07421656.2016.1164004
Goshen, I., Huss, E., & Koch, S. C. (2019). Creating an embodied phenomenological typology for describing the qualitative experience of traumatic space from continued bombings. *Journal of Loss and Trauma, 24*(5–6), 460–472. https://doi.org/10.1080/15325024.2018.1507471
Greenhalgh, P. (1997). The history of craft. In P. Dormer (Ed.), *The culture of craft* (pp. 20–52). Manchester University Press.
Huss, E. (2010). Bedouin women's embroidery as female empowerment: Crafts as culturally embedded expression within art therapy. In C. H. Moon (Ed.), *Materials and media in art therapy: Critical understandings of diverse artistic vocabularies* (pp. 215–230). Routledge.
Kaimal, G., Gonzaga, A. M. L., & Schwachter, V. (2017). Crafting, health and wellbeing: Findings from the survey of public participation in the arts and considerations for art therapists. *Arts & Health, 9*(1), 81–90. https://doi.org/10.1080/17533015.2016.1185447
Kapitan, L. (2011). Close to the heart: Art therapy's link to craft and art production. *Art Therapy, 28*(3), 94–95. https://doi.org/10.1080/07421656.2011.601728
Kikuchi, Y. (2015). The craft debate at the crossroads of global visual culture: Re-centering craft in postmodern and postcolonial histories. *World Art, 5*(1), 87–115. https://doi.org/10.1080/21500894.2015.1029139
Koch, S. C., & Fuchs, T. (2011). Embodied arts therapies. *The Arts in Psychotherapy, 38,* 276–280. https://doi.org/10.1016/j.aip.2011.08.007

Krumer-Nevo, M. (2002). M'Penelopeh l'Miri: Truma hagisha hafemineesteet l'sugiyot nashim b'metzuka kalkaleet v'hevrateet amookah v'meetmashechet [From Penelope to Miri: The contribution of the feminist approach to the issue of women in deep and continuous economic and social distress]. *Chevrah v'revacha [Society and welfare], 22*, 433–454.

Lee, J., & Miller, S. (2013). A self-care framework for social workers: Building a strong foundation for practice. *Families in Society: The Journal of Contemporary Human Services, 94*, 96–103. https://doi.org/10.1606/1044-3894.4289

Leenerts, E., Evetts, C., & Miller, E. (2016). Reclaiming and proclaiming the use of crafts in occupational therapy. *The Open Journal of Occupational Therapy, 4*(4), 13. https://doi.org/10.15453/2168-6408.1194

Lippard, L. R. (1978). Making something from nothing (toward a definition of women's "hobby art"). In G. Adamson (Ed.), *The craft reader* (pp. 483–490). Bloomsbury Academic.

Lucie-Smith, E. (1981). *The story of craft: The craftsman's role in society.* Cornell University Press.

Mainardi, P. (1982). Quilts: The great American art. In N. Broude & M. D. Garrard (Eds.), *Feminism and art history: Questioning the litany* (pp. 330–346). Harper & Row.

Miller J. J., Lianekhammy, J., & Grise-Owens, E. (2018). Examining self-care among individuals employed in social work capacities: Implications for the profession. *Advances in Social Work, 18*(4), 1250–1266. https://doi.org/10.18060/22320

Moon, C. H. (2010). Theorizing materiality in art therapy. In C. H. Moon (Ed.), *Materials and media in art therapy: Critical understandings of diverse artistic vocabularies* (pp. 1–49). Routledge.

Parker, R. (1996). *The subversive stitch: Embroidery and the making of the feminine.* Palgrave Macmillan.

Parker, R., & Pollock, G. (2013). *Old mistresses: Women, art and ideology.* I.B. Taurus.

Peled, E., & Krumer-Nevo, M. (2012). Avodat sotziyaleet femineesteet. [Feminist social work.] In M. Chovav, A. Lontel, & Y. Katan (Eds.), *Avodat sotziyaleet b'Yisrael* [Social work in Israel] (pp. 479–505). Hakibbutz hame'uchad.

Pollanen, S. (2013). The meaning of craft: Craft-makers' descriptions about craft as an occupation. *Scandinavian Journal of Occupational Therapy, 20*(3), 217–227. https://doi.org/10.3109/11038128.2012.725182

Pollanen, S. (2015a). Crafts as leisure-based coping: Craft makers' descriptions of their stress-reducing activity. *Occupational Therapy in Mental Health, 31*(2), 83–100. https://doi.org/10.1080/0164212X.2015.1024377

Pollanen, S. (2015b). Elements of crafts that enhance well-being. *Journal of Leisure Research, 4*(1), 58–78. https://doi.org/10.1080/00222216.2015.11950351

Reynolds, F. (2000). Managing depression through needlecraft creative activities: A qualitative study. *The Arts in Psychotherapy, 27*(2), 107–114. https://doi.org/10.1016/S0197-4556(99)00033-7

Reynolds, F. (2004). Textile art promoting well-being in long-term illness: Some general and specific influences. *Journal of Occupational Science, 11*(2), 58–67. https://doi.org/10.1080/14427591.2004.9686532

Riley, J., Corkhill, B., & Morris, C. (2013). The benefits of knitting for personal and social wellbeing in adulthood: Findings from an international survey. *British Journal of Occupational Therapy, 76*(2), 50–57. https://doi.org/10.4276/030802213X13603244419077

Saulnier, C. F. (1996). *Feminist theories and social work: Approaches and applications.* The Haworth.

Shimoni, S. (2016). The'oreeya me'oogenet bsadeh. [Theory anchored in the field.] In N. Tzabar Ben-Yehoshua (Ed.), *Masoret v'zrameem b'mechkar haichootanee: Tfisot, astrategiyot v'keylim mitkadmeem* [Traditions and streams in qualitative research: Perceptions, strategies, and advanced tools] (pp. 141–178). Machon Moffet.

Shiner, L. (2012). "Blurred boundaries"? Rethinking the concept of craft and its relation to art and design. *Philosophy Compass, 7*(4), 230–244. https://doi.org/10.1111/j.1747-9991.2012.00479.x

Tubbs, C., & Drake, M. (2007). *Crafts and creative media in therapy.* Slack Books.

Tubbs, C., & Drake, M. (2017). Crafts and creative media in therapy. *Occupational Therapy in Health Care, 31*(4), 376–377. https://doi.org/10.1080/07380577.2017.1360536

Yam, R. (2002). *Sod kasman shel avodot hamachat – al nashim, terapiya omanut v'omanut v'hakshareyhen* [The secrets of needlework – about women, art therapy and art and their connections]. Cherkover.

Youngson, B. (2019). Craftivism for occupational therapists: Finding our political voice. *British Journal of Occupational Therapy, 82*(6), 383–385. https://doi.org/10.1177/0308022619825807

Zehavi, R. (2015). Ma zeh bichlal craft [What is a craft anyway?]. In R. Bartal & A. Ehrlich (Eds.), *Machsahvot al craft* [Thoughts about craft] (pp. 56–83). Risling.

SECTION II

ART MATERIALS, MEDIA, AND PRACTICES IN CONTEMPORARY ART THERAPY

5

Sis, U belong here

Black Women making and taking up space

veronica precious bohanan

Calling all sistas to tha circle

I see you. I hear you. I believe you. You matter.

This chapter sheds light on Sis, U Belong Here (SUBH), a community-based art therapy program committed to creating a space for Black Women to experience themselves as healed and whole. The program is built on a generative, womanist approach that facilitates immersive and intergenerational gatherings known as sista-circles. SUBH normalizes using culturally responsive materials, such as spacemaking, rituals, and embodied practices. Despite being viewed as unconventional by art therapy purists, these materials have stood the test of time with the program's enduring presence and sustained engagement. SUBH challenges the limited constructs that assign worth, significance, and impact to art therapy materials and media, rejecting the hierarchies of fine arts.

Fortunately, art therapy constantly evolves and diversifies, with practitioners who honor their traditions and integrate cultural practices into their work. SUBH is a prime example of this innovation and adaptability, standing on the ancestral shoulders of Black Women art therapy pioneers such as Sarah McGee and Georgette Seabrooke Powell (Gipson, 2019). This chapter underscores the unique socio-cultural context of Black Women's lived experiences. It showcases how art therapy materials

DOI: 10.4324/9781032720166-7

and media can be tailored to various cultural contexts. It also illustrates how *conventional* materials and aspects of art therapy are present in the sista-circles but have been reimagined to better meet the community's needs.

SUBH is a catalyst for thrivance, creating a *safer* space for Black Women to *just be*, recognizing that safety is subjective and experienced under varying conditions and personal factors (Mental Health Commission of Canada, n.d.). This is exemplified by the expectation that Women attending the sista-circles participate but can opt out if they are at capacity. This ongoing process toward *be-ing* fosters wellness and *thrivance*, a concept Baumann (2023) defined as valuing people over output, making positive changes in the world, and sustaining culture. SUBH adopts a decolonized approach to productivity that prioritizes holistic collective care. This is demonstrated through various communal activities such as making honey jars, practicing breathwork, and ancestral veneration. In SUBH's healing-centered approach, safety and a shared sense of thriving are essential in cultivating connection and Black sistahood. This is evident in how community agreements and a Divine Feminine declaration are collectively established through engaging play, and Theatre of the Oppressed exercises—a form of participatory theater (Boal, 1975/2002). Like healing justice (Page & Woodland, 2023), a healing-centered approach focuses on communal strengths and processes rather than individual pathology and isolation (Ginwright, 2018). This is exemplified through communal activities such as making wrap dolls and felt hearts, as well as subsequent group discussions following all experiential activities. These examples are further explored in this chapter's "circle elementals" section.

Love is in the details

Growing up, Mama expressed love through details and creativity. She made both the day-to-day and special occasions meaningful. For example, she walked me to school hand-in-hand, singing, "You Are My Sunshine." When I first became a teen worker, she implemented a monthly mother-daughter date for us *working girls*, as she affectionately called us. This level of meaning-making reflects Dissanayake's (2003) concept of *making special*, which I incorporate into my practice as an art therapist.

At the end of most sista-circles, participants (referred to as *sistas who belong* or *community members*) express gratitude for the safe and welcoming space I have curated. I call what I do *spacemaking*, a concept akin to womanist *placemaking* as described by Gipson (2019). "As a survival strategy, *place making* aims to establish safety among a Black communal network based on historically shared or lived experience of oppression" (pp. 100–101). In addition, spacemaking is a thrivance strategy that accesses personal, cultural, and ancestral memories of resilience, joy, and play.

The first step toward SUBH spacemaking was selecting physical spaces throughout Chicago for our site-specific immersive experiences. Each physical space was a canvas, and each sista-circle was an experiential art medium. The venues chosen were those with a Black Woman in a leadership or operational position, demonstrating SUBH's commitment to representation.

SUBH's first home was Links Hall, a northside experimental dance and performance space—our most adaptable and spacious canvas to date. The immersive experience began upon entry. Near the studio entrance was an area where sistas removed their shoes and saged themselves for an energetic cleanse. They were then guided to form a circle with their mats, blankets, and pillows in the middle of the floor, with art materials placed at the circle's center. The bare walls displayed our manifesta and poster boards containing thought-provoking questions that sistas responded to with markers. One example of a question that sparked introspection was, "How do you reclaim parts of yourself that have been taken or given away?" The front of the room was dedicated to our communal altar, to which sistas contributed. After eight sista-circles, the 12-month agreement with Links Hall concluded.

SUBH moved south to the Pilsen neighborhood, Rootwork Gallery. While Links Hall was a malleable and spacious blank canvas, Rootwork's existing exhibitions and intimate setting created an unparalleled collaborative experience with the physical space. The gallery's commitment to investigating folk, street, and indigenous art aligned with the Black woman-centeredness of SUBH. Exhibitions such as *My Womb es mi Altar: Afro-Latinadad Visions of the Sacred* and *Intercessions: Art as Intervention and Prayer* (Rootwork Gallery, n.d.) are examples of the work highlighted in the gallery. The thought-provoking questions, previously on the walls at Links Hall, were now available to respond to on clipboards placed around the gallery. Sistas could answer the questions while walking around the gallery and engaging the artwork.

Just before COVID-19 shifted us to a virtual space, the final in-person location for SUBH was the Justice Hotel in Chicago's Edgewater neighborhood. SUBH was invited to participate in the hotel's Chicago Architecture Biennial programming that focused on conversational dinners, performances, and healing services. Most of the sista-circle activity for this location took place in the front parlor and dining room, and adjacent rooms were used for activities requiring movement.

Intersectionality

I was not only brought up *blackity black*—culturally and racially Diasporic Black—but my childhood was steeped in Black girl and womanness. I was nurtured in a matriarchal family and lived in a six-unit residential building where Black mothers formed a close-knit sistahood and supportive community. In this environment, Black culture and pride were central, so I was not inundated with White culture or fully aware of the White gaze.

Going away to college and transitioning into adulthood provided me with new experiences beyond my immediate surroundings. Self-preservation became essential, and I discovered that prioritizing decolonized care practices—over materialism—disrupted the White gaze. Therefore, SUBH is as much for me as for the sistas. In the documentary *The Pieces I Am* (Greenfield-Sanders, 2019), Toni Morrison spoke about deliberately not prioritizing the White gaze in her writing. Similarly, SUBH neutralizes the White gaze by maintaining a focus on Black Women.

Alice Walker's (1983) "In Search of Our Mothers' Gardens" details womanism and emphasizes Black Women's strength, depth, and distinctive perspective on feminism. By Walker's definition, womanism is foundational to SUBH, and sistas-circles are immersive experiences on par with Black Women's ongoing history of resistance and actively seeking freedom; therefore, intergenerational and ancestral wisdom is embedded in SUBH. My mother's role as my thought partner, who also buys and serves snacks, exemplifies the intergenerational nature of SUBH.

Additionally, we highly regard the other wise Women we lovingly refer to as *Mama,* and we have welcomed mother-daughter pairs and sistas aged 21 to 75.

Magic and the Divine

SUBH holds space for Black Women being both the strength and resilience of Black Girls Are Magic (#blackgirlmagic) coined by CaShawn Thompson (Lamar-Becker, 2022). Two beliefs can be true simultaneously; therefore, SUBH also rejects the notion that resilience is superior or more desirable than softness and ease, as tweeted by brown (n.d.):

> I dream of never being called resilient again in my life. I'm exhausted by strength. I want support. I want softness. I want ease. I want to be amongst kin. Not patted on the back for how well I take a hit. Or for how many.

The SUBH community upholds #blackgirlmagic and promotes ease while embracing an intersectional and embodied Black Divine Feminine and God of each sista's understanding. In critiquing the societal impact of White patriarchal Christianity, Cleveland (2022) discussed actively seeking a God who looked like her. This personalized representation of God promotes self-love and self-acceptance, which is central to womanism.

The concepts of the Divine Feminine and God as an internalized presence make divinity more accessible to Black Women. For example, Shange (1976) highlights finding God within oneself and loving her deeply, transcending religious boundaries. Furthermore, SUBH delves into the African Diasporic representations of the Divine Feminine, including the Black Madonna, Osun, Yemaya, Oya, Isis, Ma'at, and Mami Wata. This exploration challenges stereotypes that both demonize aggressiveness and contend that Black Women are not feminine enough. As Collins (1986) pointed out, "aggressive Afro-American women are threatening because they challenge White patriarchal definitions of femininity" (p. S17).

At a 2017 sista-circle, I introduced a working definition of the Divine Feminine and sought community approval. Later, when we transitioned to virtual gatherings in 2020, we made art about it, and the definition was further workshopped and rewritten by the collective. Reading the declaration aloud during virtual sista-circles has become a ritual that cultivates connection, vulnerability, and belonging. As Monet (2020) notes, "vulnerability is a form of healing that Black Women are often denied." For SUBH, healing is a state of being, a holistic approach to wholeness and wellness.

Belonging

SUBH's sense of belonging is rooted in a reimagined resilience that prioritizes growth and freedom rather than shrinking to avoid being silenced, controlled, or confined by stereotypes. SUBH is in an ongoing conversation with a statement made by Maya Angelou (Moyers, 1973): "You only are free when you realize you belong no place — you belong every place — no place at all. The price is high. The reward is great...I belong to myself" (n. p.). The *here* of SUBH is a play on words. We not only belong in this SUBH space, but we are also free to belong everywhere authentically because, ultimately, we are limitless. This freedom makes the White gaze ineffective.

Circle elementals

Sista-circles are built on foundational spacemaking elements that provide opportunities for creative expression, rituals, and the complete embodiment of self-love. These elements exemplify Walker's (1983) insistence that a womanist "loves herself. *Regardless*" (p. xii).

In addition to selecting venues run by Black Women decision-makers, representation is prioritized by inviting Black Women as guest facilitators and presenters. To acknowledge the legacy of Black art therapist Lucille Venture, the first person to earn a PhD in art therapy (Gipson, 2019), the names and titles of the guest art therapy facilitators are included as a vitally important cultural practice.

Informed by peace, healing, and talking circle processes, we sit in a circle because there is no hierarchy, and everyone can participate equally. Much like the Theatre of the Oppressed (Boal, 1975/2002) philosophy, there are no spectators; every sista's voice is essential. They are encouraged to leave their comfort zones and embrace new experiences; however, sistas can opt out. In addition, I offer this disclaimer, "Do what feels right to

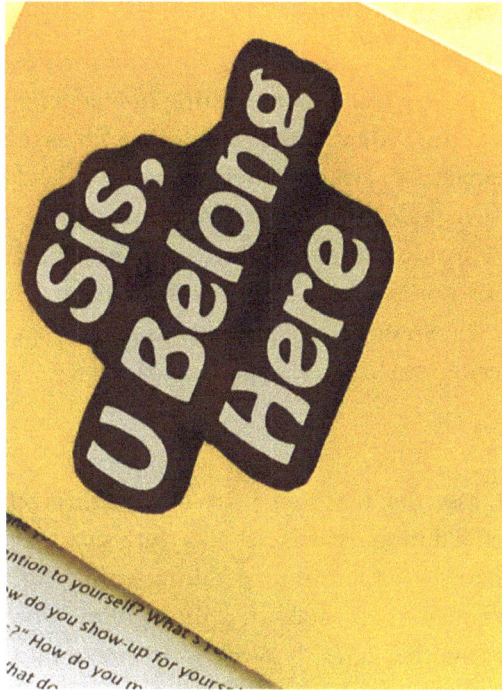

Figure 5.1 *Sis, U Belong Here* journal cover.

your spirit and trust yourself with yourself." Small journals (Figure 5.1) are provided at each sista-circle for members to take notes and document their thoughts.

Theme and focus

Each workshop has a theme specific to the season, commemorative causes of the month, or calendar year. For example, *expansion* was the 2024 theme. Along with the theme, a corresponding quote serves as a centering thought. Typically, quotes are sourced from Black cultural references, creatives, or thought leaders of the African Diaspora. For example, if we gather during a full moon, which is an optimal time for releasing anything that is not working well in one's life, members might reflect on a Toni Morrison (1977) quote, "Wanna fly, you got to give up the shit that weighs you down" (p. 179).

Community agreements

Agreements are drafted by establishing common ways of being in space together to create a safer and more trusting immersive experience. They are not fixed but rather adapt to the needs of our collective. We regularly revisit the agreements to ensure that everyone feels heard. For example, agreements have included: *Give yourself permission to Be. Here. Now.* And *Take space. Make space.* Also, a disclaimer is presented that SUBH is not therapy and does not replace seeing a licensed mental health provider. This disclaimer is my ethical responsibility as an art therapist and coincides with womanist tenets of care and transparency.

Music

Walker's (1983) assertion that womanists love music is reflected in using music as a material during sista-circles and yearly curated playlists. Music welcomes sistas to the circle and plays during artmaking. Songs primarily by Black Women artists establish a throughline for the themes and quotes, infusing another layer of Black womanness into SUBH. These playlists include artists such as Sweet Honey in the Rock, Beautiful Chorus, Mumu Fresh, Goapele, and Lizz Wright.

Opening ritual

Altar

The communal altar physically represents the diverse facets of Black Woman culture, the sacredness, resilience, optimism, and ancestral wisdom present in the sista-circle. Before sistas arrive, the altar (Figure 5.2) is set and prayed over, embodying all five natural elements through objects like a white candle, feather, glass of water, incense, plant or flowers, mirror, clear quartz crystal, and mustard seeds. The altar also features significant cultural artifacts, such as pictures of Harriet Tubman and Sojourner Truth, an afro-pick, and a book written by a Black Woman. Upon arrival, members are invited to contribute their meaningful items to the altar, transforming the altar into a co-created assemblage infused with collective energy. Even in the virtual setting, I curate an altar in my home, and members are encouraged to create their own altars, each with a minimum of a glass of water and a white candle.

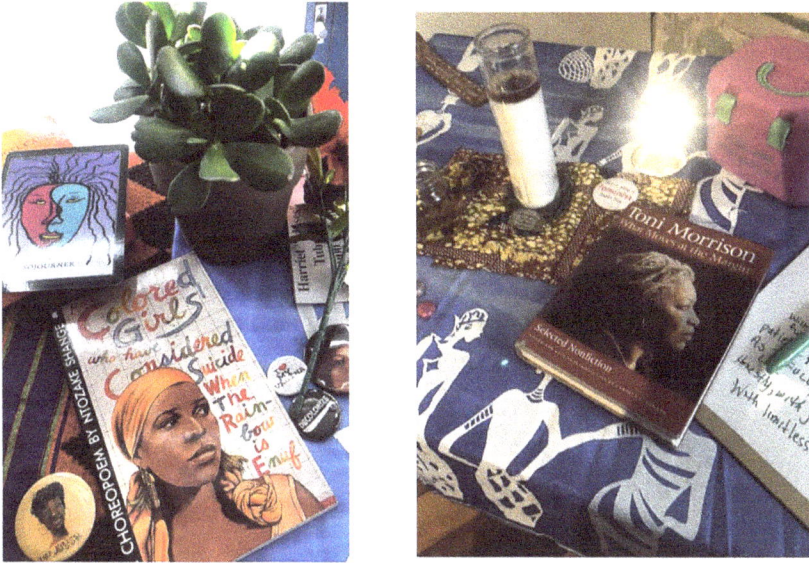

Figure 5.2 Altars in progress.

Breath as material, meditation as media

Breathwork and meditation are living extensions of the altar. These practices enable us to become fully present in our bodies and the moment. However, modifications are offered to acknowledge that connecting the breath and body can be retraumatizing for some. For Black Women, breathing is not just a physical act but a form of resistance to systemic violence, such as maternal mortality (U.S. Government, 2021) and police brutality (Crenshaw & African American Policy Forum, 2023). The COVID-19 pandemic has further underscored the importance of our breath. Also, I am acutely aware of the breath, especially at the time of this writing, due to the recent death of a loved one who was on long-term oxygen therapy.

Head blessing and ancestral veneration

Paired with breathwork and meditation, we frequently perform a spiritual head blessing ritual (Vanzant, 1992). The purpose of this ritual is to deepen our connection with our personalized higher self. Water, repetition, and intention are the primary elements of this ritual. At this pivotal moment of the opening process, sistas are invited to call forth benevolent ancestors—loved ones, personal or cultural, who are healed and well in the ancestral realm. To ground this practice, I read aloud a quote by a spiritualist:

> Venerating our ancestors is not worshiping them, but holding remembrance, reverence, and deep respect for those in our bloodline and inner circles. When we venerate our ancestors, we are helping their spirit elevate, keeping their energetic imprint & stories alive.
>
> (Isaad, 2021)

Following this, I encourage the sistas to share their ancestors' names verbally or type them in the chat for our virtual circles.

Ancestral veneration is also expressed through presentations and performances. For example, in 2019, we gathered at the Justice Hotel to remember Toni Morrison. The event included sharing our favorite Morrison quotes. In addition, there was prayer, African folklore, the channeling of Baby Suggs' monologue from Toni Morrison's book *Beloved*, and art therapist Johannil Napoleón, PsyD, guided us through an art-making activity that focused on self-trust and care. For a virtual circle in 2022, sociologist Ashley Stone also presented her dissertation research on abolitionist Ida B. Wells.

Additional circle elements are check-in questions, an arts-based experiential, group discussion, and a check-out process. Examples of these elements are below.

Body as material, image as media

Based on Augusto Boal's (1975/2002) Theatre of the Oppressed, the following exercise aims to prioritize Black Women taking up space and embodied reflection and insight. The members are given these instructions:

> Divide into three groups. Imagine being a piece of clay. Using no words, mold your bodies into group sculptures for each of the three questions. Everyone should participate in making the

sculpture cohesive, and a body part must touch or connect with at least one other member. Always ask for consent before touching.

Each group is assigned a topic.

Group 1: Misogynoir (Bailey, 2021)—Black Women's experiences with misogyny.

Group 2: Respectability politics (Higginbotham, 1993)—The unfortunate centering of whiteness as the standard of appearance and behavior.

Group 3: Emotional labor (Kelly et al., 2021)—The expectation for Black Women to provide support and care for others, even without compensation.

For each topic, the assigned group responds to each of these three questions with a collaborative sculpture:

1. What is it?
2. How do you uphold it, consciously or subconsciously?
3. How do we dismantle it?

After completing all three sculptures, each group reflects on emerging themes and ideas and chooses a series name that integrates these insights. Each small group then shares their sculptures, followed by a large group discussion about the overall experience.

Hands

Wrap dolls

On the same day we explored misogynoir, respectability politics, and emotional labor, another guest art therapist, Rochele Royster, PhD, joined us to facilitate a mini workshop on making wrap dolls using fabric and yarn (Figure 5.3). We were encouraged to use our creativity to make a doll that returned us to our inherent worth and sacredness. The room settled during doll-making, and the playlist matched the room's energy. Storytelling added nostalgia as we shared stories of playing with dolls as children.

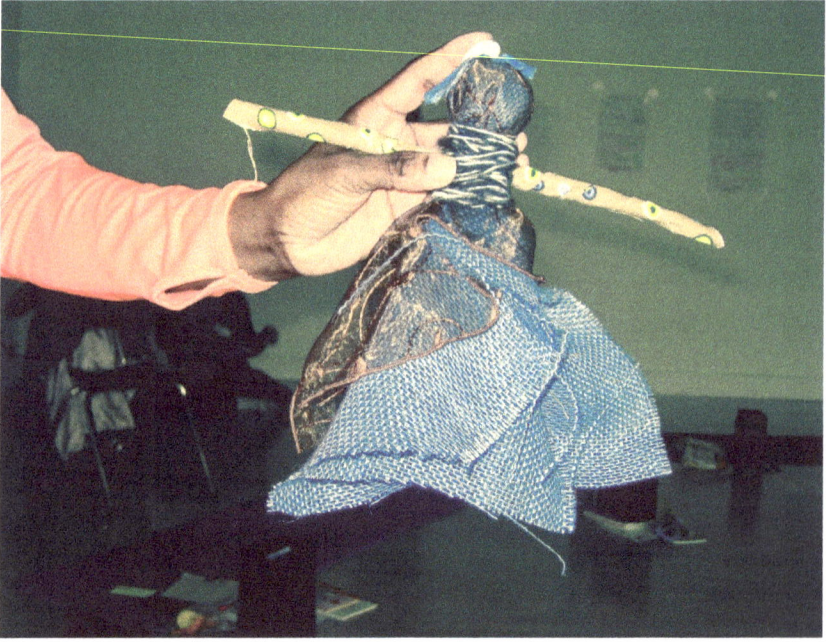

Figure 5.3 Wrap doll.

Sewing

Head-heart-womb is an accountability experiential I created to release emotional baggage. The instructions are:

1. On a slip of paper, write everything you carry in your mind, heart, and womb that no longer serves your best or highest good. Only write what you are ready to release.
2. Tear up the slip. Walk it to the trash, and do not look back.
3. On another slip of paper, write what you now choose to carry in the heart of your mind and womb.
4. Tightly fold the slip toward your heart into a small square.
5. Sew the edges of the pre-cut heart-shaped felt pieces, leaving a three-finger-width hole.
6. Fill the heart with pillow stuffing, insert the slip, and sew the hole closed.
7. When you arrive home, place your heart in a location where you will see it daily as a constant reminder of what you choose to carry.

During our group discussion, stories were shared about traumas, choices, childhood play, and family members who were quilters and seamstresses. Although many of the sistas had never sewn by hand or machine, they were committed to the process and empowered by their finished products.

Hula hoopin'

Activities like hula hoopin' encouraged movement and play. SUBH recognizes the significance of play in empowering Black Women and cultivating a sense of competence. Nicole Goss, a regular and flow arts performer in the sista-circle, was invited to facilitate a workshop on her body-positive and wellness approach to hula hoopin'. She highlighted the mental and physical health benefits of hula hoopin'. In this safer and nonjudgmental environment, sistas experimented with various sizes and weights of hoops. Several members shared that hula hoopin' reminded them of jumping Double Dutch as a child. Nicole demonstrated various hoopin' techniques and guided the group in making hula hoops with easily accessible materials like PVC pipes, a pipe cutter, and duct tape. As with sewing and doll wrapping, our hands stayed active as we decorated the hoops with duct tape.

Honey jars

Black cultural traditions are incorporated into SUBH to provide an accessible portal to art therapy. Metaphors and symbolism are utilized to encourage curiosity and discovery. This was demonstrated in 2020 during our virtual Honey Jar Series. I introduced honey as a metaphor to explore what needs sweetening, deepening, and strengthening in our lives. As part of this exploration, I led a ritual in which we created honey jars using small glass jars and various ingredients, each with its unique symbolism.

After centering ourselves and energetically cleansing the jars, we wrote our desires on a small piece of paper and placed it in the jar. We added cloves to protect our desires, cinnamon for blessings and success, gold glitter for abundance and resourcefulness, bay leaf for attraction, dried roses for self-love, and star anise for having a solid vision. Personalizing the jar with a single strand of hair or saliva was optional. Honey was added to represent sweetening and cohesiveness. The jar was sealed with green twine to signify fertility and growth. On top of the sealed jar, a candle was burned to represent sealing the intent.

I suggested placing the jar on their altar or someplace visible as a daily reminder. Everyone was encouraged to touch or shake the jar as often as they passed by it.

SoulCollage®

SoulCollage® is an intuitive, creative practice that uses collaging with the following materials: 5" × 8" matte board, a plastic sleeve, magazines, glue sticks, and scissors (Frost, 2010). A completed collage on the matte board is called a card, and multiple cards make a deck, which, for me, is like an oversized and personalized deck of homemade tarot or oracle cards. In 2021, art therapist Rev. Martina Efozdi, PhD, was invited to kick off our *Freshly Plaited Sweetgrass* virtual series with SoulCollage®. The prompt combined the nostalgic experience of Black girls getting their hair braided with the medicinal nature of sweetgrass. Once the card-making process was complete, sistas conversed with their collaged cards by embodying them. The conversation began with the official Soul-Collage® statement: "I AM One Who_____."

Check-out

We release our evoked ancestors for the closing activity while returning to our breath and reciting affirmations. Sandria Washington is a certified meditation and yoga teacher who has joined us for several in-person and virtual sista-circles. She guided us through breathwork and yoga sequences at the end of the circle. Sandria's approach is inclusive of all body sizes and abilities, making it accessible to all sistas.

And so it is…

After adjusting to sheltering in place, navigating the loss of loved ones, and receiving numerous texts and calls asking me to restart the sista-circles, I did so on Earth Day, April 22, 2020, via Zoom. The transition from in-person meetings to Zoom expanded the reach of the circles, allowing sistas to join us from anywhere in the world. Initially, my main goal was to provide a virtual platform for Black Women to discuss their experiences with new norms and transitions. Four years later, it has grown and evolved into so much more, and the community thrives.

Imbued in creativity and care, Sis, U Belong Here sista-circles are heart-centered, sacred gatherings that hold space for Black Women. SUBH's materials and media are grounded in our lived experiences, cultural traditions, and ancestral heritage, which nourishes deeper connections and understanding among ourselves. SUBH accesses joy through sistahood and reflection through rituals. This spacemaking approach favors making special and womanist placemaking.

References

Bailey, M. (2021). *Misogynoir transformed: Black women's digital resistance.* New York University Press.

Baumann, D. (2023). Thrivance is my identity: Moving beyond survival. *Journal of Ethnic and Cultural Studies, 10*(4), 1–12. https://doi.org/10.29333/ejecs/1669

Boal, A. (2002). *Games for actors and non-actors* (A. Jackson, Trans., 2nd ed.). Routledge (Original work published 1975).

brown, z. l. (n.d.). [@zandashe]. Tweets [X profile]. X, formerly Twitter. Retrieved May 18, 2021 from https://twitter.com/zandashe

Cleveland, C. (2022). *God is a Black woman.* Harper One.

Collins, P. H. (1986). Learning from the outsider within: The sociological significance of Black feminist thought. *Social Problems, 33*(6), S14–S32. https://doi.org/10.2307/800672

Crenshaw, K., & African American Policy Forum. (2023). *#Sayhername: Black women's stories of police violence and public silence.* Haymarket Books.

Dissanayake, E. (2003). The core of art—Making special. *Journal of the Canadian Association for Curriculum Studies, 1*(2), 13–38. https://doi.org/10.25071/1916-4467.16856

Frost, S. (2010). *SoulCollage® evolving: An intuitive collage process for self-discovery and community.* Hanford Mead Publishers.

Ginwright, S. (2018, May 31). Healing centered approach the future of healing: Shifting from trauma informed care to healing centered engagement. *Medium.* https://ginwright.medium.com/the-future-of-healing-shifting-from-trauma-informed-care-to-healing-centered-engagement-634f557ce69c

Gipson, L. (2019). Envisioning Black women's consciousness. In S. Talwar (Ed.), *Art therapy for social justice: Radical intersections* (pp. 96–120). Routledge. https://doi.org/10.4324/9781315694184

Greenfield-Sanders, T. (Director). (2019). *Toni Morrison: The pieces I am* (Video).

Higginbotham, E. B. (1993). *Righteous discontent: The women's movement in the Black Baptist Church, 1880–1920.* Harvard University Press.

Isaad, V. (2021, March 19). A guide for ancestor veneration for spiritual practice. *Hip Latina.* https://hiplatina.com/ancestor-veneration-spiritual-practice/

Kelly, B. T., Gardner, P. J., Stone, J., Hixson, A., & Dissassa, D.-T. (2021). Hidden in plain sight: Uncovering the emotional labor of Black women students at historically White colleges and universities. *Journal of Diversity in Higher Education, 14*(2), 203–216. https://doi.org/10.1037/dhe0000161

Lamar-Becker, S. L. (2022, September 19). The truth about #BlackGirlMagic: The origin story you didn't know. *Sesi.* https://sesimag.com/2022/09/19/black-girl-magic-the-origin-story/

Mental Health Commission of Canada. (n.d.). *Safer space guidelines.* https://www.mentalhealthcommission.ca/wp-content/uploads/drupal/2019-03/safer_space_guidelines_mar_2019_eng.pdf

Monet, A. (2020, July 1). Yes, Black girls are allowed to be soft. *Medium.* https://ashiamonetb.medium.com/yes-black-girls-are-allowed-to-be-soft-dee054974a45

Morrison, T. (1977). *Song of Solomon.* Knopf.

Moyers, B. (1973, November 21). A conversation with Maya Angelou [Video]. *Bill Moyers Journal.* https://billmoyers.com/content/conversation-maya-angelou/

Page, C., & Woodland, E. (2023). *Healing justice lineages: Dreaming at the crossroads of liberation, collective care, and safety.* North Atlantic Books.

Rootwork Gallery. (n.d.). *Home.* Facebook. https://www.facebook.com/rootworkgallery/

Shange, N. (1976). *For colored girls who have considered suicide/When the rainbow is enuf.* MacMillan.

U.S. Government Publishing Office. (2021). *Birthing while Black: Examining America's Black maternal health crisis.* https://www.govinfo.gov/content/pkg/CHRG-117hhrg44572/pdf/CHRG-117hhrg44572.pdf

Vanzant, I. (1992). *Tapping the power within: A path to self-empowerment for Black women.* Harlem River Press.

Walker, A. (1983). *In search of our mothers' gardens: Womanist prose* (1st ed.). Harcourt Brace Jovanovich.

6

CLAWING OUR WAY OUT

ART THERAPY MANICURE RITUALS AND A FEMINIST ETHICS OF CARE

Roxie Rose Ehlert

The tiny, bright glass bottles clink gently together as I delicately balance them on a makeshift metal tray, walking slowly down the blue carpeted hallway. Hands full, I carefully push the office door open with my foot, and enter the small space at the rape crisis center where I work. Sunlight streams through the sixth-story window, and the sounds of traffic drift up from the city street below. I awkwardly set my supplies down on the small round table in the corner. This little table has become a familiar, grounding oasis for me and for the people I sit across from each week.

The colors in the little bottles are yummy and exciting. Traditional bright reds and pinks are nestled next to dark blues, greens, and purples. Matte, pastel, and nude colors take up space alongside the much-needed glitter collection. Nail files, polish remover, cotton balls, decals, little jewels, and tiny rolls of tape for masking off elaborate designs fill the rest of the tray. I think Marie is going to choose something neutral, but I bring a larger collection just in case this Thursday is different.

Marie sighs heavily as she sits down. We each choose a polish from the tray (mine is never neutral) and saturate a cotton ball with nail polish remover. As we gently remove the evidence of last week's session from our fingernails, she begins to tell me about the exhaustion of her work week and about another infuriating encounter with her abusive, inappropriate boss. As we talk, she files

DOI: 10.4324/9781032720166-8

and then paints her nails neatly and precisely, quickly cleaning off her cuticles with a Q-Tip when any polish gets on them. I have less patience with my own nails and, as always, end up painting outside the lines.

In the bathroom after sessions, I inevitably end up scrubbing my hands in hot water, using the soap to help peel polish off my skin, replaying our conversations in my head. Therapy continues to happen in these micro-moments, me tumbling through feelings about patterns of exploitation as I scrub at the dried polish; Marie, weighing her tired anger, scrutinizing the imperfections in her polish application as she sits in traffic on the way home.

Why manicures matter

This is a chapter about the transformative potential of nail polish as a material in art therapy. Understood through the frameworks of queer femme identity (Brushwood Rose & Camilleri, 2003), disability justice (Piepzna-Samarasinha, 2018), and a feminist ethics of care (Morris, 2001; O'Leary, 2017; Talwar & Sajnani, 2022), the practice of art therapy manicures, in which therapists and clients paint their nails side by side in sessions, offers clients a unique body-based, relational practice for healing embodied trauma. In this chapter, I illustrate my experiences of engaging in art therapy manicures with clients at a rape crisis center. I name intersectionality as a contextual political framework necessary for culturally responsive practice (Crenshaw, 1989; Talwar, 2015), and explore how my own identity as a disabled, queer femme therapist shapes my use of manicures as an art therapy practice. I also discuss manicures in the context of other body adornment practices in art therapy, including wearable art, burlesque, drag performance, and tattooing, investigating how these kinds of ritualized embodiment practices can help heal somatic trauma. In discussing my incorporation of manicures into art therapy practice, I frame shared artmaking alongside participants as part of a feminist ethics of care that subverts traditional power dynamics. Further, I analyze how art therapy manicures provide a unique strategy for supporting marginalized clients dealing with issues like fatphobia, racism, social invisibility, misogyny, transmisogyny, body shame, and gender dysphoria. Finally, I discuss physical and practical considerations relevant to working with nail polish.

As I began to write about the transformative experiences of doing manicures with clients at the rape crisis center, I was keenly aware of the possibility that my scholarship could be dismissed due to deeply engrained misogyny that devalues and rejects traditionally feminine practices. Knowing that this work might be perceived as silly, irrelevant, or ineffective made me more determined to write about it. My commitment to understanding and sharing the therapeutic impact of this manicure practice stems from my persistent hope that art therapy will embrace its potential to become a more politicized profession in which accessible, anti-oppressive, culturally relevant creative practices are recognized as integral to healing.

In (often gendered) places like hair salons, nail salons, and other spaces centered around rituals of tending to the body, people may naturally and unselfconsciously share their stories. Doing manicures in therapy sessions evoked a kind of conversational self-disclosure that was also deeply meaningful. Integrating a soothing, accessible self-care ritual into the difficult emotional work of therapy created more ease and spaciousness for hard conversations. The novelty and simple pleasure of getting to do manicures made art therapy sessions seem less intimidating, more accessible, and more joyful for participants. Uplifting the practice of painting nails by inviting it into the context of therapy was a way of validating and honoring femininity itself. Deliberately shaping and polishing our nails together was an empowering experience of putting on a kind of metaphorical armor, gleaming digits of dexterous protection against the often-unkind world.

Where I come from

In this chapter I discuss identity broadly, and my own identity specifically, because I believe that practicing transparent, self-reflexive analysis around issues of identity is core to the practice of cultural humility, and issues of culture are deeply bound up in the materials we use in art therapy. I refer to the identities and stories of therapy participants, which reflect amalgamations of different people I have worked with over the years. Throughout the text, I use various terms to refer to people who occupy the traditional role of client, including *participants*, *care receivers*, and *people I work with*. My attempt to break from referring to people only as clients is part of an imperfect effort to problematize medical model labels that tend to pathologize people and reinforce hierarchical *us and them* frameworks for thinking about who needs care and who is well (Mullan, 2023).

I come to this writing as a disabled queer femme, and I understand the use of nail polish in art therapy through that embodied experience. Queer femme is an identity informed by queer theory, intersectional feminism, and individual self-definition. Although not all the people I worked with at the rape crisis center were queer or femme-identifying, here I offer the concept of femme as a subversive feminist framework, political orientation, relational practice, creative endeavor, and lens through which I understand gender and gender-based violence.

To be clear, art therapy manicures are not only for women, femmes, or people assigned female at birth. People of any gender can use manicures as a form of self-expression, and they can be an especially powerful act of identity-affirmation for some queer and trans people. Gender nonconforming or transfeminine people may be at risk of experiencing social scrutiny, judgment, discrimination, or violence for wearing nail polish. Therefore, conversations around gender, the meaning and experience of feminine expression, personal history, power, pleasure, sexuality, and personal safety are especially potent and necessary for these participants.

My lived experience of disability deeply informs my work, including the body-based practice of art therapy manicures. My relationship to the disability community and my commitment to disability justice principles, including interdependence, intersectionality, solidarity, collective liberation, and leadership of those most impacted (Sins Invalid, 2019, pp. 23–26), as well as values of self-determination, reciprocity, neurodiversity, mutual aid, and celebration of bodily deviance, have been formative for me as a practitioner. Disability justice frameworks inform how I understand my work with survivors of sexual violence because their bodies are profoundly impacted by the harm they have experienced.

My experiences as a disabled femme intersect with my identities as a White, middle-class, queer, anti-Zionist Jewish woman with advanced education degrees. I experience my own femmeness as a genderqueer identity, while simultaneously benefitting from cisgender and straight-passing privilege, and being subject to femme invisibility and femmephobia (Hoskin, 2017). Intersectionality is deeply nuanced and "not a finite goal;

it is an ever-shifting project—a theoretical framework necessary to tackle the viral nature of social oppressors" (Hoskin, 2017, p. 100). Living within systems of late-stage racial capitalism and White supremacy, my experiences of whiteness, education, and class privilege dramatically shape my access to safety, resources, and opportunities to thrive, especially in the field of art therapy, a largely White, class-privileged profession (Van Den Berg & Allen, 2022).

Femme strategies for reclaiming the body

There is no singular definition of femme. This "form of divergent femininity…strays from the monolithic and patriarchally sanctioned femininity…[and] provides critiques of normalcy and compulsory identity" (Hoskin, 2017, p. 99). Historically, the concept of femme was understood as an explicitly lesbian/dyke identity, in contrast to the more masculine butch. Viewed more expansively, femmes are self-identifying, including lesbians, feminine gay/queer men, trans and nonbinary people, drag queens, sex workers, and others with socially devalued identities or deviant bodies, including those marginalized by fatphobia, ableism, racism, transphobia, cissexism, and the gender binary. This understanding transcends definitions that rely on femme's opposition to a queer masculine counterpart. The perpetuation of a false butch/femme or masc/femme dichotomy often centers the queer masculine experience (Brushwood Rose & Camilleri, 2003). This flattened, binary understanding is steeped in a counterfeit narrative that risks replicating the heteronormative structures queerness seeks to disrupt.

Grounded in an enthusiastic celebration of femininity, femme reclaims all that has been dismissed and disparaged as feminine. This includes relational practices that embody values of nurturance, interdependence, deep listening, affirmation, connection, creativity, and valuing marginalized knowledge. Femme rejects the values of toxic masculinity, including misogyny, hyper-independence, violence, power-over dynamics, and emotional repression, instead centering the idea that "to be femme is to rely on each other" (Schwartz, n.d., pp. 2–3). The emotional foundation for art therapy manicures emerged from a feminist ethics of care rooted in "a recognition of interdependence, relationships, and responsibilities…[and] which criticizes notions of autonomy, independence, and individual rights as being too much based on a masculine view of people as separate from each other" (Morris, 2001, p. 13). The values of femme relational practice further nourished the bonds that grew from this creative practice.

Femme is intersectional. Not all femmes experience the same oppressions. Black participants like Marie live with the insidious trauma (Janani & Karmakar, 2023) of White supremacy and misogyny while also potentially experiencing privilege related to socio-economic class, ability, Christian dominance, and cisgender identity. I painted my nails with other clients who face fatphobia, transphobia, and poverty while simultaneously benefiting from privilege related to ability, language, and citizenship. As a feminist framework, femme requires a political commitment to ending multiple forms of oppression (Brushwood Rose & Camilleri, 2003; Mingus, 2011; Serano, 2013). Femmes subvert and destabilize traditional expectations around sex and gender, as our expressions of femininity are "culturally 'unauthorized'" and "do not approximate the ideal norm of what patriarchal femininity constitutes" (Hoskin, 2017, p. 100). Within femme's attempt to reclaim and venerate femininity is an acknowledgment that the oppressive social system of patriarchal femininity—including White supremacy, misogyny, fat phobia, transphobia, and ableism—has created a singular, impossible feminine ideal. The idealized feminine body is White, thin, cis, abled, straight, and compliant. Femme is both nuanced and subversive in the way it uplifts feminine expression but discards adherence to these oppressive ideals. Femme femininity is distinct in its autonomy and disregard for the male gaze, proudly claiming that "we do it for ourselves" (Serano, 2013, p. 68). These principles of femme agency and the rejection of male access to femme expression were central to my practice of art therapy manicures.

In the same way that many femmes experience their bodies falling outside of the norm, survivors of sexual violence may experience a sense of their bodies being different, other, outcast, or socially devalued. Many survivors struggle with issues related to self-esteem, body image, shame, and intimacy. Survivors who experience misogyny are targeted, harassed, tokenized, ignored, paid less, invalidated, judged, and objectified. They are socialized to do unpaid emotional labor for others, to minimize the space they take up, to apologize constantly, to question themselves, and to defer to people with more power and authority. Many of the people

I worked with at the rape crisis center regularly spent sessions processing their constant, daily experiences of navigating misogynist, ableist, fatphobic, and racist microaggressions. These chronic relational violations created immense suffering, and could emotionally trigger the unjust power dynamics they experienced with prior abusers. Oppression is a form of trauma (Janani & Karmakar, 2023), and my efforts to provide culturally responsive therapy included acknowledging and working with this reality.

People of all genders and sexual orientations experience and inflict sexual violence. The people I worked with at the rape crisis center were often abused by people close to them, including their parents, siblings, neighbors, teachers, friends, religious leaders, and sexual partners. Through acts of rape, ongoing child molestation, and other forms of sexual violence, therapy participants lost their sense of safety, self-worth, and belonging, as well as the ability to trust others and engage in intimacy. These acts of violation deeply injured survivors' relationships to their bodies. For some this resulted in coping through self-harming behaviors. The weekly manicure ritual provided a small, concrete opportunity for people to lovingly tend to and celebrate their bodies. Tending to our nails evoked a sense of control and resistance—sharpening and protecting the claws that act as tools for reclaiming previously stolen bodily autonomy.

Bodily adornment in art therapy

The practice of manicures in art therapy can be understood in relation to other body-centered art therapy practices, including tattooing, burlesque, drag, and other practices involving wearable art. Body adornment practices offer opportunities for creativity, joy, and celebration of the body and bodily autonomy. My investigation of literature related to these methods indicates that their use is underexplored in art therapy. While counseling and other adjacent fields have generated entire schools of praxis around somatic and body-based methods of healing from trauma, including Somatic Experiencing (https://traumahealing.org/), Sensorimotor Psychotherapy (https://sensorimotorpsychotherapy.org/), and Generative Somatics (https://generativesomatics.org/), art therapy has lagged behind. Artmaking is, at its core, an embodiment practice. As a field that holds much potential for creatively engaging the body, art therapy has the opportunity to make significant theoretical and practical contributions to somatic therapy.

Like the manicure practice, much of the art therapy literature on body adornment, including the disability fashion project Crip Couture (Yi, 2020) and Mz Mr's work with wearable art and burlesque (Gutierrez, 2021) is based on strong, intimate connections between participants. Crip Couture is a disability culture movement that "creates work for disabled people's pleasure: wearable art as objects made to serve as adornments, assistive aids, protections, armor, archive, and interlocutor of disability experiences" (Yi, 2020, para. 4). Mz Mr is a "designer-seamstress-choreographer-dancer-art therapist" (Gutierrez, 2021, p. 21) who brings expertise in costuming, jewelry, garment-making, and other wearable art to an art therapy practice centered around the creation and performance of burlesque. Within both Crip Couture and Mz Mr's work, the care provider or artist/art therapist works collaboratively with the care receiver to design highly customized wearable art. In these intentional, detailed collaborations, there is extensive dialogue on every aspect of the art piece being created, including considerations related to size, shape, weight, temperature, texture, color, movement, layers, and patterns, as well as emotional considerations, including relevant feelings, memories, experiences, and identities that inform the creation of the wearable art. This rigorous process of collaboration is a trust-building practice that, "considers…relational accountability as part of the aesthetic expression" (Yi, 2020, para. 6). In both of these examples, wearables become part of a larger expression of fashion that affirms the wearer, especially in relation to a marginalized aspect of their identity, such as disability, size, gender, or sexuality.

Customized wearables can also be part of drag performance. Drag, a form of creative expression that incorporates dance, singing, lip-synching, and political commentary to challenge dominant norms around gender and sexuality, has been used similarly in the context of art therapy, especially with queer people (Soubosky, 2021; Portelli, 2009). Because this work is often grounded in celebrating not just individuals but also communities, it can extend beyond the boundaries of clinical art therapy practices, where distinctions between "provider" and "receiver" may become less relevant.

Some art therapists have engaged with tattooing as a therapeutic art form, exploring how using permanent and nonpermanent imagery on the body can provide a sense of empowerment and self-identity. Engaging with clients around the meaning of their tattoos may be a strategy for understanding personal history, increasing rapport, building trust, and deepening therapeutic work (Alter-Muri, 2020; Moon, 2010). Tattoos offer a unique creative outlet for memorialization, individuation, special interests, identity exploration, and marking time. As with manicures, the choice to place imagery on the body is an act of asserting control of one's body, shaping how it is viewed and perceived by others.

Shared ritual and a feminist ethics of care

Being disabled is a socially vulnerable position, and being a disabled thera-pist is especially tricky, as therapy fields, including art therapy, are steeped in sanist values that encourage therapists to hide and deny their full identities (Roots & Roses, 2020). This denial serves the purpose of reinforcing false binaries between care providers and care receivers, positioning the former as inherently well, competent, and healed, and the latter as inherently ill, lacking, traumatized, or in need of cure (Ehlert, 2020). As a disabled ther-apist, the logic of a feminist ethics of care resonates deeply with my lived experience. Turning toward this feminist ethics is a matter of questioning "how care is understood and shaped by the social, economic, and politi-cal context: who provides the care, who is the recipient of care, and who has been historically and systemically left out?" (Talwar & Sajnani, 2022). Participating in the manicure ritual alongside the people I worked with challenged notions about who needs and who is capable of providing care.

By painting my own nails alongside participants who were painting theirs, I embraced my embodied creative expression, a vulnerable act that facilitated increased connection. My participation also served as an implicit acknowledgment of my own need for self-loving, self-care prac-tices, which both humanized me and disrupted medical model narratives that suggest care providers don't need care. In the context of my work with survivors of sexual violence, I struggled daily with secondary trauma experiences. Though I didn't explicitly disclose these experiences to par-ticipants, they witnessed me tending to my own body as a nourishing, grounding practice, one that supported our mutual co-regulation. The manicures became a deep act of therapeutic joining through care for the body and shared reverence for femme ritual.

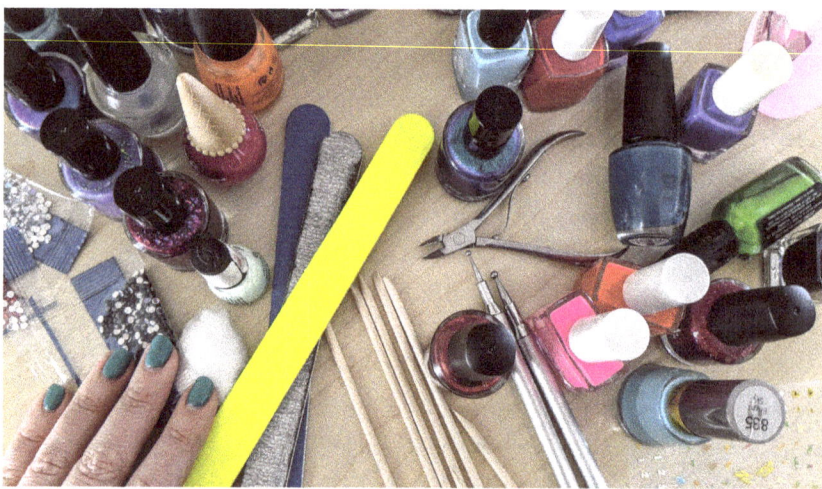

Figure 6.1 A colorful array of manicure supplies.

In its familiarity, everydayness, and shiny pop of color, nail polish became a material that helped me connect intimately with clients across markers of social difference, including race, class, sexuality, gender, size, and ability. In that small, sunny sixth-floor office, our relationships could expand beyond our therapist and client roles. We were able to be two humans keeping each other company while painting our nails. The humility, vulnerability, and authenticity that this required allowed our therapeutic work to deepen and flourish. Participants who might have been intimidated to pick up a paintbrush held the nail polish brush confidently. With tiny glass bottles in hand, conversation flowed more easily (Figure 6.1).

Material qualities and practical considerations

Nail polish is an art material that invites simple, embodied, joyful action. For many people, it recalls a childhood or adolescent act of creative self-embellishment and bodily self-expression. Some people may even recall being scrappy teenagers who used white-out or Sharpie markers to decorate their nails. Nail polish can evoke a celebratory self-aware-ness and desire to be seen in the world. It is affordable, compact to store, fun to collect, and easily found in many drug stores or grocery stores. It is commonly used by people across different racial and cultural identities, as well as across diverse socio-economic and age groups. It can offer gender-affirming self-expression for people who are typically socialized into using it, as well as for some trans, nonbinary, queer, and gender nonconforming individuals. It may be especially useful for transfeminine clients and others who experience gender dysphoria related to femininity. It can be an affirming means of self-expression for those who are subject to fatphobia, transmisogyny, and other forms of body-shaming discrimination. Nail polish is easy to use in the context of individual or group sessions, and painting nails in a group can be especially joyful.

One consideration when working with nail polish and nail polish remover is that both contain harmful chemicals and may have a toxic smell that some people are averse to, especially people with chemical sensitivities. This is an important accessibility consideration. Working outside, when possible, or working with ventilation may alleviate a negative sensory or physical experience that some participants might not tolerate. It is also possible to find less toxic nail polish brands that are made without some of the most harmful chemicals. These polishes may be preferable for some participants, in addition to having a reduced environmental impact.

We do it for ourselves

We sit side by side at the small round table in the corner, polish bottles, nail files, and cotton balls scattered in front of us. Sofia wears rings on every finger, shiny silver set with moonstone, amber, and turquoise. She pauses for several minutes after applying her final topcoat. Nails still drying, she carefully picks up a small stack of creased papers. In a steady voice, she reads me a speech she wrote for Sexual Assault Awareness Month. In her speech, which she wrote for an advocacy organization's fundraiser, she discloses her identity as an incest survivor, sharing how her brother's abuse profoundly shaped her abilities to trust other people and feel safe. When she finishes reading, she gently places her papers back on the table. One by one, she slowly rocks each hand back and forth in front of her face, softly blowing on her nails to help them dry. Sofia's long purple nails are sharpened into fierce stiletto tips. Gazing at the shiny enamel, she examines her aging hands and reflects on how powerful she felt after sharing her story.

For Sofia, this public disclosure was a way to resist the shame associated with being sexually abused and to support other survivors who wished to speak openly about their experiences. Much grief, wisdom, clarity, and emotional integration emerged for her through the many conversations we had over manicures week after week. I felt grateful that the soft, sacred space we created together could help support the birth of such a potent act of self-love and solidarity with other survivors. Through the ongoing, mundane ritual of painting our nails together, I was able to be a witness to Sofia's persistent unfolding.

As Sofia leaves the office, she asks if she can give me a copy of her speech. I am moved by her offer, and accept the gift of those victorious, crumpled papers. Clutching them, I accidentally smudge my chunky pink glitter polish. Familiar with the frequently imperfect nature of my manicures, I do my best to smooth the still-damp topcoat. The thick glitter polish takes a long time to dry, but I appreciate the way it both protects and forgives.

References

Alter-Muri, S. (2020). The body as canvas: Motivations, meanings, and therapeutic implications of tattoos. *Art Therapy, 37*(3), 139–146. https://doi.org/10.1080/07421656. 2019.1679545

Brushwood Rose, C., & Camilleri, A. (Eds.). (2003). *Brazen femme: Queering femininity.* Arsenal Pulp Press.

Crenshaw, K. (1989). Demarginalizing the intersection of race and sex: A Black feminist critique of antidiscrimination doctrine. *University of Chicago Legal Forum, 1*(8), 139–168. https://chicagounbound.uchicago.edu/uclf/vol1989/iss1/8

Ehlert, R. (2020). A little less alone: Surviving sanism in art therapy. *Art Therapy, 37*(2), 99–101. https://doi.org/10.1080/07421656.2020.1756139

Gutierrez, A. (2021). *Wearable art and the therapeutic impact of WERKING IT* [Master's thesis, School of the Art Institute of Chicago]. SAIC Thesis Repository. https:// digitalcollections.saic.edu/libraries/pdf.js/web/viewer.html?file=https%3A% 2F%2Fdigitalcollections.saic.edu%2F_flysystem%2Ffedora%2F2022–06% 2F202109_GutierrezA_MzMr_MAAT_0.pdf

Hoskin, R. A. (2017). Femme theory: Refocusing the intersectional lens. *Atlantis: Critical Studies in Gender, Culture, and Social Justice, 38*(1), 95–109. https://atlantisjournal.ca/ index.php/atlantis/article/view/4771

Janani, K. S., & Karmakar, M. (2023). Insidious trauma: A literature review. *World Journal of English Language, 13*(2), 384–392. https://doi.org/10.5430/wjel.v13n2p384

Mingus, M. (2011, August 21). Moving toward the ugly: A politic beyond desirability [Paper presentation]. Femmes of Color Symposium, Oakland, CA. https:// leavingevidence.wordpress.com/2011/08/22/moving-toward-the-ugly-a-politic- beyond-desirability/

Moon, C. H. (Ed.). (2010). *Materials & media in art therapy: Critical understandings of diverse artistic vocabularies.* Routledge.

Morris, J. (2001). Impairment and disability: Constructing an ethics of care that promotes human rights. *Hypatia, 16*(4), 1–16. https://www.jstor.org/stable/3810778

Mullan, J. (2023). *Decolonizing therapy: Oppression, historical trauma, and politicizing your practice.* W. W. Norton & Company.

O'Leary, M. E. (2017). Cripping care for individuals with psychiatric disability: Looking beyond self-determination frameworks to address treatment and recovery. *Cripping Care: Care Pedagogies and Practices, 13*(4). https://rdsjournal.org/index.php/journal/article/view/751/1838

Piepzna-Samarasinha, L. L. (2018). *Care work: Dreaming disability justice.* Arsenal Pulp Press.

Portelli, G. M. (2009). *Gender queer cabaret: How drag performance can be used as a therapeutic tool for social change* [Master's thesis, School of the Art Institute of Chicago]. https://i-share-sai.primo.exlibrisgroup.com/permalink/01CARLI_SAI/1rcln4e/alma9912819311005886

Roots & Roses (2020). Wounded healer experiences in art therapy. *Art Therapy, 37*(2), 76–82. https://doi.org/10.1080/07421656.2020.1764794

Schwartz, A. (n.d.). *Soft femme* (A. Wielenga, Illus.) [Self-published].

Serano, J. (2013). *Excluded: Making feminist and queer movements more inclusive.* Seal Press.

Sins Invalid. (2019). *Skin, tooth, and bone: The basis of movement is our people: A disability justice primer* (2nd ed.). [Self-published]. https://www.flipcause.com/secure/reward_step2/OTMxNQ==/65827; https://www.sinsinvalid.org/disability-justice-primer

Soubosky, N. (2021). *Drag as a method of expressive art therapy for LGBT+ individuals* [Master's thesis, Lesley University]. https://digitalcommons.lesley.edu/expressive_theses/519

Talwar, S. (2015). Culture, diversity, and identity: From margins to center. *Art Therapy, 32*(3), 100–103. https://doi.org/10.1080/07421656.2015.1060563

Talwar, S., & Sajnani, N. (2022). Intersectionality and the ethics of care in the creative arts therapies. *The Arts in Psychotherapy, 80*, 101944. https://doi.org/10.1016/j.aip.2022.101944

Van Den Berg, Z. D., & Allen, P. B. (2022). Specters of whiteness: Radical care for ghostly matters in art therapy. *The Arts in Psychotherapy, 80*(2). https://doi.org/10.1016/j.aip.2022.101932

Yi, C.-S. (Sandie). (2020). The crip couture manifesto. *Wordgathering: A Journal of Disability Poetry and Literature, 14*(4). https://wordgathering.com/vol14/issue4/disability-futures/yi/

7

HONORING OUR RELATIONSHIPS AND MATERIALS FROM OUR HOMELANDS

Zoë Harris (Mashpee Wampanoag), Ella Mahoney (Aquinnah Wampanoag), Michelle Napoli (Federated Indians of Graton Rancheria), Asa Peters (Mashpee Wampanoag/Narragansett), Leana Pilet (Mashpee Wampanoag), Brittney Peauwe Wunnepog Walley (Nipmuc), and Rachel Parks Winters (Cherokee Nation of Oklahoma/ᏣᏯ ᎠᏂᏴᏫᏯ)

Acknowledgments

The authors engaged in a cyclical rhythm and fluidity to represent, explore, and connect concepts in this chapter. This is an aspect of storywork, which holds our space for a multiplicity of worldviews. We are "keeping it whole" when "understanding is a layered endeavor" (Kovach, 2021, p. 24).

As context, the authors are studying and applying Indigenous methodology as a collective with Native artists to promote wellness in community. We are a Massachusetts Department of Public Health grant-supported initiative. We specifically thank Dr. Cedric Woods, Lumbee, director of the Institute for New England Native American Studies, and Jen Miller, Native Hawaiian, State Opioid Response program manager at the Bureau of Substance Addiction Services.

We center Native discourse and perspectives. We frequently include the affiliations for Native scholars as cited to contextualize and uplift the diversity of knowledge. Terms differ, change over time, and hold regard for

DOI: 10.4324/9781032720166-9

intersectionalities. We honor the ways people represent themselves, which may include terms such as Native, Indigenous, American Indian, Afro-Indigenous, Alaska Native, Native Hawaiian, First Nations, Aboriginal, Indian, etc.

Self-locating, or sharing our "self-in-relation" (Graveline, 2000, p. 361), is an ethical action that "shows respect to the ancestors and allows community to locate us through cues such as name, kinship, culture, and territory," which allows all to analyze the power dynamic present (Kovach, 2021, p. 146). To locate ourselves we represent that our stories continue living today, and that "we emerge from our ancestral interrelationships" (Kovach, 2021, p. 38), which are fundamentally with our ancestral homelands. We are an emerging collective from beyond one place. This chapter represents a polyvocality, a presentation of multiple voices and narrative forms (Sarris, 1993). Our intersectional identities and language for how to name who we are continue to be fluid as we engage in the story of our peoples beyond the interruptions and erasure from the colonial experience.

Wellness in Native communities

To locate our perspective, we discuss three constructs that formulate our cultural connectivity and revitalization as wellness and that inform our purpose and relationship with materials (Masotti et al., 2023). The three interrelated constructs are Indigenous methodology(ies), storywork, and Indigenous futurism(s). Creating, imagining, and making stories within our cultural worldviews are acts of making whole in the world (Miranda, 2013). We critically reflect on and co-construct ethics to ground our works in anti-oppressive, inclusive, and cross-cultural practices. We honor our differences as our strengths, bridging knowledge through these strengths. Like water we can flow freely, organically, and we are still powerful (Pruden, 2023). We invite multiple stories and, therefore, multiple truths, given that "we aren't always taught complete truths, because truths transform" (Yoon & Chen, 2022, p. 81).

Indigenous methodology(ies)

Indigenous methodology is built on concepts of respect and ethical relational accountability. Relational accountability is defined as "being accountable to your relations" (Wilson, 2008, p. 77). According to Kovach (2021), a Plains Cree/Saulteaux/Treaty Four member in southern Saskatchewan, Indigenous methodology is "embedded within an Indigenous paradigm and conceptual framing" (p. 31)… "to focus, make visible, and uphold Indigenous knowledge systems" (p. 43). This includes an aesthetic, ethical, and spiritual relationship between people, nature, and the cosmos (Kovach, 2021, p. 65). Indigenous methodology transforms relations and systems of power beyond what has been introduced through colonization, and centers Indigenous ways of knowing (Smith, 2012).

Indigenous methodology problematizes reductionist approaches. Uniform characterizations of Indigenous knowledge "do not work well either because the knowledge, particularly the knowledge that originates from the extraordinary, is in deep relationship to the personal and particular" (Kovach, 2021, p. 76). Within the ontology and axiology of Indigenous knowledge, there is accountability to relations "between land, sovereignty, belongingness, time and space, reality, and futurity" (Smith et al., 2019, p. xi).

Storywork

Indigenous storywork equips us to voice, listen to, and understand our stories and work collectively to become an Indigenous research community across borders (Archibald, 2008; Archibald et al., 2021). We worked diligently, slowing down our process at several points to consider and apply the seven theoretical principles of storywork, outlined by Archibald (2008), Stó:lō ̄ō/ Soowahlie First Nation, which are "respect, responsibility, reverence, reciprocity, holism, interrelatedness, and synergy" (p. xi). Eber Hampton (as cited in Archibald, 2008), Chickasaw Elder, described this iterative process as "a spiral that adds a little with each thematic repetition," where meaning is found in each turn of the spiral (p. 1). Storytelling is a culturally aligned way to create, recall, and awaken our storied memories (Archibald & Xiiem, 2018).

We show "respect through cultural protocol, appreciating the significance of and reverence for spirituality, honoring teacher and learner responsibilities, and practicing a cyclical type of reciprocity" (Archibald, 2008, p. x). We practice patience and trust to prepare for and when listening to stories (Archibald, 2008). Respecting and trusting stories involve culturally informed relationships with time and space through interrelational dimensions of storywork, "connecting on deeper levels of understanding with each other, with all living beings, with the earth and the multiverse" (Archibald et al., 2021, p. 12).

One author (E. M.) spoke to these connections:

> My Mom is the person from whom I learned how to build a relationship with a place. She looks at everything through the eyes of relationship—honoring the land and being on the land as she does her work. When her bees sting her hands (hurting from mild arthritis), she says, "They stung me there because I needed it; they sense where you need it most." Food is central too as a form of art. When I am home, I can walk down the road and pick food off the bushes as I go. Knowing what you can eat at any time feels like another way of deeply knowing a place.

Indigenous futurism(s)

Indigenous futurism(s) include "a present future beyond the imaginative and territorial bounds of colonialism" (Simpson, 2017, p. 175), with a truly emancipatory lens for what is dreamt and created (Dillon, 2012, p. 11). Indigenous artists look to "a creative space to respond to the dystopian now, grounding their survivance in contextual and relational practices" (Nixon, 2020, p. 333), engaging concepts of love and kinship as technology. Indigenous futurism includes cultural revitalization as mental health treatment, relational accountability throughout all imagining and applications, and cultural continuance with land, water, and ice-based practices from diverse Native ontologies.

Sovereignty in imagining and creating is personal and inevitably political for people navigating genocide and ongoing colonial systems. Indigenous futurism is for "everyday Indigenous peoples to restore their beings, bodies, genders, sexualities, and reproductive lives from colonial institutions… projecting decolonial love and kinship into the cosmos" (Nixon, as cited in Wikler, 2016, n.p.). *Relational-sovereign belonging* is the "honoring of self-determination while being intricately woven into relations …living in complexity, nuance, paradox, and contradiction … [and] recognizing that there is not one way of being [N]ative in the 21st century" (Tachine, 2022, p. 174).

One author (E. M.) spoke of one role model:

> My grandpa, the former medicine man of my Tribe, lost his voice box before I was born. As a quiet kid, he gave me ideas of how to communicate beyond speaking. I always draw this line back to why and when I started making art and communicating through artmaking. He taught me that there are ways to use your voice, even while silent.

Disproportionate deaths in Native communities during the COVID-19 pandemic (Center for Disease Control, 2023; Shah et al., 2020) exemplify the systemic racism Native people endure today. Given the relentless loss of our elders, youth, and the ongoing pain of Murdered, Missing Indigenous People (MMIP) (United States Department of Justice, 2021), we prioritize intersectional identity formation and cultural continuity as wellness. "Mental well-being is understood from a vantage of holism, where the individual is understood within a highly relational context, interconnected with historical and cultural contexts, and with ancestors, family, community, spirit, lands, and future generations" (O'Keefe et al., 2022, p. 12).

Relatives-materials

We purposefully engage in cultural continuity and value our cultural ways of knowing when creating. Often our creation process involves restoring honor and dignity, on our own terms, to those lost through colonial violence (Simpson, 2017). This is a profound way of healing ourselves and our communities. These values inform our aesthetic and choice of materials. Culturally connected materials are similarly bound in the complexities of relationality with the land, commerce, trade, capitalism, appropriation, and settler colonialism. Materials can serve as symbols within the story of the constructed, recognized, and imagined realms of what can be defined as art. Also true, the materials are not always what we center in our story and art.

We open an inquiry regarding the concepts of art and art materials when creating with memory and relationships to our homelands.

We also construct a culturally informed space for relationship building. Culturally informed materials in our creations embody the memory of generations of conversations with our ancestors, among other invaluable, sacred aspects. When the plants, rocks, water, and shells are part of our creations, we are creating out of love for these relatives and knowledge keepers. Basket weaver Julia Parker, Coast Miwok, and Kashaya Pomo shared,

> My elders taught me that we have to be kind to the plants. The plants were here way before we were. So, we have to learn to listen to them and we have to learn to watch them. By watching them and being respectful to them we will get good baskets.
>
> (Valoma, 2013, p. 157)

To work with our relatives in creating baskets, carvings, and paintings is to be in dialogue with generations of collective knowledge and enacting a continuous relationship between a people and place. These materials, our relatives, are our teachers, therapists, and healers. These relatives hold imprints and spirits from specific spaces and places. They hold memory and inform understanding for next steps and decision-making. While spirituality is not only an Indigenous experience, we have noted how frequently Indigenous spiritual healing practices have been appropriated via colonial frameworks. We recommend practices that engage in relational accountability are derived from one's ethical positionality and abstain from cultural appropriation (Wilson, 2008).

Adaptation is traditional: it is how Native people have survived. Access to our traditional homeland(s) and cultural practices is not always possible. Therefore, we innovate using myriad strategies and materials informed by our contemporary life. To quote singer Gregg Deal, Pyramid Lake Paiute Tribe, "While Indian, I'm also having an American experience too" (Dead Pioneers, 2023). Each Native community, and person, has a history marked with layers of colonial impact. Any relationship with our traditions continues amid these complex layers of history with our homelands.

For example, when considering place-based practices and urbanization, one author (Z. H.) shared:

> When home I can collect plants and make dye. When back in the city, I do not have access to collect those plants. Also, when in my apartment in the city, I use my kitchen sink or bathtub to soak corn husks—but then I cannot shower or do dishes—so there are trade-offs.

She (Z. H.) shared another example with the plant, staghorn sumac, which has vitamin C:

> When it is growing on the side of the road, I would only use it for dyes, and when I collect it from Nana's neighborhood, I know the plant is healthy, and so I can make tea.

Storywork with relatives-materials

For our wellness, we explore ways to sustain a community of care that centers our cultural identity formation process. As Native artists from different intersections of Tribal and Indigenous relationships, we create community where we can think and live inside the multiplicity of our cultures and forms of intelligence (Simpson, 2017). The authenticity and emotional vulnerability we bring to our group informs our path to wellness and is a form of power. We explore ways to continue our relationships with our homelands, even when we no longer have free or legal access. We hold our emerging truths as our storywork, a form of reciprocal honoring (Simpson, 2017), as we are entwined in the politics of identity and recognition.

Storytelling is a way we bind together our materials. Culturally informed materials are part of place-based practices of spiritual reconnection, honoring our collective spirit, and protecting the sacred. To know that we still belong in relationship with our homelands is a way of knowing who we are.

As a collective reflecting on the flow of one person's story to the next, we recognized the way each story connects to create a full circle (while each story is also its own full circle). Relatives-materials help facilitate these

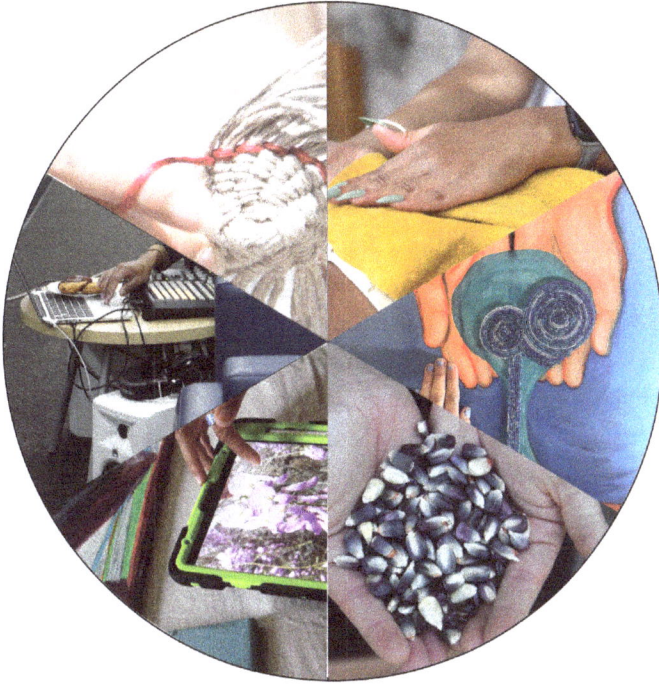

Figure 7.1 Story circle. Image designed by Zoë Harris. Photo credit: ©Dawn Colquitt-Anderson, 2022. ©Ella Mahoney, 2023. ©Tommy Lam, 2023.

circular and reciprocal relationships. Our stories are a circle of relationality: land-to-deer-to-water-to-seeds-to-plants-to-weaving-in-the-digital/ethereal-world-to-land.

Land to deer (Z.H.)

When I first moved to Chicago, I walked in the mornings at the local nature reserves, early enough so that I would get to see ahtuqak. It was always nice to see relatives because then I knew nobody in the Chicagoland area except for ahtuqak. As an urban space, Chicago is multi-Tribal. This area combines those whose ancestors originally stewarded this land and those most impacted by dislocation—but there are few Eastern Woodland people represented. Because of that, whenever I can, I wear my skins to show people where I come from. At the first pow-wow I attended in Chicago, someone came up to me and knew everything—from where I was from to who did the paintings—just by looking at my skins. Any time I wear my skins, everyone from youth to elders ask me about it. I find that colonization has done exactly what it has intended to do, since people forget that before jingle and cloth dresses, there were skins. Our Tribe has been disconnected from so much since the initial colonizers came with warfare, disease, displacement, and lateral oppression. But ahtuqak is not lost. Ahtuq is a material that transcends generations. The reason I use ahtuq is because we pass it down through our stories. I cannot use the skins without understanding how to honor the sacrifice of ahtuq. I cannot honor the sacrifice of ahtuq without understanding their own relationship with the land and water. I cannot understand the relationship ahtuq has with the earth without having *my own love for the earth. Ahtuq is not just a material; ahtuq is a story.*

Water (E.M.)

For me, water is a source of grounding. I go to the ocean when I need to clear my mind and body. As a visual storyteller, I recognize that the stories we tell about the relationships we have with the earth affect how we interact with it. I often ask myself and others, "What is your story with water?" My art and relationship with the water has become a rediscovery of myself in a place that holds so much of my and my ancestors' history.

One subject that shows up often in my work is Moshup. According to legend, Moshup was a giant who was the protector and provider of the Wampanoag people. He was so big that he would pick up whales to feed the people and kill them by slamming them against the cliffs. They say that is how the cliffs got their colors. When colonists came to the island, Moshup gave the tribe a choice to become whales or remain human and fend for themselves. In Aquinnah, we say when the fog rolls over, that's Moshup smoking his pipe. According to legend, someday he will return.

In the past few years, I have begun creating large-scale silk paintings that can move with me. This allows me to explore my relationships with stories and lets me interact more directly with legends from my ancestors. Working with Mar Parrilla, the artistic director of Danza Organica, I have learned to recognize the ways that the body speaks subconsciously through dance work. She centers the relationship with the art and what wants to come forward before giving anyone deadlines

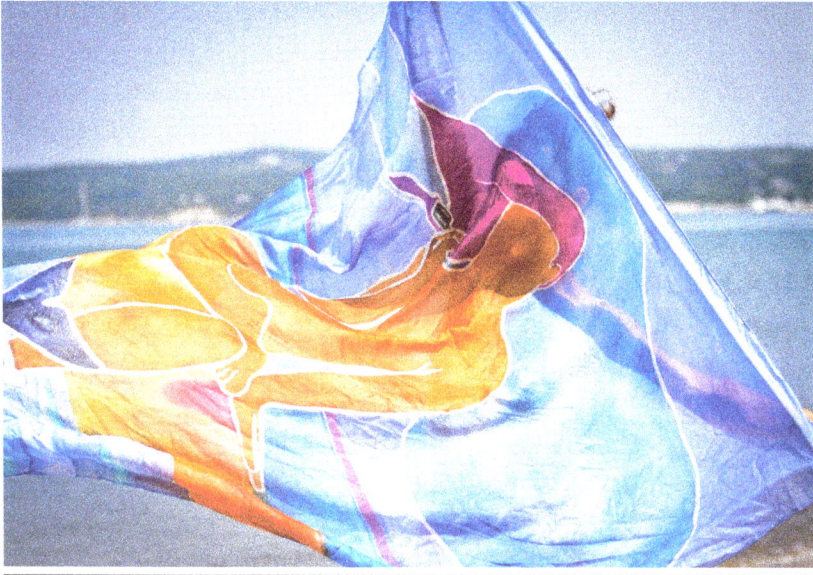

Figure 7.2 Wind, Water, Waves. Photo credit: ©Dawn Colquitt-Anderson, 2022.

or definitions. In dancing a story, we work with process to see what it will be before deciding what it will be. Working with water, the body, movement, and memory has become a process of reclamation… all that helps combat the myth that we don't exist.

Seeds (R.W.)

Ꮜ ᎢᎿᏢ ᎤᎬᏛ ᎤᏞᎥᎯᏓᎬ ᏓᏣᏫᏴ ᎢᏕᎯᏓᎬ 4M ꮔᎾᎡᎾ ᏍᏍᏯ

I can't remember a time when we didn't have a garden. My mother had us outdoors learning from plants and tending the land from what seems like birth. When we drove down the road, she would quiz my sister and me. "What tree is that? And that bush? And those flowers?" Every place I have lived I find connection to my home and family through cultivating a garden. The beauty of the plants and the food cooked from them makes me feel whole. I get a deep sense of wellness and healing when I'm outdoors walking in nature or tending to my garden.

After moving far from Oklahoma, I dreamed of having enough space to grow the three sisters: 4M (corn), Ꮝꮼ (beans), and Ꮝᏹh (squash). When the seeds arrived directly from the heritage seed bank of the Cherokee Nation, I couldn't wait to get my hands in the dirt and prepare a place for them. As I planted the seeds, I thought about the journeys they've made to get to this moment and all the caretakers ensuring the relationship with our people continues. These traditional foods are tied to Cherokee identity, and growing them is a way of continuing Cherokee history, culture, and food sovereignty no matter where we are. Watching these plants thrive in their new home and feed another generation provides me with a source of comfort and inspiration. Maybe my family and I can thrive in our new home too.

Plants (L.P.)

Sometimes I am drawn to things, and whether or not in the moment I know why it is significant, I just try to listen, be present, and notice. Sometimes, over time, I understand exactly what the significance was.

A cousin of mine reached out to me wanting to go on a hike, the first time in a while. On the hike we kept seeing this one type of plant, repeatedly. Something about this plant seemed so familiar to us; however, we did not know why. We did not know the name of the plant, nor the type, but spoke about how familiar it was. I knew this was the first time I had seen this plant in person, and I knew it was important. I observed it and took a picture.

A week later I went to tribal grounds to hold an art engagement group with some of the teachers that work for the tribe; I was beyond nervous. As soon as I got to my location, I saw a relative of mine, and felt a sense of calm seeing a familiar face. As she came over, she was speaking about how she just got done going on a walk and saw a Lady Slipper. It was in that moment I knew exactly what that plant was, when I was on the walk with my cousin. It was a Lady Slipper, the name of my grandmother, and the image I have seen for many years on her tombstone when I have visited her.

Weaving in the digital/ethereal world (A. P.)

I think of material as the creative threads of influences and musical ancestors that inspire us and give context to a new musical idea. As a saxophone player, I listen to, study, and try to embody the feel and language of jazz while also developing my own creative sensibility while playing. As a Hip-Hop producer, I eagerly stay tuned in to how the music evolves in different regions while also educating myself on Hip-Hop innovations from before my time. The musical lineage and contemporary cultural context are what make my new ideas feel relevant and potentially meaningful to listeners. Sampling in Hip-Hop is a helpful example. When I sample a recording, I am honoring and highlighting it and my relationship to it. At the same time, I'm creating something new to speak back to the recording's ideas and impact.

I am also a dedicated learner of Algonquin and Haudenosaunee social songs and dances. People in my community sing these songs in gatherings, performances, and public education spaces. I'm grateful to have heard these songs since childhood. These songs are carried and practiced by collectives much more specific and intimate than jazz and Hip-Hop. Because of that, I feel a greater weight of responsibility with the social songs and what I do with the gift of knowing them. I don't feel so inclined to remix, recontextualize, or make contributions to these social songs like I do more freely in jazz and Hip-Hop. I mostly aim to carry them as received.

The land (B.W.)

Weaving enables me to honor my ancestors while uplifting present and future generations. I have had many weaving teachers, including Nipmuc baskets themselves. There is Nipmuc knowledge about baskets, and there is Nipmuc knowledge that is baskets, and sometimes you learn about baskets from a basket!

I try to balance traditional and contemporary visuals in my work. This is true of my special effects series which includes a functional QR code basket (Walley, 2022). I had an opportunity to share my artwork in Boston, MA. Discussions with my co-curators addressed multimedia. I thought of weaving a basket with a QR code pattern that links to the video, "Ecologies of Acknowledgment" (Kanouse, 2019), which "urges its audience to go beyond merely acknowledging and instead accept the relationships and responsibilities that come with living on occupied land" (Shimshak, 2020). Certainly, a Nipmuc basket would engage in such discussions.

This basket acts like a portal via technological special effects. When aligning technology with this basket, one is transported to a digital space.

Figure 7.3 QR Code Basket in Progress. Photo credit: ©Brittney Walley, 2023.

Coded alignment revealing messages is an enduring Indigenous practice, as evidenced in patterns of celestial bodies and co-ordinated positioning of stones. Sometimes portals decay and no longer work. Misalignment occurs, technologies are lost, and encoded messages become alienated. The same could one day be true of this basket. Forgetting about QR codes may cause decontextualization of the pattern and its reinterpretation as simple geometrics. Disrupted and broken communication is represented on the reverse side of this basket through a static noise pattern.

I hope that interdimensional travelers of digital and physical landscapes return to their bodies with a deeper appreciation for their place in space and time and, of course, the land.

Conclusion

As a Native community of care, we ask that people locate *materials* in a larger context of relational accountability and respect for cultural continuity.

References

Archibald, J. [Q'um Q'um Ziiem]. (2008). *Indigenous storywork: Educating the heart, mind, body, and spirit.* UBC Press.

Archibald, J. [Q'um Q'um Ziiem], Lee-Morgan, J. B. J., & De Santolo, J. (2021). *Decolonizing research: Indigenous storywork as methodology.* Zed Books.

Archibald, J., & Xiiem, Q. Q. (2018). Indigenous storytelling. In P. Tortell, M. Turin, & M. Young (Eds.), *Memory* (pp. 233–242). UBC Press. https://www.jstor.org/stable/j.ctvbtzpfm.30

Center for Disease Control. (2023, May 25). *Risk for COVID-19 Infection, hospitalization, and death by race/ethnicity.* https://archive.cdc.gov//details?url=https://www.cdc.gov/coronavirus/2019-ncov/covid-data/investigationsdiscovery/ hospitalization-death-by-race-ethnicity.html

Dead Pioneers. (2023). Bad Indian [Song]. On *Dead Pioneers*. Hassle Records.

Dillon, G. L. (2012). *Walking the clouds: An anthology of Indigenous science fiction.* The University of Arizona Press.

Graveline, F. J. (2000). Circle as methodology: Enacting an Aboriginal paradigm. *International Journal of Qualitative Studies in Education, 13*(4), 361–370. https://doi.org/10.1080/095183900413304

Kanouse, S. (2019, August 19). *Ecologies of acknowledgment* [Video]. Vimeo. https://vimeo.com/354699007

Kovach, M. (2021). *Indigenous methodologies: Characteristics, conversations, and contexts* (2nd ed.). University of Toronto Press.

Masotti, P., Dennem, J., Bañuelos, K., Seneca, C., Valerio-Leonce, G., Inong, C. T., & King, J. (2023). The culture is prevention project: Measuring cultural connectedness and providing evidence that culture is a social determinant of health for Native Americans. *BMC Public Health, 23*(1), 741. https://doi.org/10.1186/s12889-023-15587-x

Miranda, D.A. (2013). *Bad Indians: A Tribal memoir.* Heyday.

Nixon, L. (2020). Visual cultures of Indigenous futurism. In T. Lethabo King, J. Navarro, & A. Smith (Eds.), *Otherwise worlds: Against settler colonialism and anti-blackness* (pp. 332–342). Duke University Press.

O'Keefe, V. M., Fish, J., Maudrie, T. L., Hunter, A. M., Tai Rakena, H. G., Ullrich, J. S., Clifford, C., Crawford, A., Brockie, T., Walls, M., Haroz, E. E., Cwik, M., Whitesell, N. R., & Barlow, A. (2022). Centering Indigenous knowledges and worldviews: Applying the Indigenist ecological systems model to youth mental health and wellness research and programs. *International Journal of Environmental Research and Public Health, 19*(10), 1–15. https://doi.org/10.3390/ijerph19106271

Pruden, H. (2023, April 23). *ChatReconciliACTION: Water teachings methodological reflections* [Webinar]. Kāshā. https://www.youtube.com/watch?v=sI1ohmEwRAQ

Sarris, G. (1993). *Keeping Slug Woman alive: A holistic approach to American Indian texts.* University of California Press.

Shah, A., Seervai, S., Paxton, I., Barlow, A., & Shah, T. (2020, August 12). The challenge of COVID-19 and American Indian health. *Commonwealth Fund.* https://doi.org/10.26099/m5ww-xa13

Shimshak, C. (2020, October 26). 'Ecologies of acknowledgement' calls for recognition of occupied land. *The Tufts Daily.* https://www.tuftsdaily.com/article/2020/10/ecologies-of-acknowledgement-calls-for-recognition-of-occupied-land

Simpson, L. B. (2017). As we have always done: Indigenous freedom through radical resistance. University of Minnesota Press. https://doi.org/10.5749/j.ctt1pwt77c

Smith, L. T. (2012). *Decolonizing methodologies: Research and Indigenous peoples* (2nd ed.). Zed Books.

Smith, L. T., Tuck, E., & Yang, K. W. (2019). *Indigenous and decolonizing studies in education: Mapping the long view.* Routledge.

Tachine, A. R. (2022). *Native presence and sovereignty in college: Sustaining Indigenous weapons to defeat systemic monsters.* Teachers College Press.

United States Department of Justice. (2021). Missing or murdered Indigenous persons: Legal, prosecution, advocacy, and healthcare. *The Department of Justice Journal of Federal Law and Practice, 69*(2). https://www.justice.gov/usao/page/file/1383296/dl

Valoma, D. (2013). *Scrape the willow until it sings: The words and work of basket maker Julia Parker*. Heyday.

Walley, B. [@B7.Nipmuc.Artisan]. (2022, October 28). *Special FX: Functional QR Code (Ecologies of Acknowledgement Video)*. [photo and text]. Instagram. https://www.instagram.com/p/CkRs_JnL4vf/?img_index=1

Wikler, A. (2016, November 28). Indigenous futurism: Reimagining "reality" to inspire an Indigenous future. *Exploring Indigenous Knowledge Systems.* https://blogs.ubc.ca/fnis401fwikler/2016/11/28/indigenous-futurism-reimagining-reality-to-inspire-an-indigenous-future/

Wilson, S. (2008). *Research is ceremony: Indigenous research methods*. Fernwood Publishing.

Yoon, I. H., & Chen, G. A. (2022). Heeding hauntings in research for mattering. In A. R. Tachine & Z. Nicolazzo (Eds.), *Weaving an otherwise: In-relations methodological practice* (pp. 76–91). Routledge.

8

ART FROM INSIDE

PEER ART THERAPISTS REFLECTIONS ON MATERIALS AND MEDIA IN EXPLORING COMPLEX IDENTITY SYSTEMS

Mahlie Jewell and Catherine Camden–Pratt

Acknowledgment of Country

This work was written across many Countries and has been witnessed by the ancestral place *Warrane* and the surrounding Lands of the Wangal People (Mahlie's current residence), the Lands of the Gumbaynggirr People (the place where Mahlie retreats to find peace and connection), Gundungurra Lands (Catherine's chosen home), and carrying the memory of the Lands of the Darug People on which we first met. Working, learning, yarning, and listening with each other and the Land is a privilege and an honor. The Lands on which we meet to deeply listen are as important as each of us. These Lands, rivers, oceans, mountains, trees, and all those they home and protect walk with us purposefully and have facilitated much understanding, clarity, growth, and healing. Alongside Mahlie as she moves across these Lands are her guiding ancestors from the Wiradjuri Nation, her Pop's People. They bring thousands of years of knowing and being with these Lands, and the fire and passion for change. Catherine lives with deep appreciation for and gratitude to Gundungurra Country in Darug Nation that holds her today, and Kuring-Gai Country that loved her from early childhood as she sought refuge on their earth, under their skies, with sunlight soaking her skin, moonlight holding her in the darkness, and trees welcoming her in friendship. It is part of her fabric.

DOI: 10.4324/9781032720166-10

Starting place: learning together

Catherine: A lot's happened since our early 2023 on-the-page critical conversations about peer art therapy (PATh) and art therapist Lived Experience (LE), with many changes in aspects of our respective subjectivities.

Mahlie: Understanding my/ourselves now as autistic with combination of ADHD removed many incorrect psychiatric labels, specifying complex trauma and dissociative identity disorder. More importantly we learned to crochet. We're obsessed with how it fires up the creative mind and shuts down the anxious mind simultaneously. It is magic, especially for one part/person within us who is a freeform crochet witch.

Catherine: So big, Mahls. And you live this with grace and generosity. Curiously, you came closer to us via the old DSM and my/our dissociative identity disorder—not that we both needed that to know! Love that you've discovered crocheting! Our changes? In May 2023, the day I completed ten years of work as an art therapist with people living with cancer, I was diagnosed with breast cancer. Got to love black humor—and phew for the richness of all we'd learned. I entered the medical woods with the soul-muscles and tools gained in many years of personal and professional learnings. For us, it's our multiplicity that allows us to thrive, to be here with you, with us in this chapter.

Mahlie: We understand black humor and collective internal support as survival. Voicing our experiences creates connection and representation. Important for working alongside my participants—autistic, queer, gender-diverse, disabled, non-white, chronically ill, anti-therapy, anti-colony, anti-racist, politically active humans living across spectrums of all kinds—who often require me to disclose my identities, political locations, and worldviews for them to feel safe, understood, and connected.

Catherine: We're with you! Our shared commitment to the politics of including therapist LE voices is fundamental, especially when we work like this and open ourselves to the stigmas of our profession. "Be the change we want to see" rings as true to me now as it always has. How else can therapists with LE see themselves agentically in the story unless they can see others like them? Politics is about voice and representation, and art therapy is inherently political.

We write from explicit LE, from inside, and signal our intersecting locations as art psychotherapists, peer workers, art therapy participants, and people living and working with experiences described as autistic, neurodivergent, queer, chronically ill, and complex trauma. Mahlie is a First Nations person in a continuously colonized society and accesses government medical, housing, and disability services. We are challenged by both commonly accepted language that pathologizes ways of being and own our seeming complicity with its use (Eastwood, 2020, 2021, 2022; Mullan, 2023). Where possible, we choose other words and ways of naming experiences.

This chapter explores mutuality, safety, informed consent, and therapists celebrating diverse communication through materials and media. Through the lens of our respective LE, we focus on those living in complex identity systems. These systems are creative, intelligent, skillful responses to complex trauma, and are commonly pathologized under dissociative disorders categories (American Psychiatric Association, 2013; World Health Organization, 2022). Our ongoing critical conversations and chapter focus are political, challenging the stigmatization that has led to a dearth of autonomous, critical art therapist LE voices (Huet & Holttum, 2016; Roots & Roses, 2020; Woods & Springham, 2011).

Art therapists have researched and written extensively about trauma-related dissociation (e.g., Drass, 2012; Lev-Wiesel, 2005; Sagan, 2019; Thayer-Cox & Cohen, 2005) with examples from participant narratives to explicate their ideas, void of LE co-authorship. Ford et al. (2021) was co-produced with LE co-authors centered. While not about complex trauma, Roots and Roses (2020) wrote anonymously about their LE, with Woods and Springham (2011) co-producing an article informed by Woods's LE. The limited LE voices in academic literature not mediated by a therapist's voice may signpost the implicit clinician/participant power imbalance.

Acknowledging the well-documented exploration of media and materials in art therapy across various approaches (e.g., Malchiodi & Perry, 2014; Moon, 2010; Rubin, 2016), we briefly discuss harm where participants are not active and supported in making their own choices. We also consider the ways in which relationship, connection, worldview, and co-learning in PATh can expand the participant/therapist alliance and lead to deep and meaningful work.

Through our artwork, we signal how specific materials, colors, and media reveal diverse languages and can expertly communicate complex identity systems.

Peer Art Therapy

The PATh framework integrates professional training in peer support with clinical training in art psychotherapy. It actively values and draws on therapists openly disclosing mentalized LE while working alongside participants. PATh creates strong, mutual, therapeutic alliances and creates connection and community between participants and art therapists through Intentional Peer Support's four core tasks: connection, worldview, mutuality, and working toward (Intentional Peer Support, 2019; Jewell & Camden-Pratt, 2021; Mead & MacNeil, 2006). In making art-alongside participants, having mentalized their LE through exploration of media and materials, peer art therapists (PAThR) disrupt the dominating therapist/participant hierarchy and embody these core tasks (Jewell & Camden-Pratt, 2023).

The PATh framework locates behaviors and processes as intelligent responses and seeks to understand their meanings. The relationship is mutual and consensual; both PAThR and participant articulate their LE. For many people living *complex identity systems*, open disclosure and self-identification within the therapy space can be unsafe (e.g., Jacobson et al., 2015) due to high levels of discrimination and stigma. PATh can provide people with safer spaces to explore and understand themselves, and with experiences of connection, being believed, and encountering people as skilled professionals living complex identity systems.

Mentalizing LE, media, and materials

Within complex identity systems, parts/people hold and have access to specific experiences and understandings, and their expression. There are complex internal politics and at times multiple ideologies, wants, needs, and convictions. This can be simultaneously tumultuous, resourceful, and supportive. It is unhelpful to assume that all parts/people within a system have the capacity and ability to understand the needs of others in the system and to respond effectively, as assumed by Thayer-Cox and Cohen (2005). Arriving at the place where it is possible to hold inner common goals and/or respect the autonomy of particular parts/people in specific contexts, is exhausting. Co-consciousness (Fisher, 2017; West, 1997) requires becoming conscious of parts/people existing, then connecting with who they each are, the experiences they hold, and their roles in the system/s.

This lived complexity is intensified by stigmatized narratives that disrespect, misrepresent, and minimize. Who and how parts/people can be present in the therapy needs to be held respectfully by the therapist; not all parts choose to actively participate. Pathologizing ideas about *switching* and *fronting* minimizes and disrespects the intelligence of complex identity system. Therapist terms like *progress*, *healing/recovery*, and *reaching therapy goals* can be triggering for people with complex trauma due to their experiences of medical colonization and medical standards for symptom remission, often including the treatment goal *integration of parts* (Balsara et al., 2024). Depending on how integration is conceptualized (Fisher, 2017; Steele et al., 2016) and whether it is based on the participant's or therapist's agenda, integration might not be the participant's goal for therapy.

Herstorical they-stories with materials

Catherine: While a student in art therapy training in 2009, teachers told our class that finger-painting was best not used with adults unless the intention was regression. Clay was a no-no for survivors of sexual assault and those with "severe mental disturbance" (Sherwood, 2004, p. 12). Well, that shut us down. We live/d with a so-called dissociative identity disorder, we were a survivor of familial and nonfamilial sexual assault (we didn't know a time with bodily integrity), and an artist using clay and finger-painting. These views, expressed by teachers and with backing in the literature, othered our experiences and silenced our voices. Fortunately, I later discovered counterpoint views in the literature. Using our fingers to paint was not and is not regression; it enables us to express knowledges held within our system. Yes, always from within our Littlies Team and younger parts. This is a way they communicate and isn't to be pathologed. How else can a little one speak? Especially those who have no verbal language? It's crucial art therapists examine judgmental language used to conceptualize the content a multiple/plural/person with a complex identity system explores in therapy. The term regression invites misunderstanding of the part/person in a multiple system and their neurodevelopmental stage. Peer art therapists are invited to deeply examine and unpack their worldviews, judgments, and internalized stigma. I remember your experiences with clay, Mahlie. There is no one-size-fits-all approach to media and materials.

Mahlie: At university, I understood my challenges associated with claywork and messy artmaking to be a result of my trauma. Now, with my autistic neurotype identified, I understand them as sensory processing challenges. Although they are difficult to pull apart (like you, I have no memory of a trauma-less existence), I know that our younger parts/people all dislike skin-contact with particular sensory profiles (slimy, wet, sticky) but actively seek other sensory encounters (fluffy, rough, sparkly) for stimming. Like you, our Littles are way more tactilely oriented artists because of their neurodevelopmental stages. They are not regressing; they are appropriately responding as themselves. It is vital that they be encouraged to choose the materials that work for them at their neurodevelopmental level.

Catherine: The Littles Team says goodbye

In PATh, mentalization (the process of perceiving and interpreting our own and others' mental states) is fundamental. Without it, the PAThR risks processing their own psychological/emotional material with therapy participants (Intentional Peer Support, 2019; Jewell & Camden-Pratt, 2021, 2023; Mead & MacNeil, 2006). The PAThR, in modeling mentalization, demonstrates the possibility of moving toward connection with and across complex systems.

When I was diagnosed with breast cancer in May 2023, I had worked with many people living with cancer and read extensively (e.g., Fenner et al., 2024; Waller & Sibbet, 2005; Winlaw, 2023). Our discussion here is from a LE co-conscious voice, and as mixed-media artists. Being multiple, we had various responses across our system from initial discovery of the lump through diagnosis, surgery, radiotherapy, and ongoing treatment. We processed these experiences using reflective writing, 5Rhythms dance (Roth, 1999), and artmaking, as well as in talking psychotherapy. With inner permission, we share our artmaking and mentalization from a team within our system. Media and materials supported this sense-making and our moving toward connection with, and understanding of, my and our lived experience of cancer.

Our system is rich and diverse in age, gender, and preferred ways of communicating (including muteness), with alliances/teams often not mutually supportive or in immediate agreement. We refer to ourselves as Catherine & Co—like a dance company, not a corporation. The Littlies Team (TLT) members, ranging in age from babyhood through ten years, each hold separate lived experiences, their own names, and specific functions within our system. The moment I/Catherine sensed and then felt the lump, TLT sprang into action, welcoming the lump and tending it, loving it. After all, they decided, there's no need to be mean to something that grows in the body.

I jump forward over many experiences prior to and during treatment, and much inner communication with and across my system, including with TLT and all our other parts/people, to Figure 8.1.

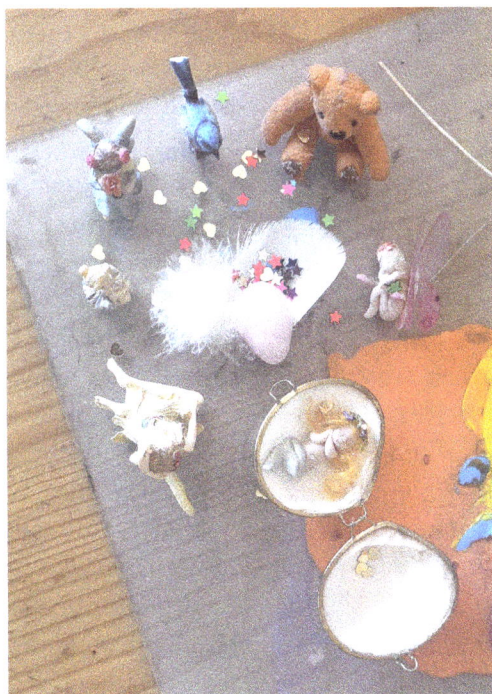

Figure 8.1 Camden-Pratt/The Littlies Team (2023). Goodbye. Figurines, mixed-media.

Six weeks after surgery to remove the tumor, a friend asked me, "Do you feel like it's gone?" I was surprised I couldn't answer immediately. After a few moments I said, "Truth is, I'm not sure." I *should* have felt tumor-free. Cognitively, I knew it had been removed and could see my physical improvement daily, felt pleased at the outcome. Yet I hadn't answered *yes*. Sharing this with another friend, she asked me, "How does your breast feel now?" And I cried. Each of TLT tumbled out, seen then quickly gone, not the time and place. On and off, I had been experiencing an undertow. I recognized this at-odds-with-the-surface, viscous and opaque, visceral dragging beneath my daily tasks, an unseen gathering current, the increasing build-up of internal pressure. It wasn't an emotion—that would have been too easy to identify. It was the body's materiality. The day after this new question, the undertow pushed through, gained my attention. I have long learned to notice this communication, to stop, to pay attention, allow this felt sense to come forward, and then gently ask, "Who's here?" if I don't immediately know. Then wait, listen, engage, and communicate with the part/person/s who emerge. I learned how to do this many years ago with my psychotherapist and am also informed by my training in somatic psychotherapy, my doctoral somatic research (Camden-Pratt, 2003, 2007), and co-parenting my own children. Becoming co-conscious is painstakingly hard work, built over time. While there are useful strategies for engaging verbally with parts (Fisher, 2017), what is most effective for me and for us is using art and mixed-media to communicate between ourselves.

I sat quietly, listening, waiting, open to hearing, to knowing. The body as material. Parts come forward—LC, TPPG, B, TSO, TB, TF, TGITC (initials respect their privacy). Each is bereft. They didn't want the lump to go, didn't understand why the lump had to go. They had surrounded the lump with love and warmth, cradling them. And they weren't at all ready for the lump to no longer be there under their care. Where had their new friend gone?

Prior to surgery, I communicated across my system about aspects of the treatment I knew would be harder for some. I hadn't anticipated that TLT would miss and grieve the tumor. To them, it wasn't an *it* or *a tumor*; it was a living, breathing, growing part of us. I apologized, listened to each of their sadnesses. I talked with each of them, age appropriately, about the tumor and asked them what they needed.

Figure 1 is their response. Using figurines, we worked quickly, eagerly. They knew what they needed: to say goodbye, to come together to fare-well the lump. There was no disagreement about creating the ritual circle. (TPPG had read about this in a book they love and suggested it.) The lump is lovingly represented with a pink crystal and its movement from presence to absence by the feather, signaling its flight into freedom (suggested by TF and B who know about nature's capacity to heal). Glittery hearts and stars hold this transformation. Each part of TLT is represented, those who speak and those who choose not to, and an older part/person TGITC who wanted to join them. No tumor to be rid of, instead a new friend to be farewelled.

Figurines allowed easy communication of feeling states and their res-olution and facilitated in-team co-operation. It was essential everyone in TLT have their say and none to be silenced by divergent neurodevelop-mental skills.

Through making the installation we experienced collective physical, emotional, and psychological relief. Mentalizing this collective process across my system enables me to work with participants who also live complex identity systems. Embodied knowledge of the importance of cross-system/co-conscious communication is not an academic under-standing or approach to working with people with dissociation and trauma; it is an inside-out knowing that can only be lived and brings congruence to my working with these kinds of identities. Our experien-tial grasp of the materiality of the body across complex identity systems is fundamental to how I work with participants.

Mahlie: the protection of E

Our system is referred to as *The Sharehouse* and parts/people are referred to as *Housemates*—a more descriptive insight into our specific lived expe-rience. E is a young part/person who holds severe, prolonged trauma that activated our body in distressing ways at the time of artmaking. E presents a different set of needs than others in our Sharehouse. She is hyperaware of our body, has extreme sensory challenges connected to autism/ADHD and co-occurring tic disorder. She is hyperlexic but often nonspeaking and nonengaging internally or externally—which does not mean noncommunicative, nonunderstanding, nonobservant, nonempa-thetic or nonintelligent (Kedar, 2012)—as she experiences all humans as unsafe. Not all Littles have the same attachment styles.

Understanding E's specific neurodevelopmental and trauma experiences is crucial to working alongside her. She requires our art psychotherapist to be patient and work in nontraditional ways to ensure safety and engagement when therapy with E stalls and is challenging. Our art psychotherapist is a cisgender woman and a *Mother*, a significant activation for us. This needs to be responded to actively and our psychotherapist works collaboratively with the part/person who cares for E within our Sharehouse. Therapy spaces with E require considerable structure, routines, rules, and use of clearly articulated prompts to aid her in understanding, remaining engaged, and avoiding distress. Side-by-side artmaking with our art psychotherapist supports E's understanding and connection, as does describing experiences and feelings using emotion cards, popular media, and the natural world.

The protection of E (Figure 8.2) is a system map that—through color, line, and shape—allows Housemate responses to be mentalized. This aids in our understanding of system roles and resources. Each color in the artwork is representative of a Housemate within the Sharehouse, depicting relationships that are fluid and specific to the situation being explored.

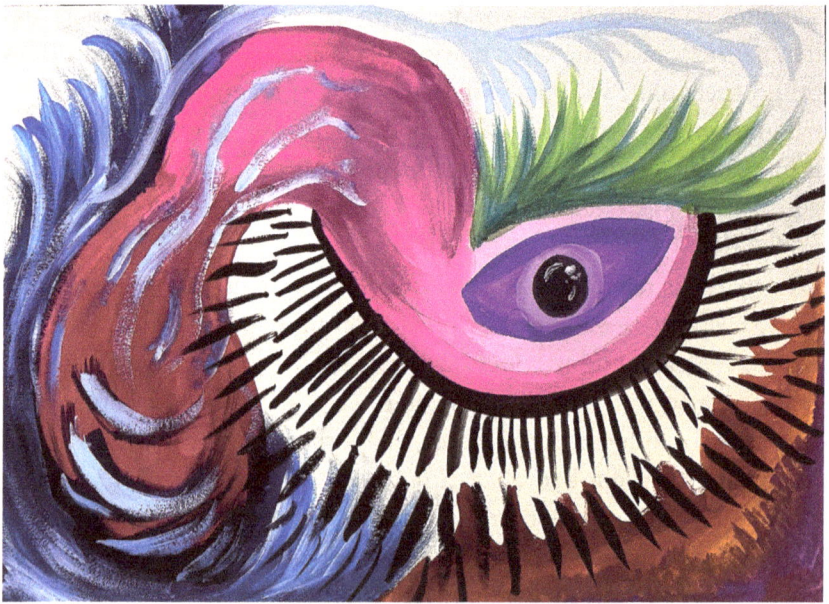

Figure 8.2 Jewell (2024). The protection of E. Gouache on heavy card.

Through them, we see the relational lines of E's experiencing of her memories and how each Housemate is responding, or not responding, to her increased needs and distress. For us, it is incorrect to assume that our system is always functional, helpful, kind, and supportive. Reaching internal common goals is often the subject of therapy sessions. Our art psychotherapist has developed a strong knowledge of our color language. At the time of artmaking, the common goal was to hold and protect E's rights to be silent and withdraw from the therapy space when she needed to. It is essential that this be held and respected by those around her, internally and externally. It is crucial that our psychotherapist sees E's boundaries as valid and respects them, even when this conflicts with the desires of other Housemates or stalls therapy.

There have been many experiences in our life that are unspeakable and unprocessable in language or thought. White people developed and sustain pathological terms (Mullan, 2023) such as *complex trauma* and *generational trauma* to describe this; First Nations/Indigenous people often refer to these traumas as *soul wounds* (Duran, 2006). Surrounding many soul wounds is silence. *Selective mutism* has personally followed us throughout life, and we have been deemed failures at talk therapy when asked to acknowledge, communicate, and process hundreds of intensely traumatic experiences in colonial ways.

Many autistic and traumatized people receive a pathologizing diagnosis of *alexithymia*, described as "difficulties in recognizing and distinguishing between different emotions and bodily sensations, difficulties in expressing emotions" (Kinnaird et al., 2019, p. 80). It is assessed based on dominating Western neurotypical communication practices. As an art psychotherapist, we work with people who are diagnosed as alexithymic and yet create deeply expressive, emotive, and meaningful artwork using color, shape, and line.

Color is our first and preferred language, and synesthesia is strongly identified in autistic neurotypes (Van Leeuwen et al., 2019) as a communication method. It is important to avoid universal color theories that are presumptive and constructed through White supremacy (Wierzbicka, 2008), and instead to be curious about colors being connected to emotions difficult to articulate via verbal language. As a person who experiences a multiple identity profile, color is how we internally locate who is present. We can internally ask, "What color are you?" and we will receive a response that leads to prospective identification of a Housemate. We often use deductive reasoning (Evans, 2005), asking "What emotional label-words DON'T fit with that color?" (Abukhodair et al., 2024) when knowing what "does fit" is too difficult. Application and attributes also have significance. Is the experience a metallic watercolor across a ridged page, a thick gouache on unrelenting packing cardboard, or a pigment glitter ink on a thirsty paper towel? We are speaking, communicating, expressing; you are unable to understand us because we do not share a common language. Alexithymia feels like an invalidation of our language.

Supporting participants' living complex identity systems

Mahlie: We became aware of the shared use of color identification when working with people living complex identity systems to create system maps. Color was often important to the identity of parts/people. Understanding color as an identification system can inform the therapist about "who is in the room" or who was involved in an experience, without having to use a communication method (such as speech) that may feel unsafe or overwhelming, or unavailable to that part/person.

Catherine: Respecting differing identification systems supports participant agency in communications with their therapist and relies on the therapist being willing to understand and view these communications as valid. As a participant, our therapist being aware of who is in the room is extremely important for us, including the therapist using their specific name and knowing their age, gender, capacity, function, and grouping location in our system. As a peer art therapist, our inside-out knowing supports participants in the unspoken, intersubjective space through holding participant identities in their wholeness and, when helpful, using appropriate mentalized transparency. Being able to apply a variety of identification systems (e.g., color, symbols, figurines, and fabrics) to communicate parts is key to facilitating the development of co-consciousness.

Mahlie: Art therapists understand that trauma memory is implicitly stored in the body, rather/more explicitly than in the cognitive mind. My hope is that this means we are inherently skilled at encouraging and respecting participants' diverse communication styles. Direct verbal engagement with trauma memory can cause re-traumatization. When a participant's stated goal is to process an experience, I suggest we tap into pre-verbal language and ask, "What color is it? What shape is it? What kind of line is it?" instead of "Tell me what happened."

Catherine: Yes! These questions allow the experience to present itself in a way that might at first feel unfamiliar but can generate curiosity and fresh perspectives. Many people living complex trauma develop specific ways of telling their story, for example, sometimes with a blunt, logical, verbal storyline, seemingly dissociated from emotion, or being unable to verbalize a narrative, remaining externally silent while internally busy/chaotic/distressed.

Mahlie: Art therapy taps into pre-verbal knowing and communication. Practicing "What color is it?" process over and over, interspersed with narrative conversations about our connections to colors and their wider implications (e.g., "What other experiences have felt blue?") may be less distressing and provide an alternative approach.

Catherine: This relates to how I work with figurines/symbols. Engaging with figurines either in or outside the sand tray allows separate identities and their specific experiences and functions to be made visible/speak. When a part/self cannot or chooses not to speak, using figurines/symbols gives the participant and therapist an opportunity to communicate, making it possible to build relationships with these parts. A powerful aspect of using figurines/symbols is the capacity to move them around physically, to change the story as new insights emerge. Working with communication across a system, this capacity to add, move, and create worlds using additional studio materials facilitates co-consciousness. Developing the capacity for co-consciousness supports the participant becoming increasingly available to themselves, understanding who's in the room in their day-to-day lives, and the therapist's increasing awareness of the participant's specific identity system.

Mahlie: And working the ways we describe has the potential to invalidate a part/person who would prefer a direct narrative approach rather than a symbolic one, so consent and choice are essential. Any process needs to be used only with a part/person's prior knowledge, ongoing consent, and active engagement.

Catherine: This respectful approach is central to working with trauma, and to building trust across complex identity systems, both within the participant and within the therapeutic relationship.

Resting place: sharing worldviews of curiosity and possibility

Our shared artwork (Figure 8.3) is an example of art-alongside. Mahlie's Sharehouse started painting as we talked across Zoom and sent their artwork (left side) from Wangal Land so Catherine could respond with artwork. Gundungurra Country under their feet, Catherine & Co responded with alchemical golden co-consciousness as their foundation (right side). Our collective artwork makes tangible our heart-connected solidarity, allyship, professional courage, and honoring conversations across identity systems and ways of knowing.

Through art from inside, we demonstrate the exploration, connection, and growth possible for participants living complex identity systems when diverse art languages are used for communication within art therapy. Art therapists can provide an alternative to talk therapies through the languages of materials and media, with deep respect and curiosity for what is, and how it is, expressed. Our LE examples document finding a safer and more accepting space, internally and in therapy, for feeling understood, respected, and celebrated. We provide insight into ways of working that skilled art therapists can take up. As PAThRs with intelligently ordered creative identity systems that are frequently pathologized in mental health discourse, we urge conversations in our profession that both destigmatize therapist LE and recognize that it is a rich resource for participants and for our profession.

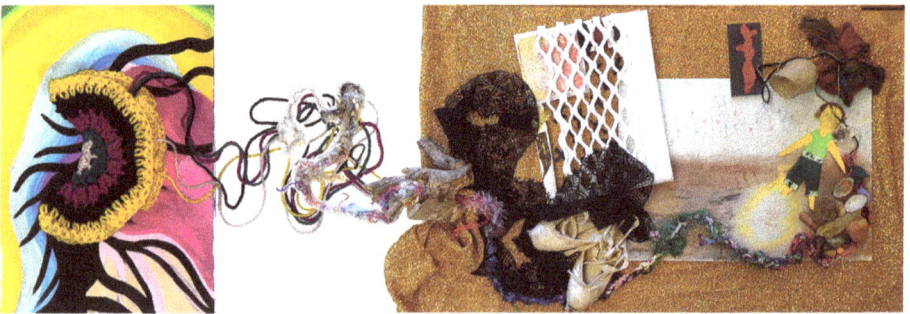

Figure 8.3 Jewell and Camden-Pratt (2024). 'I see you, I hear you, I believe you.'

References

Abukhodair, N., Song, M., Pekçetin, S., & DiPaola, S. (2024). Designing a wheel-based assessment tool to measure visual aesthetic emotions. *Cognitive Systems Research, 84.* https://doi.org/10.1016/j.cogsys.2023.101196

American Psychiatric Association. (2013). *American Psychiatric Association: Diagnostic and statistical manual of mental disorders* (Vol. 5). American Psychiatric Association.

Balsara, C., Garcia, S., Coetzee, S., Belaunzaran, M., & Villalba-Alvarez, C. (2024). Psychotherapy and non-pharmacologic treatment of Dissociative Identity Disorder. In H. Tohid & I. H. Rutkofsky (Eds.), *Dissociative identity disorder: Treatment and management* (pp. 213–231). Springer.

Camden-Pratt, C. E. (2003). Daughters of Persephone: Legacies of maternal 'madness' [Doctoral thesis, Western Sydney University]. ResearchDirect Library. http://handle.uws.edu.au:8081/1959.7/20751

Camden-Pratt, C. E. (2007). Creative arts and critical autobiography: Challenges of blending the deeply personal and the academic. In J. Higgs, A. Tichen, D. Horsfall, & H. B. Armstrong (Eds.), *Being critical and creative in qualitative research* (pp. 248–260). Hampden.

Drass, J. M. (2012). *Exploring the use of art therapy to treat trauma and dissociation in patients with borderline personality disorder: A literature-based study.* Drexel University.

Duran, E. (2006). *Healing the soul wound: Counseling with American Indians and other native peoples.* Teachers College Press.

Eastwood, C. (2020). White privilege and art therapy in the UK: Are we doing the work? *International Journal of Art Therapy, 6*(3), 75–83. https://doi.org/10.1080/17454832.2020.1856159

Eastwood, C. (2021). Resisting cultural devouring in a third, art-based space: Opre Roma! Shades of Noir. https://shadesofnoir.org.uk/ journals/content/resisting-cultural-devouring-in-a-third-art-basedspace-opre-roma

Eastwood, C. (2022). Snaky crazy lady and the air head princess: 'Colourblind' intersectionality and normative unconscious process in psychodynamic art therapy practice. In J. Collier & C. Eastwood (Eds.), *Intersectionality in the arts psychotherapies* (pp. 103–118). Jessica Kingsley.

Evans, J. S. B. T. (2005). Deductive reasoning. In K. J. Holyoak & R. G. Morrison (Eds.), *The Cambridge handbook of thinking and reasoning* (pp.169–184). Cambridge University Press.

Fenner, P., Crane, T., Byrne, L., Scottney, F., Boatman, T., & Schofield, M. J. (2024). The impact of group art therapy in post-acute cancer care: A longitudinal qualitative study. *The Arts in Psychotherapy, 87.* https://doi.org/10.1016/j.aip.2024.102122

Fisher, J. (2017). *Healing the fragmented selves of trauma survivors: Overcoming internal self-alienation.* Routledge.

Ford, E., George, N., Holland, E., Maher, S., Maree, L., Naylor, K., Rossel, K., & Wake, J. (2021). Seven lived experience stories of making meaning using art therapy. *International Journal of Art Therapy, 26*(1–2), 65–72. https://doi.org/10.1080/17454832.2021.1893771

Huet, V., & Holttum, S. (2016). Art therapists with experience of mental distress: Implications for art therapy training and practice. *International Journal of Art Therapy, 21*(3), 95–103, https://doi.org/10.1080/17454832.2016.1219755

Intentional Peer Support Core Materials. 2019. IPS. Follow Up at https://www.intentionalpeersupport.org/?v=6cc98ba2045f

Jacobson, L., Fox, J., Bell, H., Zeligman, M., & Graham, J. (2015). Survivors with dissociative identity disorder: Perspectives on the counseling process. *Journal of Mental Health Counseling, 37*(4), 308–322. https://doi.org/10.17744/mehc.37.4.03

Jewell, M., & Camden-Pratt, C. (2021). Advocating therapist lived experience: Towards an Australian peer art therapy model (PATh): Signposting the pivotal role of art therapy education. *Journal of Creative Arts Therapies, 16*(2), 17–38. https://www.jocat-online.org/a-21-camdenpratt-jewell

Jewell, M., & Camden-Pratt, C. (2023). Creating "art-alongside" in Peer Art Therapy (PATh) groups: Nurturing connection and trust and responding to power dynamics. *International Journal of Art Therapy, 28*(1–2), 38–50. https://doi.org/10.1080/17454832.2023.2175002

Kedar, I. (2012). *I do in Autismland: Climbing out of autism's silent prison.* Sharon Kedar.

Kinnaird, E., Stewart, C., & Tchanturia, K. (2019). Investigating alexithymia in autism: A systematic review and meta-analysis. *European Psychiatry, 55,* 80–89. https://doi.org/10.1016/j.eurpsy.2018.09.004

Lev-Wiesel, R. (2005). Dissociative identity disorder as reflected in drawings of sexually abused survivors. *The Arts in Psychotherapy, 32*(5), 372–381. https://doi.org/10.1016/j.aip.2005.02.003

Malchiodi, C. A., & Perry, B. D. (2014). *Creative interventions with traumatized children* (2nd ed.). Guilford Publications.

Mead, S., & MacNeil, C. (2006). Peer support: What makes it unique. *International Journal of Psychosocial Rehabilitation, 10*(2), 29–37.

Moon, C. H. (2010). *Materials & media in art therapy: Critical understandings of diverse artistic vocabularies.* Routledge.

Mullan, J. (2023). *Decolonizing therapy: Oppression, historical trauma, and politicizing your practice.* W.W. Norton & Co.

Roots & Roses. (2020). Wounded healer experiences in art therapy. *Art Therapy, 37*(2), 76–82. https://doi.org/10.1080/07421656.2020.1764794

Roth, G. (1999). *Sweat your prayers: Movement as spiritual practice.* Newleaf.

Rubin, J. A. (Ed.). (2016). *Approaches to art therapy: Theory and technique* (3rd ed.). Routledge.

Sagan, O. (2019). Art-making and its interface with dissociative identity disorder: No words that didn't fit. *Journal of Creativity in Mental Health, 14*(1), 23–36. https://doi.org/10.1080/15401383.2018.1499062

Sherwood, P. (2004). *The healing art of clay therapy.* ACER Press.

Steele, K., Boon, S., & van der Hart, O. (2016). *Treating trauma related dissociation: A practical, integrative approach.* W. W. Norton & Company.

Thayer-Cox, C., & Cohen, B. M. (2005). The unique role of art making in the treatment of dissociative identity disorder. *Psychiatric Annals, 35*(8), 695–697. https://doi.org/10.3928/00485713-20050801-11

Van Leeuwen, T. M., Van Petersen, E., Burghoorn, F., Dingemanse, M., & Van Lier, R. (2019). Autistic traits in synaesthesia: Atypical sensory sensitivity and enhanced perception of details. *Philosophical Transactions of the Royal Society of London B Biological Sciences, 374.* https://doi.org/10.1098/rstb.2019.0024

Waller, D., & Sibbett, C. (2005). *Art therapy and cancer care.* Open University Press.

West, C. (1997). *The experience of co-consciousness and switching in dissociative identity disorder: A multiple case study.* (Publication No. 9809609) [Doctoral dissertation, Saybrook University. ProQuest Dissertations and Theses.

Wierzbicka, A. (2008). Why there are no 'colour universals' in language and thought. *Journal of the Royal Anthropological Institute, 14*(2), 407–425. https://doi.org/10.1111/j.1467-9655.2008.00509.x

Winlaw. K. (2023). A healing journey: Using a daily visual journal practice to process the emotional experience of early breast cancer. *Journal of Creative Arts Therapies, 18*(2), https://www.jocat-online.org/a-23-winlaw

Woods, A., & Springham, N. (2011). On learning from being the in-patient. *International Journal of Art Therapy, 16*(2), 60–68. https://doi.org/10.1080/17454832.2011.603697

World Health Organization. (2022). International Classification of Diseases 11th Revision. https://icd.who.int/en

9

PLASTIC MANDALA

ECO-ART AS COMPASSIONATE ACTION

Eunhae Jung

I live on Jeju Island, my chosen home. It is Korea's largest island located south of the Korean Peninsula. Jeju is a volcanic island with a tall mountain in the middle and over 350 *oreum* (small volcanic hills). It also has many forests, lava tube caves, and, of course, is surrounded by the ocean. Jeju is Korea's most beloved vacation destination and is becoming increasingly popular among tourists from other East Asian countries. The island is famous for its natural beauty but suffers from excessive tourism, over-development, and the continuing destruction of its natural habitat.

Jeju is also famous for the presence of the highly respected Haenyeo (dive women). Primarily elderly women in their 70s and 80s, they have been diving all their lives, without equipment, to collect seafood. They are known for their close-knit community, communal diving culture, and care of the ocean. However, the tradition is facing looming extinction due to the gentrification of sea villages and the destruction of the marine ecosystem, among other factors (UNESCO, 2023).

Jeju has many environmental problems, including ocean trash. Because it is a tourist island, the government hires workers to do regular beach cleanups, and several volunteer groups also collect trash. Still, there is so much of it.

I often go to Hamdeok Beach to swim in its sapphire-colored water, walk on its white sand, and watch sunsets. I have also brought my art therapy clients on many occasions to play with the sand, safely burn a trauma art piece, or scream out loud what they have buried in their hearts. Whenever I am there, I try to pick up trash. However, after a storm has come and gone, the beach is covered in massive amounts of trash, looking like a scene from an apocalyptic movie. I want to give up. I am disillusioned not just by the amount of trash but also by how people try to ignore the mountain of waste as they crowd together on a small patch of relatively clean sand to take selfies or wedding photos.

Eco-art and eco-art therapy practices

I have been practicing as an eco-artist for the last ten years. In 2019, I began a project called *Plastic Mandala* (Jung, 2021) in which I, with the help of collaborators, collect micro-plastics from the beach, sort them by color, install them in a circular pattern for gallery and museum exhibits, and dismantle them at the end of each exhibition. I do not consider Plastic Mandala to be an art therapy project. However, the eco-art I have been practicing for a decade on Jeju Island is informed by, and based upon, core elements of art therapy. These elements include: (1) an ethics of care, (2) emphasis on the multi-layered meanings of materials and the process of engaging with them, and (3) compassionate action that seeks to reduce suffering or, if impossible, to sit with it.

Ethics of care

An ethics of care refers to approaching ethical problems with attention to their relational and contextual natures (Gilligan, 1982). In art therapy, there is a third space between therapist and client where creativity and art-based exploration occur. Entering the relational space with our clients with the intention of perceiving the poetry of their lives (Moon, 2002) is a practice of care ethics.

An ethics of care can also be extended to include the natural environment. Wright et al. (2023) believe that including nature as a meaningful component of therapy is less challenging for art therapists than for many verbal therapists due to art therapy already including a third element— engagement in art—as part of its framework. Harper and Fernee (2022) propose an "ethics of care for outdoor therapists to include all of nature—human and non-human—as vital parts of an ecosystem in dire need of dignified care" (p. 3).

Kim (2023), an eco-feminist, argues that people experience sadness and mourning at the sight of environmental destruction not merely as emotional responses, but also from a sense of duty to care for our kin, which includes the fauna, flora, water, air, and other environmental elements. Moreover, she argues that we can create community solidarity through which developing hope is possible. Hope, Kim writes, "does not mean the joy that comes from knowing that something is going well.…but from the ability to muster oneself for something meaningful and good" (p. 22). Likewise, it is possible to turn the pain and grief of environmental harm into art, which can create room for hope—not false hope, but hope based on an ethic of care.

Emphasis on materiality and meaning

The most critical aspect of *Plastic Mandala* is the physicality of the material—plastic trash that kills life. An emphasis on the significance of materials requires multidimensional considerations of its socio-politico-cultural context (Moon, 2010). It is the material in *Plastic Mandala* that separates it from many other contemporary artworks addressing environmental issues. While artists may convey warning messages about the climate crisis through their art, they often do so without considering the harmful environmental impact of the art materials and processes they use.

One example is *Ice Watch*, a 2014 project by Olafur Eliasson, in which the artist had arctic ice chunks from Iceland delivered to art venues in Europe, like the Place du Pantheon in Paris and Tate Modern in London. Olafur allowed the ice to melt so that viewers could have a tactical connection with the destruction of nature (Eliasson, 2014). However, questions arose about the carbon footprint from transporting the ice (the equivalent of 52 flights from London to Iceland) and its impact on living beings and the surrounding environment. The artist and his team attempted to mitigate the damage and balance the project's carbon footprint by donating money for tree planting (Judah, 2018).

From the perspective of Deep Ecology, which considers all the earth's organisms to be related to, and dependent on, each other

(Naess, 1973), and from an ethics that extends caring to all beings, *IceWatch* demonstrates the limits of ecological art that is anthropocentric, that is, made by and for humans (van Niel, 2021). *IceWatch* is but one example among many contemporary art projects that address environmental issues while also causing environmental harm.

It is an awkward position for environmentally conscious visual artists. Some artists have given up artmaking altogether because they find it untenable to participate in an art scene mired in a capitalist system that bears responsibility for the climate crisis. It is as if artists are recognizing that "the master's tools will never dismantle the master's house" (Lorde, 1984/2007, p. 112).

Compassionate action

In art therapy, the purpose of making art about pain and suffering is clear: either to reduce the pain or to sit with it. The art therapist's compassionate action is not simply empathy; it is action toward the relief of suffering. The central *art* of such work is not located in the final art produced but in the "relational aesthetics" (Moon, 2002, p. 140) formed and experienced throughout the process of making art in relationship with the client.

Many art therapists who explore nature art therapy, eco-art therapy, or nature-based therapy pay homage to Andy Goldsworthy's land art (Manthe, 2017). I find land art to be poetic, beautiful, and moving. However, I question whether a pristine, wild nature site exists anywhere on the planet at this point in history. Micro-plastics have been found in Arctic snow (Katz, 2019). Garbage is scattered around the Himalayas. Seabirds protect their eggs in nests made with plastic threads. We are in the Anthropocene epoch, an era in which human disturbance has become the most significant force affecting the planet (Swanson et al., 2015).

Tsing (2015), an anthropologist, asks how we can continue life amid destruction. Neville (2014) asks about the place of therapy in a world that is in a state of emergency. The place of therapy, eco-art, and eco-art therapy is amid destruction-in-progress. Art therapists can begin where contemporary art has often stopped. In art therapy, we not only raise awareness and provoke dialogue, but we also create holding spaces for pain, grief, mourning, and hope.

A healing process

I led a 12-week art therapy group combining indoor and outdoor art-making, following the 12 stages of the mandala as elaborated by Fincher (2009). The themes of the final mandala were transcendental ecstasy, returning home, a good death, and a new beginning. I knew the perfect site to create this mandala—by the ocean. I gathered my group at Hamdeok Beach soon after dawn, when tourists do not crowd the beach and the early morning light is other-worldly. There, we drew giant sand mandalas and waited for the tide to come and take the mandalas away. It was a perfect way to finish the cycle and end the group.

As I repeated this group over several years and sometimes led a stand-alone sand mandala workshop, I took on a stewardship role at this site. Drawing the sand mandalas always began with sweeping the sand with a broom woven from branches. Sweeping the sand had a dual purpose—to clean the beach and to prepare our canvas for drawing.

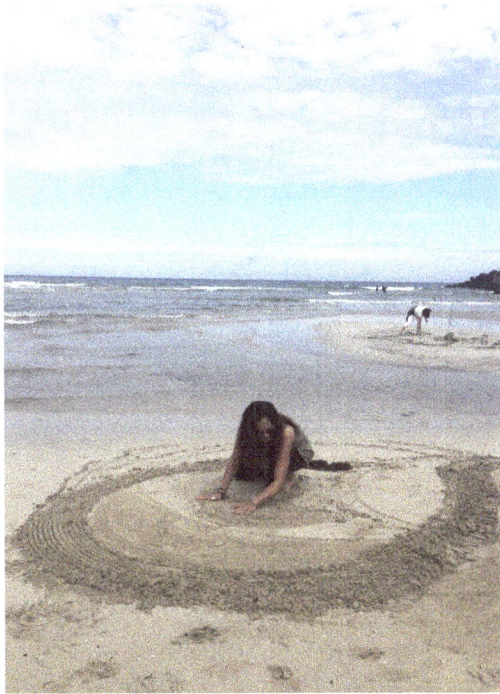

Figure 9.1 Sand mandala workshop at Hamdeok Beach, Jeju, 2017.

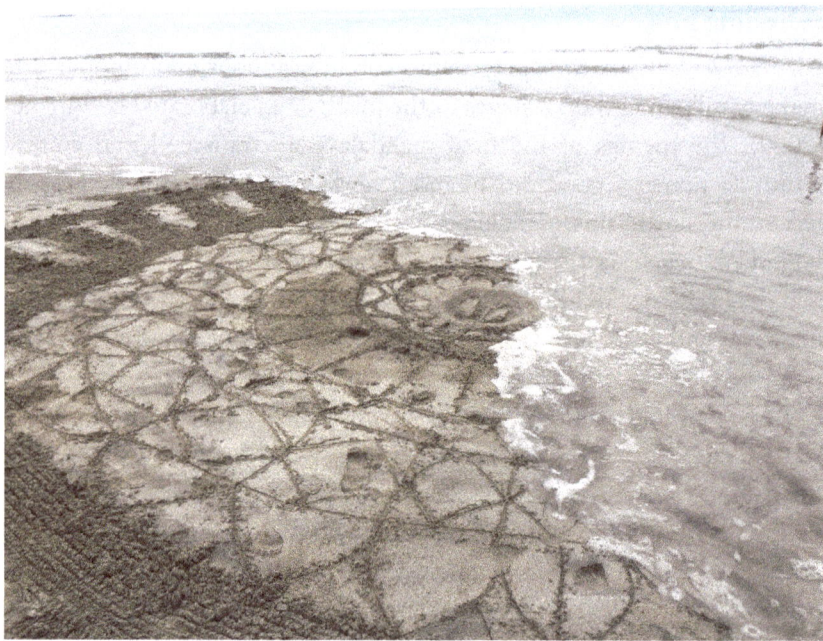

Figure 9.2 Disappearing Mandala, Sand mandala workshop at Hamdeok Beach, Jeju, 2017.

My relationship with the ocean, especially with Hamdeok Beach, completely changed when my father passed away. He died in Toronto, and as a first-generation immigrant to Canada, he had always wanted to be buried back home in Korea. His ashes were returned to Korea and placed beside his father's ashes at a gravesite in Seoul. While transporting his ashes from a carrying box to an urn, I took a pinch of his ashes to bring to Jeju. He loved swimming at Hamdeok Beach whenever he visited me, and I thought he would love to be part of the ocean, as free-spirited as he was. On a cold November morning, I swam into deep water and sprinkled a pinch of his ashes on the water's surface. As I did so, I swear I heard him laughing. At that moment, my relationship with the ocean completely changed. The ocean became my father.

I continued returning to the beach to collect trash as I had done before. However, I was no longer doing it to maintain a clean 'canvas,' but rather because I felt a kinship with the ocean. Around that time, I noticed brightly colored micro-plastic forming a trail along the

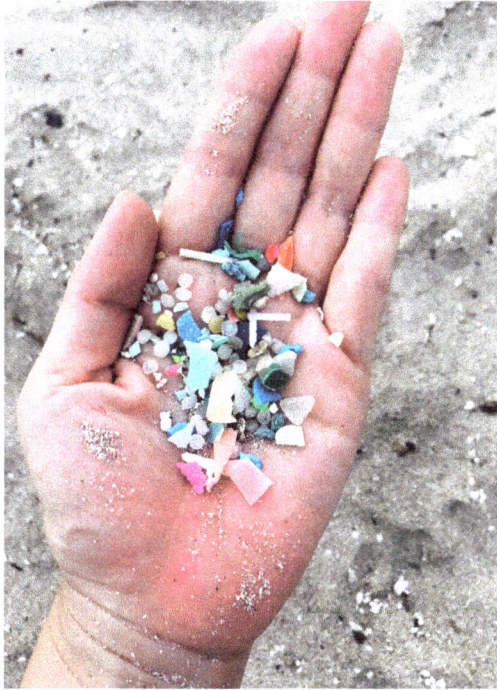

Figure 9.3 Small and micro-plastic found in the sand, Hamdeok Beach, 2010.

coastline at low tide and under a thin layer of sand. They came in various colors, sizes, and thicknesses.

I also found many identically shaped, opaque white beads. I had no idea what they were until I came across a foreign news report about plastic spills in the ocean. I learned that these lentil-sized plastic beads are called *nurdles*. They are pre-production plastic pellets that can be turned into clear water bottles and cups. I also learned that they enter the ocean in many ways, mainly during transportation (Baurick, 2021).

For instance, on May 20, 2021, a fire broke out on the deck of the *M/V X-Press Pearl* cargo ship while it was anchored off the west coast of Sri Lanka. Everyone on board was rescued, and no one was hurt, but 1680 tons of plastic nurdles were released into the ocean. The plastic covered a 50 km (31 mile) stretch of the beach months after the fire (de Vos et al., 2022). All ocean plastic threatens marine ecology, but plastic nurdles are especially deadly because they look like fish eggs and are often mistaken for food by seabirds, fish, and other wildlife (Knight, 2022). To my knowledge, there has been no report or warning about plastic nurdles in Korea, but they have arrived on the shores of Jeju Island.

I started to collect the nurdles and other small pieces of plastic without planning to make art with them. However, I had been creating sand mandalas for years, so making a mandala with plastic was the first thing that came to mind when I was invited to participate in a group exhibition with an ocean theme. With the help of friends and community members, I assembled these small plastic pieces into a circle, symbolizing the earth, the ocean, and the cycle of life. Since then, I have repeatedly collected, sorted, installed, and dismantled tiny bits of plastic into mandala forms. Approximately 350 people have participated in creating the *Plastic Mandala* over the course of five years.

Beauty and pain; empathy and grief

Over the course of seven years I have been repeatedly asked variations of this question: "Why don't you glue them or melt them to make something like a whale?" From the beginning, I had no plan of making permanent artwork because my inspiration came from making sand mandalas that disappeared with the tide. The only permanent aspect was the material itself, the plastic, and the fact that we cannot be rid of it. *Not* altering the material was my most significant artistic decision in creating *Plastic Mandala*. By not making any symbolic or physical changes to the material, I wanted people to see the material for what it is—a deadly threat to life. I had hoped viewers would respond as they typically do when seeing others in pain, that is, with empathy, grief, and mourning. However, arousing such a response was difficult because the plastic beads were so pretty.

When I find a particularly colorful piece of plastic in the sand, I often think, "Wow, it's pretty!" Then, I quickly reproach myself. "How can I call this pretty?" However, this was the initial response from almost everyone who collected plastic from the sand, helped assemble a mandala, or viewed the finished installation at an exhibition. After repeatedly hearing the word *pretty*, I began to think that perhaps the planet's plastic disaster is not just due to the convenience of plastic, but also due to its appeal. Perhaps humans are not so different from Australian satin bowerbirds that collect shiny blue objects, often plastic, for their nests, preferring its vivid color and glossy surface (Siossian, 2018).

When the Plastic Mandala was installed in an exhibition setting, the most challenging question revealed itself to me. Can eco-art be both beautiful and painful? Can eco-art evoke empathy and grief even though people tend to anticipate seeing beauty in art exhibitions?

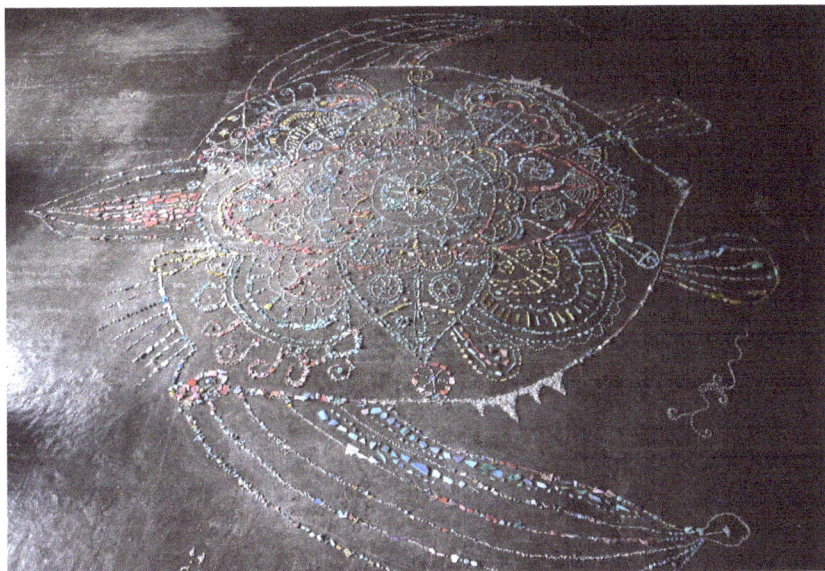

Figure 9.4 Plastic Mandala: Eco-art of mourning and blessing, Dolharebang Gallery, Jeju, 2020.

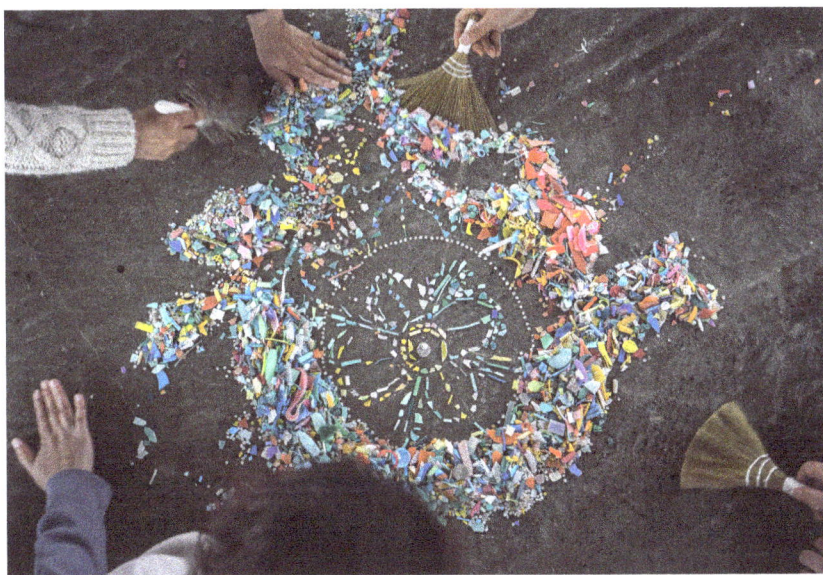

Figure 9.5 Dismantling of Plastic Mandala, Dolharebang Gallery, Jeju, 2020.

Han (2018) argued that contemporary notions of beauty can be characterized as smooth and self-reflective, as people surround themselves with mirrors and mirror-like apparatuses such as selfies, social media, and art. From reflective sculptures, like Chicago's famous *Cloud Gate* by Anish Kapoor (Martinique, 2019), to currently popular immersive media exhibitions of old masters, such as Van Gogh, Monet, and Matisse, people mostly do not look at the artworks *per se*, but look at themselves in the work (Wiener, 2022). Immersive exhibitions perfectly exemplify what Han (2018) calls smooth beauty. The texture, brushstrokes, and patina of the original works are missing, and in their place are smooth surfaces that operate as backdrops for Instagram-worthy photos.

Visual spectacle versus reality

Along with Plastic Mandala, in 2022, I also exhibited "Tears of the Ocean" at the National Asian Culture Center as part of an international group exhibit titled Aqua Paradise. This work, comprised of 400 tiny glass bottles containing micro-plastics, aimed to convey pain and evoke empathic responses from viewers. However, hung from the high ceiling in the darkened gallery and lit with a dramatic spotlight, the artwork looked like a fancy chandelier made of 400 glittery objects.

While installing the work, the curator asked me, "Where did you get these tiny bottles?" I told her I bought them online from China. She replied, "No." Deeply puzzled, I asked, "What? No?" She continued, "To complete the story, they must be salvaged from the ocean. That is what I'm going to tell people." It was not a suggestion but an announcement of the narrative she planned to apply to the work.

The exhibit was a huge success, attracting more than 50,000 viewers (Choi, 2022). I even received an award from the Ministry of Culture, and Tears of the Ocean became a popular 'photo zone'. However, I felt like the artwork was a total failure. I had not intended to create a photo zone. I was not trying to make a good narrative. I was trying to say, "Look! These micro-plastics are here. They are deadly. We need to stop this!" The message was delivered, but the responses were not what I expected. I wondered, "Is there no place for sadness, pain, or mourning in art exhibitions?"

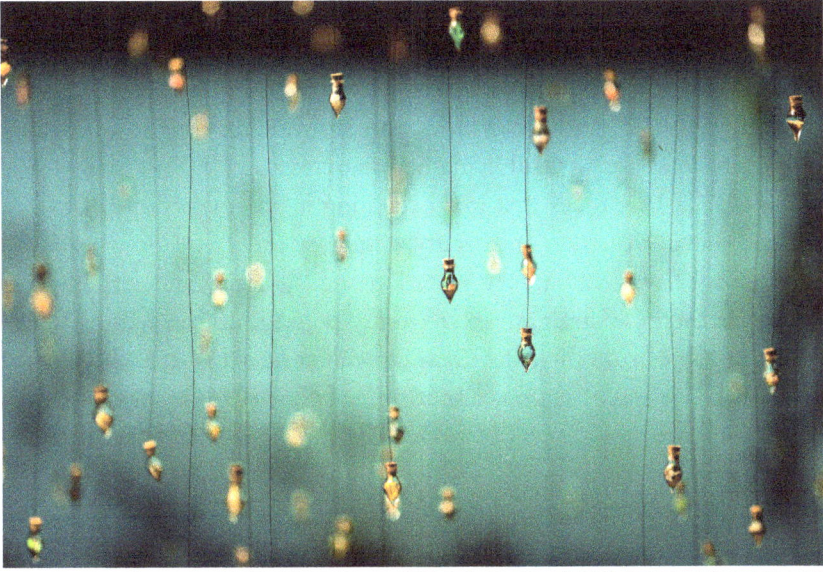

Figure 9.6 Eunhae Jung, *Tears of the Ocean*. National Asian Culture Center, Gwangju, Korea, 2022.

I once went to an art museum to see an exhibition of media art about the ocean. It consisted of a video projection showing the ocean at night, accompanied by an audio recording of ocean waves. Before entering the installation room, there was an announcement saying that the piece was meditative and warning us that the space would be dark, so not to panic. The audience members were released after about 20 minutes of watching and listening. As I was coming out of the room, my eyes connected with the eyes of a friend, and we both burst into laughter. We thought the exhibit was hilarious because the real ocean was only ten minutes away from the museum. Why watch a video of the ocean when the actual ocean was close by? What is the point if you do not feel the wind, taste the salty air, and have your hands and feet in the sand? However, that might have been the point. When I am at the beach, I often hear, "Do not touch the sand. It's dirty!"

"I don't think I will die." A teenage client who spent most of his waking hours playing computer games told me this once. He said these words while inserting a wired heart into a black eagle sculpture made with foil and masking tape. I asked him what he meant by his comment. He said he thought body parts would be replaced in the future, as he was doing with his sculpture, and that there would be external storage for brain memory. While ecological destruction is rapidly increasing, humans are trying to overcome the cumbersome nature of being alive, which always includes suffering, aging, and dying. But isn't the life cycle the one thing that unites humans with all living beings on earth?

Harari (2019) argues that it is becoming increasingly difficult to distinguish between fiction and reality as history progresses because of the illusions we have created, such as nations, gods, money, and corporations. However, there is a straightforward test to determine if something is real. It is the test of suffering. If something can suffer, it is real. If it cannot suffer, it is not real. A nation cannot suffer. Money cannot suffer. AI cannot suffer. A narrative cannot suffer. But people suffer. Animals suffer. Our planet suffers.

Today, people are living with the current crisis of environmental destruction. Some people believe technology will save us. Some people think the only way out of the climate crisis is the extinction of our species. Many people become numb at the sight of ecological destruction and fall back on romantic notions of nature or view nature through its visual spectacle that replaces reality with its representation (e.g., a soundscape of ocean waves), which Baudrillard (1994) called "simulacra" (pp. 1–2). However, the fact is that we have only what we have. There is no other earth. The waters may be filled with trash, but no other ocean exists. We live on earth, where life and death coexist, where life-in-flourish and life-in-extinction intermingle.

Relationship between the signifier and the signified

The work's title, *Plastic Mandala*, leads or misleads viewers to think of the practice of creating sand mandalas in Tibetan Buddhism. In Tibetan sand mandalas, grains of colored sand are used to create intricate mandala patterns, which may take days or weeks to complete. When the mandala is finished, the work is dismantled by sweeping the sand. It is one of the highest tantric practices of Tibetan Buddhism, and each mandala is the sacred home of a deity who represents and embodies the enlightened qualities of the Buddha. For lay Tibetan people, seeing the mandala is a great blessing because they believe it leaves within them an impression of enlightenment that goes deep into their subconscious (Bryant, 2003).

The Tibetans also believe the sand used to create the mandala contains blessings. Thus, when the mandala is complete, the sand is distributed to those witnessing the ritual, and the rest is poured into a nearby river or sea. They trust that the grains of sand, now blessings, will reach all sentient beings through the one ocean that connects us all (Chittister, 2011).

The similarity between *Plastic Mandala* and Tibetan sand mandalas ends at the superficial level of placing the grains in a circular format and sweeping them up when finished. But the aspect I attempted to emulate was the sand becoming a blessing. In Tibetan villages, it is common to see a Tibetan turning a prayer wheel or a metal cylinder containing a scroll with a printed mantra on it. The belief is that turning the wheel is equivalent to reciting the script (Marin, 1987). Also, everywhere, from windy hills in the Himalayas to yoga studios in the West, there are prayer flags with written scripture on them. Tibetans hang prayer flags because they believe the wind will carry the mantra to the world (Borkar, 2018). In these examples, there is no clear division between the symbol and what the symbol represents.

Plastic Mandala operates in a similar realm, whereby the symbolic and the physical overlap. However, unlike the Tibetan mandala, in which pouring the sand is pouring blessings into the ocean, *Plastic Mandala* operates in the opposite way. Plastic and micro-plastic are taken out of the ocean as penance, environmental activism, and compassion-in-action.

Sometimes with a group of people, and more often by myself, I am on my knees, crawling while slowly caressing the sand, searching for plastic. Children are screaming, young couples are having simulated picnics (for staged photos), and several couples are taking wedding photos. The visitors to the beach seldom talk to me. When they do speak to me, they mostly say, "Su-go-ha-sip-ni-da." This can be roughly translated as, "You are doing good work." Then, they return to their activities.

These bodily positions of kneeling and crawling were not intentional. They were the most accessible postures for my aching back and bad eyesight. But they became part of a performance art piece or a prayer in action. I can understand why, in all religious traditions, prayer involves kneeling on the ground. It becomes an embodied prayer.

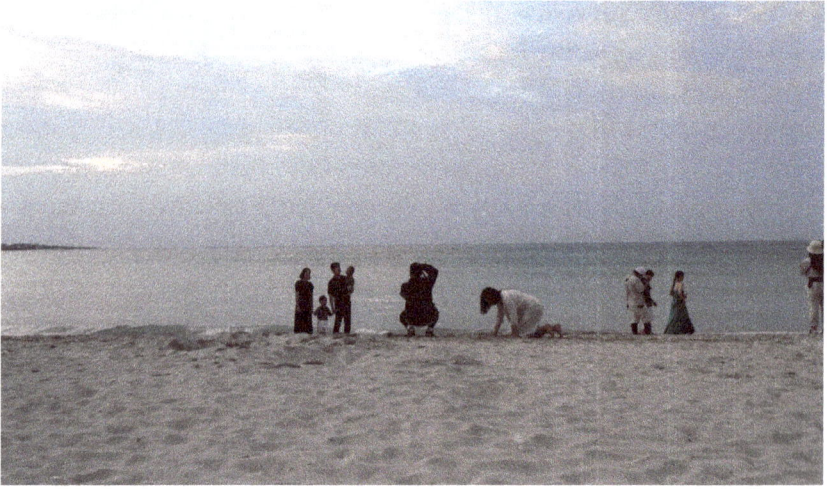

Figure 9.7 Crawling on knees to find micro-plastic, Hamdeok Beach, 2023.

The messy middle

Regarding the climate crisis, one voice says technology will solve it all. The other says we are doomed; we will all die. The voice in the messy middle acknowledges that we are both offenders and victims. This messy middle is where we must stand if we want to make any impact on the current situation. This messy middle is where we come into a third space with nature and its grandeur, beauty, tragedy, saltiness, and trash. Also, the messy middle is where we practice healing because it is the only ground for creative action that is not divided by what we want to see and what we are.

Haraway (2016) has advocated for "staying with the trouble" (p. 10), which calls for learning to live with trouble in times of climate emergencies instead of focusing on a trouble-free future, and Tsing (2015) has asked that we explore the possibility of living among the earth's ruins. Along with these standpoints, turning suffering into poetic visual expressions so that we do not ignore either beauty or pain is what art therapists do best.

References

Baudrillard, J. (1994). *Simulacra and simulation* (S. Glaser, Trans.). University of Michigan Press (Original work published in 1981).

Baurick, T. (2021, February 1). A new crop of nurdles is washing up in New Orleans, renewing calls for cleanup, penalties. *Nola.* https://www.nola.com/news/environment/a-new-crop-of-nurdles-is-washing-up-in-new-orleans-renewing-calls-for-cleanup/article_820710fc-64cc-11eb-85ce-93b2793068d5.html

Borkar, N. (2018, March 23). 8 Things you should know about Tibetan prayer flags before hanging them up. *India Times*. https://www.indiatimes.com/lifestyle/self/8-things-you-should-know-about-Tibetan-prayer-flags-before-hanging-them-up-257899.html

Bryant, B. (2003). *The wheel of time: Visual scripture of Tibetan Buddhism*. Snow Lion Publications.

Chittister, J. (2011, September 20). The mandala: Why do monks destroy it? *HuffPost*. https://www.huffpost.com/entry/mandala-why-destroy-it_b_970479

Choi, K. (2022, August 21). ACC '아쿠아 천국' 관람객 5만명 돌파 '인기' [Aqua Paradise at ACC attracted more than 50,000]. *Jeon-nam Ilbo*. https://jnilbo.com/68328852306

de Vos, A., Aluwihare, L., Youngs, S., DiBenedetto, M. H., Ward, C. P., Michel, A. P. M., Colson, B. C., Mazzotta, M. G., Walsh, A. N., Nelson, R. K., Reddy, C. M., & James, B. D. (2022). The M/V X-Press Pearl nurdle spill: Contamination of burnt plastic and unburnt nurdles along Sri Lanka's beach. *ACS Environmental Au, 2*(2), 128–135. https://doi.org/10.1021/acsenvironau.1c00031

Eliasson, O. (2014). *Ice Watch, 2014*. https://olafureliasson.net/artwork/ice-watch-2014/

Fincher, S. (2009). *The mandala workbook: A creative guide for self-exploration, balance*, and well-being. Shambhala.

Gilligan, C. (1982). *In a different voice: Psychological theory and women's development*. Harvard University Press.

Han, B. (2018). *Saving beauty*. Polity Press.

Harari, Y. (2019). *Twenty-one lessons for the 21st century*. Vintage.

Haraway, D. J. (2016). *Staying with the trouble*. Duke University Press.

Harper, N. J., & Fernee, C. R. (2022). Unpacking relational dignity: Pursuit of an ethics of care for outdoor therapies. *Frontiers in Psychology, 13*. https://doi.org/10.3389/fpsyg.2022.766283

Judah, H. (2018, December 14). Was Olafur Eliasson bringing 30 icebergs to London a sustainability own goal? *Frieze*. https://www.frieze.com/article/was-olafur-eliasson-bringing-30-icebergs-london-sustainability-own-goal

Jung, E. (Director). (2021). *Plastic mandala*. [Video]. Jeju Foundation for Arts and Culture. https://www.youtube.com/watch?v=kjd1t9OWC2I

Katz, C. (2019, August 15). Tiny pieces of plastic found in Arctic snow. *National Geographic*. https://www.nationalgeographic.com/environment/article/microplastics-found-in-arctic-snow

Kim, H. (2023). 우리는 지구를 떠나지 않는다. [We won't go to outer space]. In Moon Trees Ecofeminism Research Center (Eds.), 우리는 지구를 떠나지 않는다: 죽어가는 행성에서 에코페미니스트로 살기 (pp. 13–29). Chagbi Publication. https://www.changbi.com/BookDetail?bookid=4292

Knight, T. (2022, May 27). *Noxious nurdles - the plastic pellets threatening marine wildlife*. Fauna & Flora. https://www.fauna-flora.org/opinion/noxious-nurdles-the-plastic-pellets-threatening-marine-wildlife/

Lorde, A. (2007). *The master's tools will never dismantle the master's house. Sister outsider: Essays and speeches*. Crossing Press, pp. 110–114 [Original work published 1984].

Manthe, L. (2017). Nature art therapy: Preliminary research findings. *ATOL: Art Therapy OnLine, 8*(10). https://doi.org/10.25602/GOLD.atol.v8i1.439

Marin, D. (1987). On the origin and significance of the prayer wheel according to two nineteenth-century Tibetan literary sources. *Journal of the Tibet Society, 7*. https://himalaya.socanth.cam.ac.uk/collections/journals/jts/pdf/JTS_07_02.pdf

Martinique, E. (2019, May 10). Reflections on Cloud Gate, Chicago's shiny bean. *Widewalls*. https://www.widewalls.ch/magazine/cloud-gate-chicago-bean-anish-kapoor

Moon, C. (2002). *Studio art therapy: Cultivating the artist identity in the art therapist*. Jessica Kingsley Publishers.

Moon, C. (2010). *Materials and media in art therapy: Critical understanding of diverse artistic vocabularies.* Routledge.

Naess, A. (1973). The shallow and the deep, long-range ecology movement. A summary. *Inquiry,16*(1–4), 95–100. https://doi.org/10.1080/00201747308601682

Neville, B. (2014). Arts and health as an ecopsychological practice: Developing a conversation. *Journal of Applied Arts & Health, 5*(2), 273–280. https://doi. org/10.1386/jaah.5.2.273_1

Siossian, E. (2018, October 6). Satin bowerbirds fall victim to plastic waste, wildlife experts urge mindfulness. *ABC Mid North Coast.* https://www.abc.net.au/news/2018-10-06/satin-bowerbirds-falling-victim-to-plastic-waste/10215078

Swanson, H. A., Bubandt, N., & Tsing, A. (2015). Less than one but more than many: Anthropocene as science fiction and scholarship-in-the-making. *Environment and Society: Advances in Research, 6*, 149–166. https://doi.org/10.3167/ares.2015.060109

Tsing, A. L. (2015). *The mushroom at the end of the world.* Princeton University Press.

UNESCO (2023, October 12). *The haenyeo: Guardians of Jeju Island's coastal legacy.* https://www.unesco.org/en/articles/haenyeo-guardians-jejus-coastal-legacy

Van Niel, F. (2021). Ice art ethics: On Olafur Eliasson's Ice Watch. In I. Halland (Ed.), *Ung Uro: Unsettling climates in Nordic art, architecture and design* (pp. 59–68). Cappelen Damm Akademisk. https://doi.org/10.23865/noasp.127.ch5

Wiener, A. (2022, February 10). The rise of "immersive" art: Why are tech-centric, projection-based exhibits suddenly everywhere? *The New Yorker.* https://www.newyorker.com/news/letter-from-silicon-valley/the-rise-and-rise-of-immersive-art

Wright, T., Blakeman, V., Andrew, T., & Labovitch, S. (2023). A qualitative evaluation of an outdoor arts therapies group. *International Journal of Art Therapy, 29*(2), 109–118. https://doi.org/10.1080/17454832.2023.2229893

1O

Transgender joy as community art in a "Trans Refuge State"

Owen Paul Karcher and G. Nic Rider

The vibrancy, creativity, and resilience of the transgender community cannot be overstated. Amid an increasing onslaught of attacks on our existence (Ciesemier, 2023; Human Rights Campaign, 2023; Reed, 2024), our communities come together in various ways to envision joy and move toward authentic alignment (Kichler, 2022). Our communities do this through mutual care networks, referrals, clothing swaps, dance parties, meal trains, fundraising, grants for transition needs, storytelling, embodying resistance to oppression, vigils, art, and creating networks of support for folks traveling for access to healthcare, among the myriad other ways we creatively push the bounds of what is possible by envisioning what we haven't seen before.

The authors invited transgender people seeking gender-affirming healthcare to respond to the following prompt: "Using lines, shapes, and colors, create a picture of what trans joy looks like." We also invited them to share what gender-affirming care means to them and what they want healthcare providers to know about better supporting transgender people. Though the materials were limited by the contexts where the project took place—a medical center, a therapy office, and a community Pride festival—participants created vibrant swirls of color, used an abundance of symbols, and responded with hopeful messages of love, growth, aliveness, and community.

DOI: 10.4324/9781032720166-12

The authors are two transgender individuals who strive to increase access to gender-affirming care and support transgender people in our roles as therapists and researchers. Owen (he/they) is a transmasc/gender-fluid, neurodivergent, White, currently physically abled, transpersonal art therapist, author, spiritual/somatic practitioner, and manager of the M Health Fairview Comprehensive Gender Care (CGC) Program in Minneapolis, Minnesota. He has worked with transgender and gender-diverse people for two decades as a community organizer, therapist, researcher, and peer. They believe queer and trans people are inherently beautiful, creative, resilient, and deserving of love, dignity, and liberation.

Nic (they) is a non-binary/trans masc, queer, immunocompromised Asian American counseling psychologist, sex therapist, researcher, and educator. They are the director of the National Center for Gender Health and an associate professor and licensed psychologist at the Institute for Sexual and Gender Health, which are both within the University of Minnesota Medical School. Their work examines social and structural factors impacting the lives of sexual and gender-diverse communities and explores how these communities (re)define and (re)explore healing, resilience, and liberation.

The CGC is situated within a large academic medical institution called M Health Fairview and includes specialists from a wide range of disciplines, including mental health, voice therapy, surgery, and primary care. The mission of the CGC is to provide accessible, interdisciplinary, and integrated gender-affirming care for people of all ages. The program's vision is to center the voices of transgender and gender-diverse people, to be historically accountable and trauma-informed, to translate leading-edge research into compassionate care, and to address health disparities through advocacy. The relevant components of CGC to this project are the surgical services at the Clinic and Surgery Center and the psychological services offered at the Institute for Gender and Sexual Health.

Project context and aims

We came to this project with the desire to challenge and shift away from the deficit-oriented, negative, shallow stories about trans and gender-diverse communities. Although some narratives reflect accurate realities, others are myths or spread misinformation (Billard, 2024;

Erickson-Schroth & Jacobs, 2017; Feder, 2020; Lepore et al., 2022). We wanted to embrace and share the hope we were holding onto so dearly, as hope is a necessity not only for changing the narrative about trans and gender-diverse people but also for strategizing in relation to social change. As Freire (1994/2014) said, "I am hopeful, not out of mere stubbornness, but out of an existential, concrete imperative… my hope is necessary, but it is not enough. Alone, it does not win. But, without it, my struggle will be weak and wobbly" (p. 2).

We knew we needed community. Our goal was to focus on collective participation and liberation by inviting and welcoming transgender and gender-diverse people of all ages to engage in a project that would make the implicit more explicit, especially related to trans joy and gender-affirming care. We intentionally asked trans people to use their own voices through imagery grounded in their own experiences, which is consistent with the practices of other Queer art therapists who design their work for LGBTQ people (Anderson, 2021). Our intention was to stimulate hope, which is crucial to gender-affirming care. We wanted participants to reflect on positive experiences, celebrate structural change and social protections, and imagine a future to strive for, so that we all might thrive, not simply survive.

We invited participants to express their hopes for liberatory, gender-affirming care and trans joy through contributing to a large map representing Minnesota. This collaborative project was meant to elicit a collective image of resilience, convey a sense of welcome to this recently dubbed "trans refuge" state (Finke, 2023), and reflect the reality that many transgender people are traveling to Minnesota from surrounding states for healthcare, as shown by increasing demands for our services. They are traveling from states that have created barriers to well-being by proposing and passing laws restricting access to medically necessary, lifesaving health care and involvement in public life. About half of transgender and gender-diverse patients in this country travel outside their home state to access gender-affirming surgeries, creating additional financial burdens for them (Downing et al., 2022).

Mapping resources and employing visual maps to track anti-trans healthcare and legislation has been a project of trans activists and communities for years. Sharman (2021a) explains that queer and trans people have long shared tips for navigating health systems, calling this practice "one of the queer and trans community's superpowers and core survival strategies" (p. 111). Sharman prompts readers to map their experiences with the U.S. healthcare system and to think about the history, underlying assumptions, and implications of the system for LGBTQ+ health. This mapping can help transgender people contextualize their experiences with healthcare within a long history of resistance and resource sharing (Mingus, 2015).

Artmaking, systems change, and trans well-being

We chose an arts-based method because of the potential of the arts to foster empowerment, build connections through collaboration, create "narratives of action" (Mulligan et al., 2008, p. 50), and creatively challenge cis- and heteronormative systems of power within the healthcare system (Zappa, 2017). Mulligan et al. (2008) challenge researchers to be precise in their use of the term 'community' and in their investigations of *how* art functions to build a stronger sense of community. Their study found that arts participation can offer a sense of narrative, purpose, agency, and a means of "building and re-building a sense of community and identity" (p. 64). Expressive arts therapies can be a method of illuminating and challenging the ingrained and individualistic pathologization of marginalized people in the medical industrial complex. By using disability, queer, and social justice frameworks, expressive arts allow for connection and shift power dynamics to uplift the voices of marginalized groups (Sayre, 2022). The invitation to consider trans joy within a medical setting was based on our critique of the individualistic and often isolating experience of accessing care in large medical structures, and our hope that taking part in the project would enable participants to feel more connected to each other and the broader community. Joseph (2006) writes about mural making as a strategy for building community and involving patients in art-based activism. While not technically a mural, the project was a collaborative image that served similar purposes.

Background of project development

On December 3, 2022, we arrived at the Minneapolis city capital building to witness a historic milestone. Surrounded by stakeholders, including us, Major Jacob Frey signed Executive Order 2022–04 protecting gender-affirming health care in Minneapolis, Minnesota. It was a small victory, and everyone in that room as well as the activists outside knew they still had work to do. Another win came on March 8, 2023, when Governor Tim Walz held a signing ceremony for Executive Order 23–03, the trans refuge bill for the state of Minnesota. The signing of both executive orders into law means that trans and gender-diverse people in or relocating to Minnesota are welcome, their right to health will be protected, and they will be treated with dignity. These rights stand in stark contrast to changes in laws across the nation that limit or ban gender-affirming care even though several court cases have affirmed that transgender people should not be discriminated against on the basis of their gender identity (Medina et al., 2021).

In April 2023, as the weather started to warm enough that Minnehaha Falls had thawed and was flowing strong, we walked along the creek path, finding inspiration from the budding trees and emerging spring greenery of the urban forest plants. We have found that both of us tend to feel the most grounded when breathing in the fresh, crisp air, listening to the birdsong and flow of the water. The purpose of the walk was to plan a potential Twin Cities Pride project that would center "community defined evidence" (Martinez et al., 2010; Timm-Bottos, 2017) of trans joy and resilience. With the signed executive orders still fresh in our minds, we discussed ideas for how to support transgender and gender-diverse people in our community and our work, and how to build a stronger sense of community. We also talked about how people from different social locations (e.g., people of color, people with disabilities, people living in states with legal restrictions on healthcare) have varied access to gender-affirming care.

Given the longstanding history of transgender people being forced to develop their own healthcare resources (Sharman, 2021b), we discussed what trans people have learned over time. We also acknowledged the pervasiveness of trauma and its inhibiting impact on our collective imagination (Imarisha, 2015), while also envisioning what might be possible if we could remove such limitations. We developed the idea for a collective project that could resource and welcome trans people and simultaneously educate cisgender healthcare professionals about what trans people actually want from gender-affirming care.

Material considerations

Our material selection was influenced by the settings we chose for this project, the time limitations of therapy sessions, and the wait times for consultation appointments. Our choices needed to meet several criteria. The media needed to be accessible to people with a range of abilities, be self-explanatory, not too messy, nontoxic, and easily transportable. We chose to use a variety of materials that were relatively easy to manipulate and allowed for affective expression through bright, saturated colors. We used Posca paint pens, colorful markers, colored pencils, glitter glue sticks, and thick printmaking paper to ensure participants could saturate the paper surface with paint without compromising the structure of the paper. For those less comfortable with mark making, we had an abundance of stickers and made sure to include culturally relevant imagery and symbols for transgender and nonbinary communities. These included a variety of animals, flags, uplifting phrases, rainbows, and nature imagery.

According to the Media Dimension Variables model, which describes characteristics of art processes, our media choices had low complexity, and were simple and unstructured (Kagin & Lusebrink, 1978). We also considered the Expressive Therapies Continuum (Lusebrink & Hinz, 2020), a theoretical model that identifies various ways people interact with media. We chose materials that elicited perceptual and affective engagement, but selected paint pens rather than liquid paints to allow for the expression of joy through bright colors and vibrant materials, while also allowing for control over unwieldy emotional experiences that might arise if materials were too fluid or messy. When transgender people access medical care, they often experience minority stress; that is, they anticipate mistreatment and/or have experienced it in the past (Hendricks & Testa, 2012; Testa et al., 2015). Many transgender people delay care to avoid mistreatment and discrimination (James et al., 2016), and need to employ coping strategies to mitigate stress while seeking medical care. For that reason, our choice of paint pens was particularly supportive of participants who would be entering medical appointments and would need their protective strategies to be intact for communicating their needs with providers. In addition, we considered the physical well-being of all participants by choosing materials that were nontoxic and safe to use.

In addition to deliberately selecting media, we also intentionally created prompts that focused on trans joy and on what participants hoped providers might know about gender-affirming care. We chose these prompts rather than asking open-ended, experience-based questions that might evoke complaints or memories of negative interactions within healthcare settings. We used relatively small sheets of paper and limited drawing materials to encourage a sense of containment and to limit emotional dysregulation (O'Neill Haaga & Schwartz, 2022). We did not want people to have to process strong, unpleasant feelings immediately prior to medical consultations or amid a large public gathering.

The printmaking paper was cut in the shape of puzzle pieces, which when put together created the shape of the state of Minnesota. We determined the size of the puzzle pieces based on the amount of time participants would likely have to wait for their appointments, or to stop at the Twin Cities Pride table. The puzzle pieces were meant to symbolize participants' belonging to a larger whole and to reinforce a sense of community. This emphasis on collectivity was particularly important because the patients accessed care at different sites, but all sites were part of an effort to coordinate gender-affirming care across a large medical system.

Surgery clinic setup

In the surgery clinic waiting room, we set up a multi-use cart with art supplies, release forms, and envelopes in which patients could place their completed artwork and release forms. The cart was chosen for ease of transporting the materials to and from the patient waiting area, simplifying clean-up, and serving as an inviting, organized, and accessible display of material options. The waiting area and treatment rooms appear sterile and lifeless, so even just the presence of colorful art materials and imagery transformed the environmental ambiance. The vibrant project flyers, created using digital design software, displayed rainbows and Pride flags, along with invitations for patients to contribute their ideas and imagery. Two small canvases that had the prompts written on them and one larger canvas containing an outline of the state of Minnesota were leaned against the wall. The larger canvas would eventually provide the surface on which the art was displayed once the project was complete.

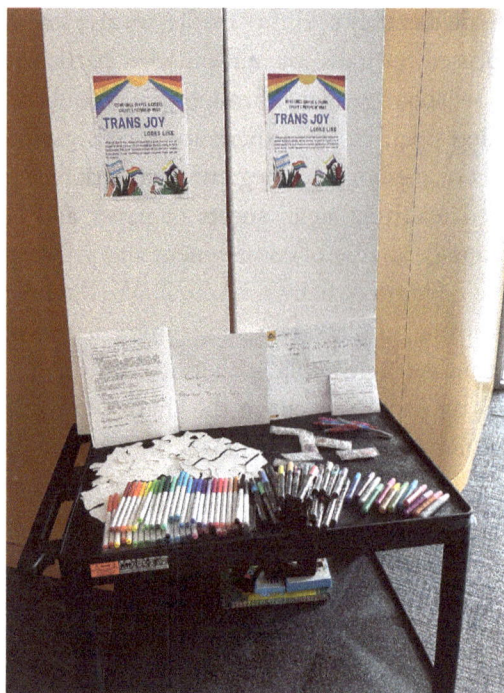

Figure 10.1 Surgery clinic art project setup.

Patients were invited to contribute to the project while they waited for appointments to meet with surgeons. Several patients said they enjoyed engaging in the art process while they waited, and a few continued their artmaking even after they were led to the examination rooms.

Institute for Sexual and Gender Health setup

In the waiting area for the Institute for Sexual and Gender Health, there is a corner that regularly contains child-friendly art supplies, coloring pages, and dry erase boards. Patients across the lifespan often used materials from this area to create something while waiting for their appointments, which made it a convenient location for our project materials. Right next to the existing artmaking space, we set up the same art supplies, flyers, canvases with prompts, release forms, large canvas with an outline of the state, and envelopes for patients to place their artwork. As a result of our project, the area became a site of interaction, storytelling, smiling, and laughter, in contrast to the typically quiet waiting room.

Several patients said they liked the idea of a *by and for* trans community collaborative art and advocacy project, and how it filled them with joy to see it displayed and in progress in the clinic.

Twin Cities Pride setup

The project continued at Twin Cities Pride, where we displayed the artwork made by patients on large canvases and invited Pride attendees to contribute their own artwork and responses. The central canvas displayed the map with the imagery and puzzle pieces, the left canvas showed the responses to what participants wanted providers to know, and the right canvas held the responses to what gender-affirming care meant to them. Twin Cities Pride Festival welcomes 400,000–500,000 attendees to Loring Park in Minneapolis over the course of three days (Strom, 2023). It is an exuberant event for people of all ages who are there to celebrate the resiliency and vibrancy of the LGBTQ+ community, build connections, reflect on the community's shared history, and access needed resources. The Living Well Park area provides attendees with an opportunity to learn about local health systems as well as available services that are specific to the LGBTQ community.

M Health Fairview, a university-health services collaboration in Minnesota, commanded a large area within Living Well Park. It consisted of an entrance and three large tents where various community programs had information tables. The CGC and the LGBTQ employee resource group set up a stage where scheduled speakers gave presentations about different gender-affirming services, including voice therapy and vocal cord surgery, top and bottom surgeries, and sex therapy. To the right of the stage, CGC set up three tables in a U shape for attendees to make art and learn about the gender care program. Art materials were on the tables, the large canvas with the map was behind the back table, and the two canvases with the art and writing prompts were on easels on either side of the tables. A team of volunteers, most of whom work for the CGC, set up the space each day and attended to the tables and art processes.

Artists ranged in age from about four to sixty, and had various responses to the prompts. Their responses ranged from sharing their experiences with trying to access or provide care, to joy and laughter while playing with

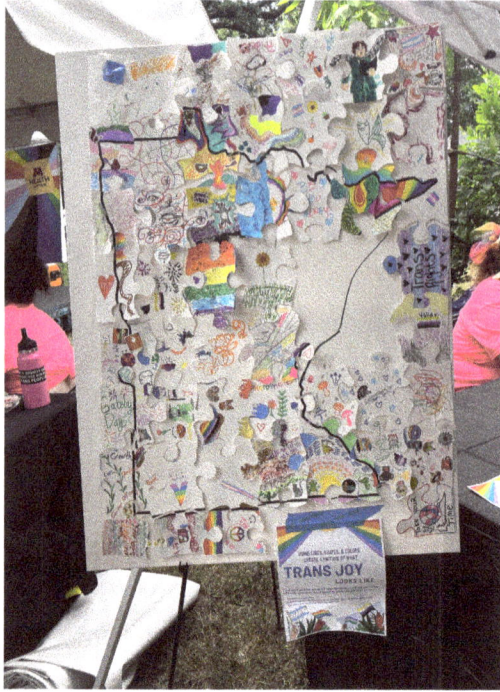

Figure 10.2 Art project at Twin Cities Pride.

the materials, to questions about how they could access services. While attendees created their imagery, they heard about the gender-affirming services available within M Health Fairview, asked providers questions about options for care, viewed the artwork, and read the responses from transgender patients and other Pride attendees.

Results

By the end of Twin Cities Pride, all 56 puzzle pieces were transformed into vibrant, whimsical, interconnecting symbols of resilience, strength, joy, and beauty. Most participants combined all the materials to create their imagery and most of the pieces were filled to the edges with color. We observed a range of symbols including, but not limited to, animals (e.g., koala, dinosaur, dog, butterfly, squirrel, snail, frog), organic content (e.g., flowers, pumpkins, mushrooms), hearts, stars, and identity pride flags. Each of the pieces had at least two colors. Most contained several colors that intersected, and the vast majority incorporated multiple

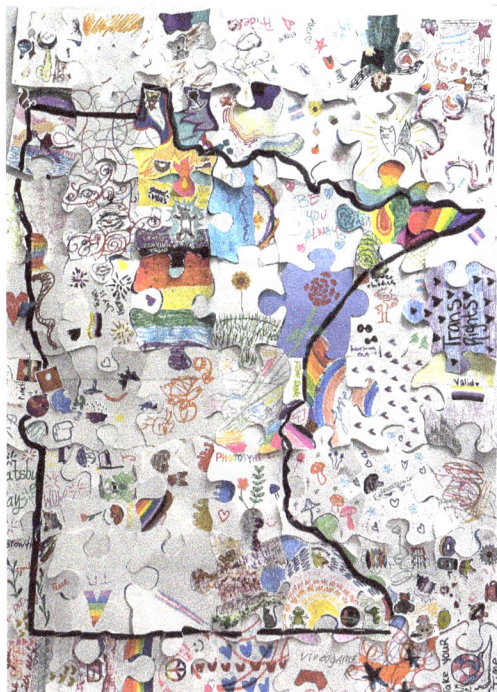

Figure 10.3 Canvas depicting trans joy.

materials. We noticed that on the outline of the state of Minnesota, within individual puzzle pieces and as part of the whole composition, the imagery, colors, and shapes often extended toward and beyond edges. Notably, two images depicted the word *growth* on the outside of the Minnesota borderline. The most frequent words to represent trans joy across all puzzle pieces were *love*, *growth*, *community*, *rights*, *equality*, *pride*, *wow*, *trans*, *joy*, *power*, and *staying*.

What gender-affirming care means

Participants also had the opportunity to respond with written comments to our prompt about what gender-affirming care means to them. In general, there were two interrelated themes: *Lifesaving* and *Aliveness*.

Scholars, medical experts, and activists emphasize that gender-affirming healthcare is lifesaving for a variety of reasons, including improved quality of life, decreased suicidality, and increased sense of safety. This was also represented in written responses. For example, one participant disclosed that the care they received eliminated their suicidal thoughts. Another participant wrote "gender-affirming care means saving lives." Additional contributions included love, support, and radical joy.

Aliveness characterizes the comments and the observed affective responses of participants who indicated that gender-affirming care enabled them to be their authentic selves and feel a sense of freedom and rejuvenation. For example, we noticed increased laughter, animation, and playfulness as participants grabbed the writing utensils, engaged with the prompt, and shared their stories. They described social gender affirmation (e.g., having pronouns respected, exploring gender expression) and medical interventions (e.g., hormone therapy, surgeries) that were life-affirming or life-giving. For example, one participant wrote, "It's nothing less than what provides me the ability to exist as I am. My care has made possible a life I thought wasn't possible." Images of growing plants, water, and hearts were repeatedly included with the comments, which also served as symbolic representations of what is needed to sustain life.

What providers need to know

For the prompt about what patients would like providers to know, the general themes were *communication* and *comfort*. Participants wanted providers to know that communication and comfort were important to them. Multiple people noted that trans individuals are the experts of their own lived experiences and identities. As such, providers should listen to trans people and create a space where trans people feel safe and heard.

Providers should also avoid making assumptions about patients' comfort or discomfort, and instead engage in conversations about how patients are experiencing (or not experiencing) and defining (or redefining) comfort for themselves and in their healthcare. Oftentimes, to be privileged is to expect comfort. It is important that providers think critically about the complexities of power and privilege, and that they consider and address power dynamics present in their work with patients.

Lessons learned

For half of the first morning of Twin Cities Pride, the weather caused logistical challenges. We had to secure the easels with zip ties and bungee-cords due to the high winds and rain that poured down. The puzzle pieces swirled in a gust of wind before we were able to securely weigh them down or attach them to the canvases. The materials we brought to attach the pieces to the canvases proved insufficient, and the pieces kept falling off, so we had to use a combination of different tapes. Painter's tape ended up being the most effective. In retrospect, we realized it would have been helpful to test methods of adhesion and to be prepared for inclement weather prior to setting up the project outside.

Conclusion

This chapter describes a collaborative art project between patients of a CGC program and participants at a large Pride festival in Minneapolis. The authors sought to elicit positive feelings of joy and welcome as transgender participants reflected on what trans joy and gender-affirming care meant to them. Most participants used multiple drawing materials to create their images, filled them with multiple colors, and centered themes of growth. The drawing materials, stickers, and glue were accessible for people of various ages, and the small puzzle pieces were sized according to time and space constraints.

As advocates for gender-affirming care have been asserting for years, participants indicated that gender-affirming care is lifesaving and helps them transition into an enlarged sense of aliveness. Suggestions for providers included listening to their patients and viewing them as the experts of their own healthcare experiences, advocating for increased access to care, and understanding that not all trans people are the same. The aims of this project were to offer an experience that brought joy to transgender participants and to raise awareness about what transgender people want when seeking gender-affirming care.

References

Anderson, M. (2021). Queer ethos in art therapy. In L. Leone (Ed.), *Craft in art therapy: Diverse approaches to the transformative power of craft materials and methods* (pp. 218–236). Routledge.

Billard, T. J. (2024). The politics of transgender health misinformation. *Political Communication, 41*(2), 344–352. https://doi.org/10.1080/10584609.2024.2303148

Ciesemier, K. (Host). (2023, April 27). Why and how trans hate is spreading. [Audio podcast episode]. In *At liberty podcast*. ACLU. https://www.aclu.org/podcast/why-and-how-trans-hate-is-spreading

Downing, J., Holt, S. K., Cunetta, M., Gore, J. L., & Dy, G.W. (2022). Spending and out-of-pocket costs for genital gender-affirming surgery in the US. *JAMA Surg, 157*(9), 799–806. https://jamanetwork.com/journals/jamasurgery/fullarticle/2793977

Erickson-Schroth, L., & Jacobs, L. A. (2017). *"You're in the wrong bathroom!": And 20 other myths and misconceptions about transgender and gender-nonconforming people.* Beacon Press.

Feder, S. (Director). (2020). *Disclosure* [Film]. Netflix.

Finke, L. (2023, March 24). *Trans refuge bill passes off the house floor.* Minnesota House of Representatives Legislative News and Views. https://www.house.mn.gov/members/profile/news/15575/36792#:~:text=%2D%20This%20morning%2C%20the%20Minnesota%20House,of%20gender%2Daffirming%20health%20care

Freire, P. (2014). *Pedagogy of hope: Reliving pedagogy of the oppressed* (R. Barr, Trans), Bloomsbury Publishing (Original work published 1994).

Hendricks, M. L., & Testa, R. J. (2012). A conceptual framework for clinical work with transgender and gender nonconforming clients: An adaptation of the Minority Stress Model. *Professional Psychology: Research and Practice, 43*(5), 460–467. https://doi.org/10.1037/a0029597

Human Rights Campaign. (2023). *LGBTQ+ Americans under attack: A report and reflection on the 2023 state legislative session.* https://hrc-prod-requests.s3-us-west-2.amazonaws.com/Anti-LGBTQ-Legislation-Impact-Report.pdf

Imarisha, W. (2015, February 11). Rewriting the future: Using science fiction to re-envision justice. *Bitchmedia.* https://bitchmedia.org/article/rewriting-the-future-prison-abolition-science-fiction

James, S. E., Herman, J. L., Rankin, S., Keisling, M., Mottet, L., & Anafi, M. (2016). *The Report of the 2015 U.S. Transgender Survey.* National Center for Transgender Equality. https://transequality.org/sites/default/files/docs/usts/USTS-Full-Report-Dec17.pdf

Joseph, C. (2006). Creative alliance: The healing power of art therapy. *Art Therapy, 23*(1), 30–33. https://doi.org/10.1080/07421656.2006.10129531

Kagin, S. L., & Lusebrink, V.B. (1978). The expressive therapies continuum. *The Arts in Psychotherapy, 5,* 171–180. https://www.sciencedirect.com/science/article/abs/pii/0090909278900315

Kichler, R. (2022). "What has kept me alive": Transgender communities and support. *Journal of Homosexuality, 69*(14), 2463–2482. https://pubmed.ncbi.nlm.nih.gov/34264806/

Lepore, C., Alstott, A., & McNamara, M. (2022). Scientific misinformation is criminalizing the standard of care for transgender youth. *JAMA Pediatrics, 176*(10), 965–966. https://jamanetwork.com/journals/jamapediatrics/article-abstract/2795567

Lusebrink, V. B., & Hinz, L. (2020). Cognitive and symbolic aspects of art therapy and similarities with large scale brain networks. *Art Therapy, 37*(3), 113–122. https://doi.org/10.1080/07421656.2019.1691869

Martinez, K., Callejas, L., & Hernandez, M. (2010). Community-defined evidence: A bottom-up behavioral health approach to measure what works in communities of color. *Emotional Behavioral Disorders in Youth, 10*(1), 11–17. https://nirn.fpg.unc.edu/wp-content/uploads/Community-Defined-Evidence.pdf

Medina, C., Santos, T., Mahowald, L., & Gruberg, S. (2021). Protecting and advancing health care for transgender communities. *Center for American Progress.* https://www.americanprogress.org/article/protecting-advancing-health-care-transgender-adult-communities/

Mingus, M. (2015, February 6). Medical industrial complex visual. *Leaving evidence.* https://leavingevidence.wordpress.com/2015/02/06/medical-industrial-complex-visual/

Mulligan, M., Scanlon, C., & Welch, N. (2008) Renegotiating community life: Arts, agency, inclusion and wellbeing. *Gateways: International Journal of Community*

Research and Engagement, 1, 48–72. https://epress.lib.uts.edu.au/journals/index.php/ijcre/article/view/591

O'Neill Haaga, M., & Schwartz, J. (2022). Understanding media: Laying the groundwork for art-making. In M. Rastogi, R. P. Feldwisch, M. Pate, & J. Scarce (Eds.), *Foundations of art therapy theory and applications* (pp. 32–75). Academic Press.

Reed, E. (2024, March 25). *Anti-trans legislative risk assessment map: March 2024 update.* Erin in the morning. https://www.erininthemorning.com/p/anti-trans-legislative-risk-assessment-cd3

Sayre, D., (2022). Care work and social justice in creative arts therapy: Putting queer performance theory and disability justice in conversation with drama therapy. *The Arts in Psychotherapy, 80*, 1–6. https://www.sciencedirect.com/science/article/abs/pii/S0197455622000612?via%3Dihub

Sharman, Z. (2021a). *The care we dream of: Liberatory & transformative approaches to LGBTQ+ health.* Arsenal Pulp Press.

Sharman, Z. (2021b). Regrowth in ruins: Abolitionist dreams for health system transformation. In Z. Sharman (Ed.), *The care we dream of: Liberatory & transformative approaches to LGBTQ+ health* (pp. 135–158). Arsenal Pulp Press.

Strom, D. (2023, June 23–25). *2023 Pride festival info: Twin Cities Pride Festival changes & vendor information June 23–25, 2023* [PowerPoint slides]. Twin Cities Pride. https://tcpride.org/wp-content/uploads/2023/01/2023-TCPride-Festival-Vendor-Info-Session-v1.pdf

Testa, R. J., Habarth, J., Peta, J., Balsam, K., & Bockting, W. (2015). Development of the gender minority stress and resilience measure. *Psychology of Sexual Orientation and Gender Diversity, 2*(1), 65–77. https://doi.org/10.1037/sgd0000081

Timm-Bottos, J. (2017). Public practice art therapy: Enabling spaces across North America. *Canadian Art Therapy Association Journal, 30*(2), 94–99. https://doi.org/10.1080/08322473.2017.1385215

Zappa, A. (2017). Beyond erasure: The ethics of art therapy research with trans and gender-independent people. *Art Therapy, 34*(3), 129–134. https://doi.org/10.1080/07421656.2017.1343074

11

SOCIO-POLITICAL STRESS AND ARTMAKING

CLOTHING, IDENTITY, AND SOCIAL CHANGE

Michelle Kendrick Hartney

In the United States, socio-political stress has become a significant source of depression and anxiety, stemming from a myriad of causes. From the looming threat of climate change to the tumultuous struggle for democracy and the disruptive impacts of a global pandemic, the collective psyche has grappled with uncertainty and upheaval (Suzuki et al., 2023). Compounding this stress has been the erosion of human rights, including the overturning of Roe versus Wade and legislative assaults on transgender rights (Tordoff et al., 2022).

Over the past decade, my interdisciplinary art practice has been focused on exploring socio-political issues, particularly examining the intersections of racism and misogyny within the American healthcare system. Through various art mediums, with a particular emphasis on clothing and social practice, I've delved into topics about gender-affirming care, contraception, pregnancy, obstetric abuse, postpartum PTSD, and maternal mortality. Several of my projects facilitate cathartic or activist experiences for others to engage in, whether through direct involvement in the creation of the artwork or by integrating community voices into the final piece. Collaborative public art projects play a crucial role in fostering community engagement and addressing challenges arising from the increasing influence of social conservatism, especially as state-sponsored social programs and services continue

 DOI: 10.4324/9781032720166-13

to be defunded (Robertson & Vinebaum, 2016). It is important for art therapists to consider their socio-political engagement with clients, especially those clients most affected by the erosion of human rights in the United States. In this chapter I discuss collaborative community projects that use clothing as a lens through which to interrogate pressing social issues.

Clothing, beyond its obvious utilitarian function, acts as a conduit through which people navigate the complexities of identity, safety, and societal perception (Tajuddin, 2018). Garments can serve as armor, shielding from physical harm or providing a sense of security. Yet, paradoxically, clothing can also mark people as targets for discrimination or other kinds of harm because of societal norms, stereotypes, or perceptions (Ferguson, 2024). Clothing acts as a medium through which humans express the diverse spectrum of their identities, ranging from gender and sexuality to culture and personal style (Tajuddin, 2018). It also conveys societal markers of wealth, prestige, intelligence, and power or, conversely, challenges and subverts these constructs (Adam & Galinsky, 2012). In this intricate dance between the material and the symbolic, clothing is a potent vehicle for shaping and reshaping personal narratives, challenging norms, and advocating for inclusivity and authenticity. In a therapeutic setting, clothing can be a means to explore the significance of identity (Yi, 2020).

Mending: an act of love

For several years, I've been working on a project that serves as a testament to the profound potency of clothing as both a medium of expression and a means for healing. *Mending: An Act of Love* is a collaborative series that emerged from the deeply personal experience of altering my transgender child's baby clothes to align with their gender identity. When my child started identifying as a girl, they embraced hyper feminized clothing for several years. I altered their baby clothes to mirror their evolving identity by adding lace or intricate embroidered patterns to their garments. Months into the project, after several years of identifying as a girl, my child started using they/them pronouns and expressing themselves with clothing that was more gender neutral. The alterations I had made to their baby clothes no longer reflected their current gender identity, mirroring the fluidity many people experience with gender and providing me with another lesson about the futility of labels. As their identity continued to shift, so did the embellishments I made to their clothing. I started asking my child how they would have liked their baby clothes to look, which turned this project into a collaboration between the two of us.

When preparing to install the altered clothing for an exhibition, I unraveled a Texas state flag and turned the fibers into a clothesline. I suspended the clothesline from two Texas star finials, then used clothes pins to hang my child's garments on it. Texas has attempted to enact some of the most inhumane laws in the country related to transgender people, including Governor Abbott's attempt to classify gender-affirming care as child abuse (Day & Harper, 2022).

The experience of altering my child's baby clothes inspired me to create a workshop so other families with transgender children could experience the healing benefits of this practice. The workshop offers a safe space for families to alter their transgender children's garments to align with their child's gender identity. Through this process, parents can express their love for their child, heal guilt about how they handled their child's

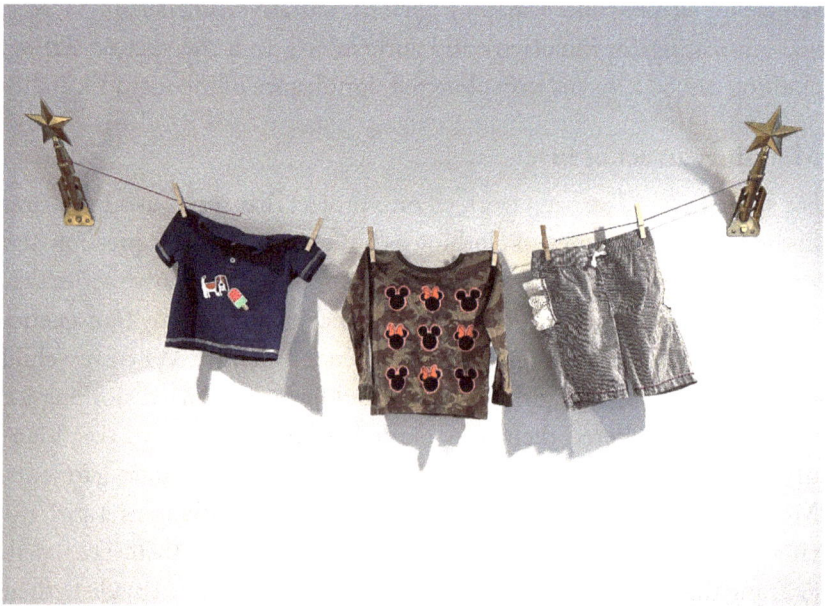

Figure 11.1 *Mending* (2020–2023), Artist's child's baby clothes, embroidery floss, appliqué, lace, Texas flag finials, unraveled Texas state flag.

gender identity, and affirm their child's authentic self. Historically, health professionals have often aimed to "correct" or "fix" queer individuals, contributing to a collective sense of trauma within the queer community (Hardy & Monypenny, 2019) and highlighting the need for alternative forms of care outside the medical model. By offering a platform for self-expression, empathic connection, healing, and unity, these workshops contribute to the likelihood that parents will accept and support their children, which, in turn, has been shown to improve mental health outcomes for transgender people (Jin et al., 2020).

These workshops underscore the symbolic power of clothing as a vehicle for self-expression, protection, vulnerability, and healing. Given the alarming number of anti-LBGTQIA+ bills in the United States—479 at the time of this writing (Choi, 2024)—projects like *Mending: An Act of Love* take on even greater significance. It becomes increasingly crucial for families of transgender children to find spaces of acceptance and support for themselves and their kids.

Unplanned parenthood

While some garments can be used as tools of expression, defiance, or protection, few garments in American culture carry deeper significance than the wedding gown. It embodies notions of purity, promise, and tradition. Laden with layers of meaning, wedding dresses evoke romanticized ideals of matrimony, serve as symbols of love and commitment, and represent the beginning of a new chapter in life. Wedding dresses also carry a complex narrative shaped by patriarchal norms and power dynamics. Historically, marriage has served as a vehicle through which husbands have exerted control over women, dictating societal roles and expectations regarding child-rearing and domestic responsibilities (Ross, 1991). Wedding dresses serve as a symbol of the ways patriarchal structures have historically constrained women within the confines of marriage and family life.

Vintage wedding dresses played a central role in *Unplanned Parenthood*, the collaborative mixed-media installation I developed that delves into the history of birth control and its intersection with racism in the struggle for reproductive justice in the United States. This project is centered around the stories of mothers who wrote letters to Margaret Sanger, the founder of Planned Parenthood. Though many people aren't aware of the controversies associated with Sanger, she supported eugenics and forced sterilizations of those the state deemed unfit, and accepted speaking engagements with the KKK (Stewart, 2020). However, she also published a book called *Motherhood in Bondage*, which included a selection of the 250,000 letters she received in the 1920s from desperate mothers asking for information about birth control. At the time, news about reproductive healthcare was deemed obscene, and disseminating information about it was punishable by law (Belluck & Ploeg, 2023). Some mothers wrote that they would rather die than be pregnant again. Many were living in extreme poverty, had abusive husbands, had survived over a dozen pregnancies, and/or had suffered multiple miscarriages and stillbirths (Sanger, 1928). *Unplanned Parenthood* was centered around the stories of these mothers who longed for reproductive justice.

Select letters from the collection were hand-written by volunteers from across the country and embroidered onto fabric cut from vintage wedding dresses. The embroidery was completed at sewing circles that were held at universities, museums, and galleries around the United States, and by dozens of volunteers who sewed letters at home. The collaborative nature of the project infused each embroidered letter with collective energy and a sense of solidarity.

Throughout history, sewing circles and quilting bees have been a means for people to connect, share stories, and discuss social and political issues (Brown, 2020). Quilts were created by enslaved people in the United States to reveal their stories of suffering and hardship (Fry, 1990). Suffragettes organized quilting bees to raise funds and strategize about how to secure voting rights (LaBar, 2021).

Just as quilting circles have historically been a vehicle for change and solidarity, *Unplanned Parenthood* sewing circles offered a place for participants to grieve the reversal of Roe versus Wade. The project started several months before the supreme court leak regarding the case of Dobbs versus Jackson and gained momentum after the court voted to strip away the constitutional right to abortion, discarding nearly five decades of established precedent. Several of the sewing circles held discussions with representatives from the American Civil Liberties Union who shared their legal expertise and extensive knowledge about the rapidly shifting laws regarding abortion bans. Many participants shared their stories, or the stories of their mothers who were forced to bear children. One of the volunteers disclosed that her father was Dr. David Gunn, the first doctor murdered by anti-abortion extremists. A sewing circle was held at Weinberg/Newton Gallery in Chicago on the thirtieth anniversary of his death. The sewing circle gave Dr. Gunn's daughter an opportunity to grieve, alongside others, the murder of her father and to honor the work he did and the lives he changed.

Once *Unplanned Parenthood* volunteers finished their embroidery, I suspended the fabric from porcelain backings, evoking the fragility of women's rights. I also incorporated imagery from wedding cakes and other articles of clothing like lingerie into the finished piece. Many of the embroidered scraps of wedding dresses hang from vintage meat hooks, symbols of the brutality of the patriarchy. I also sewed rosary beads onto several of the pieces as a reminder of the enduring influence in the United States of Christianity

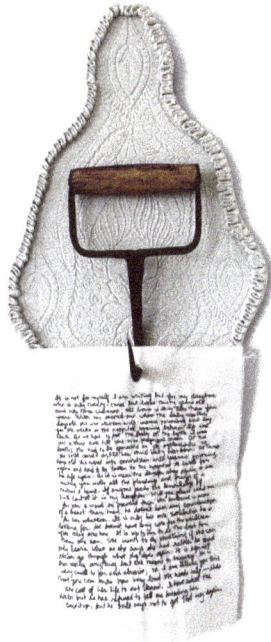

Figure 11.2 *Unplanned Parenthood 3*, 2023, porcelain, vintage wedding dress fabric, vintage meat hook, embroidery floss.

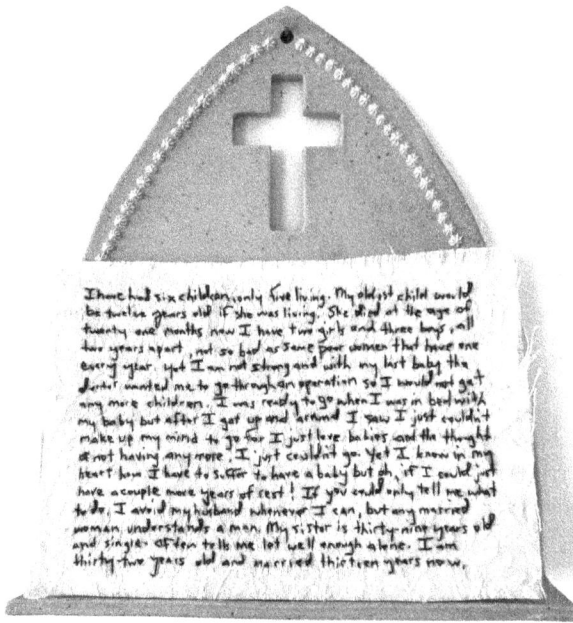

Figure 11.3 *Unplanned Parenthood 6*, 2023, porcelain, vintage wedding dress fabric, embroidery floss.

and the roles religious institutions have played in shaping societal norms and controlling the bodies of women and trans folks (Whitehead & Perry, 2019). Just as these dresses carry the stories and memories of past unions, they also bear witness to the generations of people who fought for the right to control their own bodies and destinies, including women of color who have historically faced intersecting forms of oppression (Smith, 2020).

Limited access to abortion is a significant socio-political issue affecting nearly half of the states in this country (Choi & Cole, 2024). It has direct implications for mental health outcomes, particularly for people living in states with abortion bans (Steinberg, 2024). This reality should be considered when providing support to clients in these areas. Social action art therapy is inherently participatory and collaborative (Golub, 2005) and public art projects focused on storytelling through sewing can offer a space for healing and community building. Engaging with art and hearing others' stories can help create new cultural narratives and

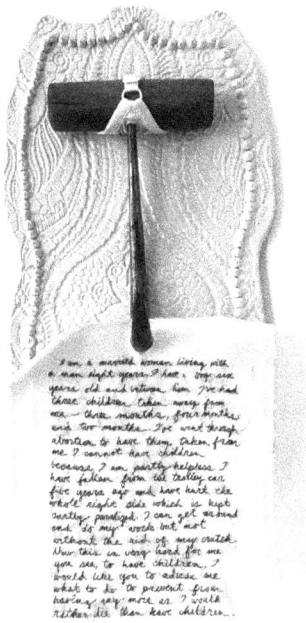

Figure 11.4 *Unplanned Parenthood 9*, 2023, porcelain, vintage wedding dress fabric, vintage meat hook, bra strap, embroidery floss.

foster social change (van Laar, 2019). Sewing serves as "a metaphor for repair, connection, and storytelling" (Ferranto, 2023, p. 222), offering therapeutic benefits to those involved (Wolk & Orr, 2023). Using needle and thread to document history allows participants to listen to stories in a more personal and intimate environment, while the rhythmic, bilateral movements of stitching can be a calming way to process emotions (Leone, 2020).

Mother's right

Mother's Right is an installation and performance piece created to raise awareness about maternal mortality, postpartum PTSD, and the impact of racism on U.S. maternal health outcomes. For this project, I worked with a group of volunteers, including midwives, doulas, mothers, and college students. We sewed 1,200 hospital gowns, one for every person who died from pregnancy or childbirth-related causes in 2013.

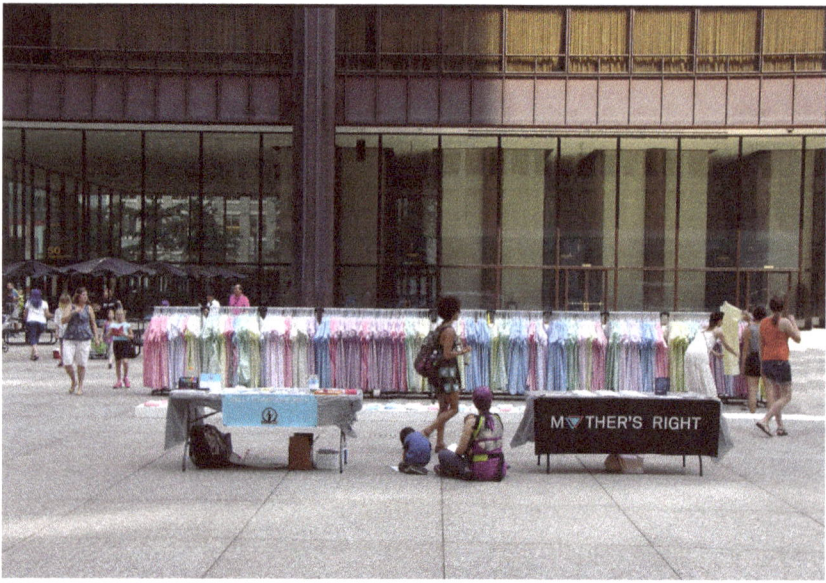

Figure 11.5 *Mother's Right*, 2015, 1,200 handmade hospital gowns.

The fabric for the gowns was screen printed with small images of the plant derivatives of drugs that have been given to pregnant people throughout history, often to the detriment of both those who have received the drugs and their babies.

The hospital gowns not only represent the deaths of those who died during childbirth, but also serve as commentary on the institutionalization of childbirth in the United States, which has had both positive and negative influences on maternal health outcomes (Shajarizadeh & Grépin, 2022). The history of hospital gowns is intertwined with the evolution of healthcare practices and societal attitudes toward illness and childbirth. Hospital gowns, as we know them today, have undergone significant transformations over time, reflecting changes in medical technology, hygiene standards, and cultural perceptions of modesty and privacy (Kaur & Brar, 2017). Hospital gowns often evoke feelings of vulnerability, loss of control, and lack of privacy among patients (Morton et al., 2020). They are symbolic of the institutionalized nature of maternal healthcare, which has significantly changed the way people give birth (Peahl & Howell, 2021). The pathologizing of childbirth

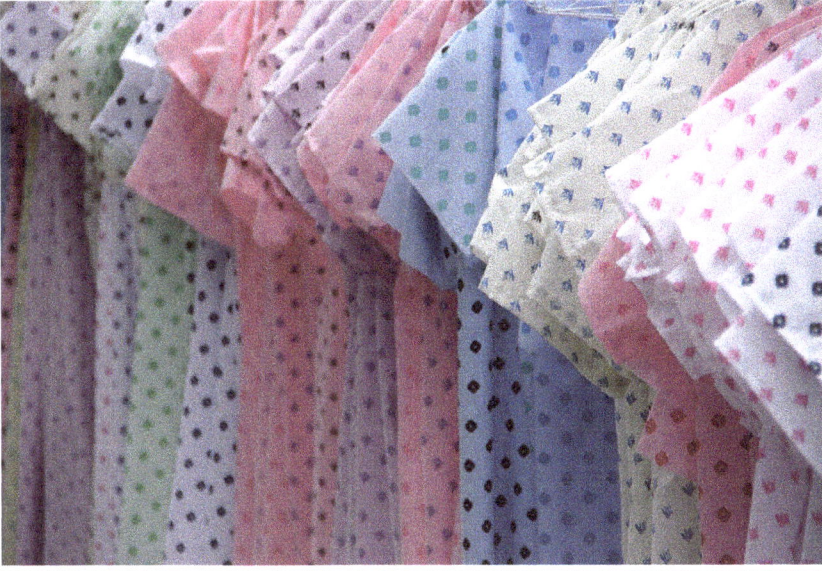

Figure 11.6 *Mother's Right*, detail of hospital gowns.

often leads to unnecessary medical interventions (Johanson et al., 2002) that are not backed up by evidence-based medicine. The rising prevalence of C-sections in the United States is alarming due to the substantial risks associated with this major surgical procedure (Ledbetter, 2023) and its impacts on postpartum recovery, making it challenging for birthing people to care for their newborns effectively (Li et al., 2021).

Mother's Right incorporates a performance that engages the audience and invites volunteers to stand facing each other and fold all 1,200 gowns into triangles, appropriating the flag folding ceremony used at the funerals for former military service members. This ritual performance symbolically highlights the fact that many people come out of childbirth with postpartum PTSD, presenting the same psychological symptoms as those who have fought in wars (Martínez-Vazquez et al., 2021). Obstetric violence, one of the causes of postpartum PTSD, is a form of medical abuse that disproportionately affects marginalized communities (Grilo Diniz et al., 2018) and is finally being acknowledged in the medical community (Garcia, 2023). Just like with abortion access, medical and healthcare institutions often prevent birthing people from fully exercising their rights to choose, as well as to receive, safe and necessary healthcare (Torrealba & Champagne, 2020). Postpartum depression in the United States has increased from 9.4% in 2010 to 19.3% in 2021 (Getahun et al., 2022). Many people who have given birth feel more conscious of other people's judgment and carry the weight of conforming to narrow definitions of motherhood, which can negatively impact their mental health. Art-based interventions can help reduce depression and anxiety in postpartum patients (Qian et al., 2023), as well as assist in processing birth experiences, mediating stress, and transitioning into new parenthood (Hogan, 2018).

In the spring of 2021, the *Mother's Right* gowns and performance were showcased at the Association of Women's Health Obstetric and Neonatal Nurses convention to shed light on racism within maternal healthcare. This performance entailed the ironing of a black armband onto the gowns, symbolizing the disproportionate number of Black people in 2020 who lost their lives while giving birth. Spanning across two days, the performance sparked numerous conversations among nurses directly involved in caring for women during difficult and life-threatening childbirths. Childbirth disproportionately affects marginalized communities, particularly Black and Indigenous birthing people, who face higher rates of maternal mortality compared to their White counterparts (Njoku et al., 2023). Structural racism within the healthcare system, including biases among healthcare providers and disparities in access to quality care, exacerbates these disparities (Harrigan-Farrelly, 2022).

Black, pregnant, and detained

In the spring of 2021, I was commissioned by the Refugee and Immigrant Center for Education and Legal Services (RAICES) to work on a collaboration with photographer Akilah Townsend and participants who identified as women and who shared their experiences as pregnant individuals detained by the U.S. Immigration and Customs Enforcement (ICE). This project, named *Black, Pregnant, and Detained*, was created for RAICES' Mother's Day campaign, which was aimed at raising awareness about the surge in ICE detentions of pregnant women, particularly under the policies enacted during the Trump administration. In stark contrast to the guidelines established in 2016 by the Obama administration, which reserved detention for pregnant immigrants only under

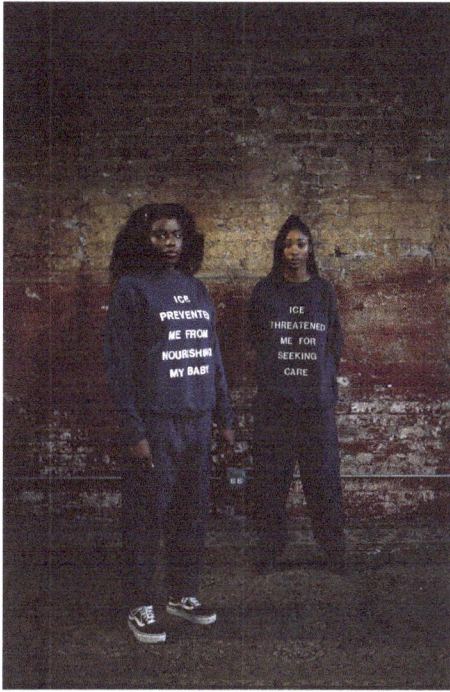

Figure 11.7 Black, Pregnant and Detained, 2021, embroidered garments.

extraordinary circumstances, ICE arrested over 4,000 undocumented pregnant individuals between 2016 and 2021 (Sullivan, 2021).

RAICES, along with various immigration advocacy groups, lodged a complaint with the Department of Homeland Security regarding the treatment of pregnant immigrants in detention centers, highlighting instances of pregnant detainees being deprived of essential medical attention. These accounts served as the foundation for the project, which was created by RAICES as part of their efforts to raise awareness about the detainment of pregnant people.

Collaborating with RAICES and women directly affected by ICE detentions, I created a series of garments adorned with embroidered quotes extracted from their testimonies. Their words were embroidered onto sweat suits, replicas of the garments they were required to wear as detainees. Akilah Townsend photographed the women wearing the garments I had embellished. Through embroidering the women's words onto these garments, we sought to reclaim agency and dignity for people whose voices had been silenced and whose bodies were subjected to the oppressive forces of patriarchy and systemic racism. The garments became a means for bearing witness to injustices faced by pregnant individuals detained by ICE.

On July 9, 2021, shortly following the complaint RAICES and several other agencies filed against the government, a significant milestone was achieved when the Biden administration announced measures to bar ICE from detaining pregnant or nursing individuals, except under "exceptional circumstances" (Sullivan, 2021). This development marked a crucial step forward in the fight for reproductive justice and human rights. Through this project we harnessed the power of clothing not only as a means of expression, but also as a vehicle for advocacy and social change.

To create a more profound impact, it is essential for art therapists to engage more deeply in activist work. By doing so, they can work toward transforming the systemic issues that underpin their clients' struggles. Arts activism in community settings can complement therapeutic practices and offer transformative healing (Frostig-Newton, 2011).

Conclusion

As art therapists and artists navigating the complexities of the socio-political landscape and its potential intersections with art and activism, may we continue to harness the power of creativity to illuminate truths, inspire change, and forge a path toward a more just and compassionate society. It is important for art therapists to consider the role socio-political issues play in their clients' lives, and incorporate arts activism into their practices. When clothing is used as a medium in a therapeutic setting, it can be a potent symbol of resistance and resilience, serving as a canvas for storytelling, reclaiming agency, and challenging oppressive norms. From the embroidered quotes adorning replica detention center garments to the transformation of hospital gowns into symbols of systemic injustices within the American healthcare system, clothing becomes a powerful tool for amplifying marginalized voices and advocating for social change. In the face of uncertainty and upheaval, art remains a beacon of hope, offering solace, healing, and a call to action for a world where all voices are heard, valued, and celebrated.

References

Adam, H., & Galinsky, A. D. (2012). Enclothed cognition. *Journal of Experimental Social Psychology, 48*(4), 918–925. https://doi.org/10.1016/j.jesp.2012.02.008

Belluck, P., & Ploeg, L. (2023, May 16). What to know about the Comstock act. *The New York Times.* https://www.nytimes.com/2023/05/16/us/comstock-act-1978-abortion-pill.html

Brown, P. (2020, December 16). Gone but never forgotten in a quilt. *The New York Times.* https://www.nytimes.com/2020/12/16/arts/design/quilt-art-women-injustice.html

Choi, A. (2024, January 22). Record number of anti-LGBTQ bills were introduced in 2023. *CNN.* https://www.cnn.com/politics/anti-lgbtq-plus-state-bill-rights-dg/index.html

Choi, A., & Cole, D. (2024, April 26). See where abortions are banned and legal—and where it's still in limbo. *CNN.* https://www.cnn.com/us/abortion-access-restrictions-bans-us-dg/index.html

Day, S., & Harper, K. (2022, February 28). Transgender Texas kids are terrified after governor orders that parents be investigated for child abuse. *The Texas Tribune.* https://www.texastribune.org/2022/02/28/texas-transgender-child-abuse/#:~:text=In%202019%2C%20Abbott%20and%20Paxton,of%20parents%20of%20transgender%20children

Ferguson, D. (2024, March 23). Medieval Christian misogyny shapes how we judge women today, says scholar. *The Guardian.* https://www.theguardian.com/education/2024/mar/23/medieval-christian-misogyny-shapes-how-we-judge-women-today-says-scholar

Ferranto, J. (2023). Vulva education through fiber arts: The +cunt project. *Art Therapy, 40*(4), 220–224. https://doi.org/10.1080/07421656.2023.2206778

Frostig-Newton, K. (2011). Arts activism: Praxis in social justice, critical discourse, and radical modes of engagement. *Art Therapy, 28*(2), 50–56. https://doi.org/10.1080/07421656.2011.578028

Fry, G. (1990). *Stitched from the soul: Slave quilts from the antebellum South.* University of North Carolina Press.

Garcia, L. M. (2023). Obstetric violence in the United States and other high-income countries: An integrative review. *Sex Reproductive Health Matters, 31*(1). https://doi.org/10.1080/26410397.2024.2322194

Getahun, D. Oyelese, Y., Peltier, M., Mensah, N., Avila, C., & Fassett, M. (2022). Trends in postpartum depression by race/ethnicity and pre-pregnancy body mass index. *American Journal of Obstetrics and Gynecology, 228*(1). https://doi.org/10.1016/j.ajog.2022.11.248

Golub, D. (2005). Social action art therapy. *Art Therapy, 22*(1), 17–23. https://doi.org/10.1080/07421656.2005.10129467

Grilo Diniz, C. S., Rattner, D., Lucas d'Oliveira, A. F. P., de Aguiar, J. M., & Niy, D. Y. (2018). Disrespect and abuse in childbirth in Brazil: social activism, public policies and providers' training. *Reproductive Health Matters, 26*(53), 19–35. https://doi.org/10.1080/09688080.2018.1502019

Hardy, S., & Monypenny, J. (2019). Queering queer spaces: Journey of a creative arts program for trans, non-binary, and gender creative youth. *Voices: A World Forum for Music Therapy, 19*(3). https://doi.org/10.15845/voices.v19i3.2687

Harrigan-Farrelly, J. (2022, February 7). For Black women, implicit racial bias in medicine may have far-reaching effects. *U.S. Department of Labor Blog.* https://blog.dol.gov/2022/02/07/for-black-women-implicit-racial-bias-in-medicine-may-have-far-reaching-effects

Hogan, S. (2018). *The birth project: Using the arts to explore birth.* Arts & Humanities Research Council, UK. https://www.derby.ac.uk/media/derbyacuk/assets/departments/business-services/documents/65835-The-Birth-Project.pdf

Jin, H., Restar, A. Goedel, W. C., Ogunbajo, A., Biello, K., Operario, D., Kuhns, L., Reisner, S. L., Garofalo, R., & Mimaga, M. J. (2020). Maternal support is protective against suicidal ideation among a diverse cohort of young transgender women. *LGBT Health, 7*(7), 349–357. https://doi.org/10.1089/lgbt.2020.0219

Johanson, R., Newburn, M., & Macfarlane, A. (2002). Has the medicalization of childbirth gone too far? *The BMJ.* https://doi.org/10.1136/bmj.324.7342.892

Kaur, R., & Brar, P. (2017). Design and development of novel patient garments: A review paper. *International Journal of Home Science, 3*(2), 553–555. https://www.homesciencejournal.com/archives/2017/vol3issue2/PartI/3-2-102-512.pdf

LaBar, L. (2021). Maine quilts: 250 years of comfort and community. *Down East Books.*

Ledbetter, A. (2023, July 21). C-section rates are way too high. We need to hold doctors and hospitals accountable. *Scientific American.* https://www.scientificamerican.com/article/c-section-rates-are-way-too-high-we-need-to-hold-doctors-and-hospitals-accountable/#:~:text=A%20study%20of%20194%20World,million%20unnecessary%20surgeries%20every%20year

Leone, L. (2020). *Craft in art therapy: Diverse approaches to the transformative power of craft materials and methods.* Routledge.

Li, L., Wan, W., & Zhu, C. (2021). Breastfeeding after a cesarean section: A literature review. *Midwifery, 103.* https://doi.org/10.1016/j.midw.2021.103117

Martínez-Vazquez, S., Rodríguez-Almagro, J., Hernández-Martínez, A., Delgado-Rodríguez, M., & Martínez-Galiano, J. M. (2021). Long-term high risk of postpartum post-traumatic stress disorder (PTSD) and associated factors. *Journal of Clinical Medicine, 10*(3), 488. https://doi.org/10.3390/jcm10030488

Morton, L., Cogan, N., Kornfält, S., Porter, Z., & Georgiadis, E. (2020). Baring all: The impact of the hospital gown on patient well-being. *British Journal of Health Psychology, 25.* https://doi.org/10.1111/bjhp.12416

Njoku, A., Evans, M., Nimo-Sefah, L., & Bailery, J. (2023). Listen to the whispers before they become screams: Addressing Black maternal morbidity and mortality in the United States. *Healthcare (Basel), 11*(3), 438. https://doi.org/10.3390/healthcare11030438

Peahl, A. F., & Howell, J. D. (2021). The evolution of prenatal care delivery guidelines in the United States. *American Journal of Obstetrics and Gynecology, 224*(4), 339–347. https://doi.org/10.1016/j.ajog.2020.12.016

Qian, J., Sun, S., Wang, M., Sun, X., & Yu, X. (2023). Art-based interventions for women's mental health in pregnancy and postpartum: A meta-analysis of randomized controlled trials. *Frontiers in Psychiatry, 14*(1112951). https://doi.org/10.3389/fpsyt.2023.1112951

Robertson, K., & Vinebaum, L. (2016). Crafting community. *Textile, 14*(1), 42–473. https://doi.org/10.1080/14759756.2016.1084794

Ross, C. (1991). Marriage and the sense of control. *Journal of Marriage and Family, 53*(4), 831–838. https://doi.org/10.2307/352990

Sanger, M. (1928). *Motherhood in bondage.* Brentano's.

Shajarizadeh, A., & Grépin, K. A. (2022). The impact of institutional delivery on neonatal and maternal health outcomes: Evidence from a road upgrade programme in India. *BMJ Global Health, 7*(7). https://doi.org/10.1136/bmjgh-2021-007926

Smith, B. (2020, July 20). Until Black women are free, none of us will be free. *The New Yorker.* https://www.newyorker.com/news/our-columnists/until-black-women-are-free-none-of-us-will-be-free

Steinberg, J. (2024). Mental health symptoms when abortion access is restricted. *JAMA*, *331*(4), 289–291. https://doi.org/10.1001/jama.2023.26816

Stewart, N. (2020, July 21). Planned Parenthood in N.Y. disavows Margaret Sanger over eugenics. *The New York Times*. https://www.nytimes.com/2020/07/21/nyregion/planned-parenthood-margaret-sanger-eugenics.html

Sullivan, E. (2021, July 9). Biden will end detention of most pregnant and postpartum undocumented immigrants. *The New York Times*. https://www.nytimes.com/2021/07/09/us/politics/pregnant-postpartum-immigration-biden.html

Suzuki, S., Hoyt, L. T., Yazdani, N., Kornbluh, M., Hope, E. C., Hagan, M. J., Cohen, A. K., & Ballard, P. J. (2023). Trajectories of sociopolitical stress during the 2020 United States presidential election season: Associations with psychological well-being, civic action, and social identities. *Comprehensive Psychoneuroendocrinology, 16*, 3–6. https://doi.org/10.1016/j.cpnec.2023.100218

Tajuddin, F. N. (2018). Cultural and social identity in clothing matters: "Different cultures, different meanings." *European Journal of Behavioral Sciences, 1*(4), 21–25. https://doi.org/10.33422/EJBS.2018.07.63

Tordoff, D. M., Wanta, J. W., Collin, A., Stepney, C., Inwards-Breland, D. J., & Ahrens, K. (2022). Mental health outcomes in transgender and nonbinary youths receiving gender-affirming care. *JAMA Network Open, 5*(2). https://doi.org/10.1001/jamanetworkopen.2022.0978

Torrealba, D. B., & Champagne, F. (2020). *Therapeutic arts in pregnancy, birth and new parenthood*. Routledge.

van Laar, C. (2019). Seeing her stories: Finding a place in the landscape of art therapy literature. *Australian and New Zealand Journal of Arts Therapy, 14*(1), 15–25.

Whitehead, A. L., & Perry, S. L. (2019). Is a "Christian America" a more patriarchal America? Religion, politics, and traditional gender ideology. *Canadian Review of Sociology, 56*(2), 151–177. https://doi.org/10.1111/cars.12241

Wolk, N., & Or, M. B. (2023). The therapeutic aspects of embroidery in art therapy from the perspective of adolescent girls in a post-hospitalization boarding school. *Children (Basel), 10*(6). https://doi.org/10.3390/children10061084

Yi, C. S. (2020). The crip couture manifesto. *Wordgathering: A Journal of Disability Poetry and Literature, 14*(4). https://wordgathering.com/vol14/issue4/disability-futures/yi/

12

DRAWING CONNECTIONS

COMICS IN ART THERAPY PRACTICE

Rakshanda Khan

Comics as a medium for art therapy

Comics have been defined as a combination of sequential text and images that convey information, evoke meaning, and express emotion through multimodal visual and word-based literacies (Jacobs, 2007; McCloud, 1994; Rifkind et al., 2019). They have been effectively used as educational, informational, reflective, and storytelling mediums within communication, journalism, research, public health, education, law, and art therapy, among other professions (Botzakis et al., 2017; Czerwiec et al., 2015; Fernandez & Lina, 2020; Green & Myers, 2010; Huxtable et al., 2022; McCreight, 2018; Moretti, 2023; Phang, 2023; Speigel et al., 2013; Wisenthal, 2017). Comics have been used to narrate and advocate for lived experiences related to loss, illness, disability, and pathology (Czerwiec et al., 2015; Finlay, 2019; Fishman, 2015; Scavarda & Moretti, 2024). They also aid in representing and supporting the expression and processing of emotional, medical, and physical challenges (Haines & Standing, 2015; Hershler et al., 2021; Lucas-Falk, 2010; McCreight, 2018; Phang, 2023).

In enabling the describable and inexpressible to join on the page so that disparate yet interconnected visceral experiences can co-exist, comics allow for a more genuine encounter with disability, illness, and underreported lived experiences (Thaller, 2017). They are ideally suited to portray

 DOI: 10.4324/9781032720166-14

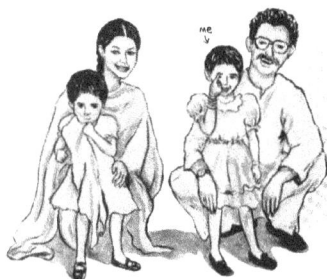

I AM A NEUROTYPICAL CISGENDER FEMALE, SOUTH ASIAN SETTLER, AND IMMIGRANT TO TKARONTO, CANADA, WHO WAS BORN IN KARACHI, PAKISTAN.

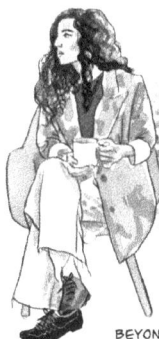

MY CHILDHOOD IN THE '80S AND '90S WAS FILLED WITH LONG, HOT SUMMERS SPENT ABSORBED IN COMICS.

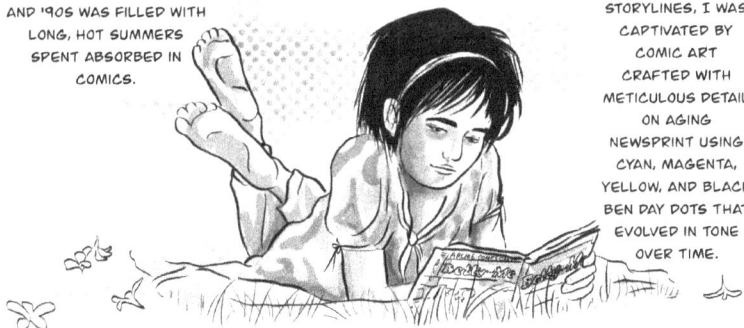

BEYOND THE STORYLINES, I WAS CAPTIVATED BY COMIC ART CRAFTED WITH METICULOUS DETAIL ON AGING NEWSPRINT USING CYAN, MAGENTA, YELLOW, AND BLACK BEN DAY DOTS THAT EVOLVED IN TONE OVER TIME.

I DEVELOPED MY ILLUSTRATION SKILLS BY COPYING THE COMIC CHARACTERS AND THE PRECISION WITH WHICH THEY APPEARED ON EACH PANEL.

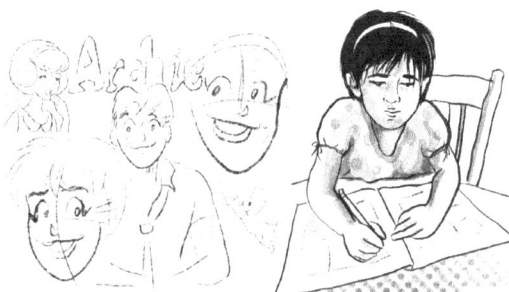

DESPITE MY LOVE FOR COMICS, THE WORLDS THEY DEPICTED RARELY MIRRORED MY OWN EXPERIENCES.

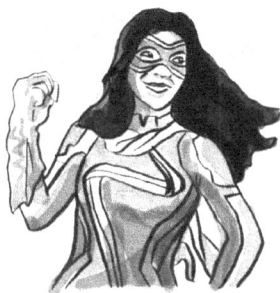

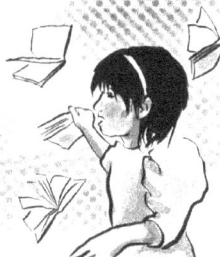

IT NEVER CROSSED MY MIND THAT A PAKISTANI SUPERHERO LIKE KAMALA KHAN (MS. MARVEL) WOULD ONE DAY EMERGE WITHIN THE COMIC UNIVERSE.

I GRADUALLY BEGAN CRAFTING MY OWN COMICS, PORTRAYING THEMES AND ELEMENTS FROM MY LIFE THAT I DIDN'T SEE REPRESENTED ELSEWHERE

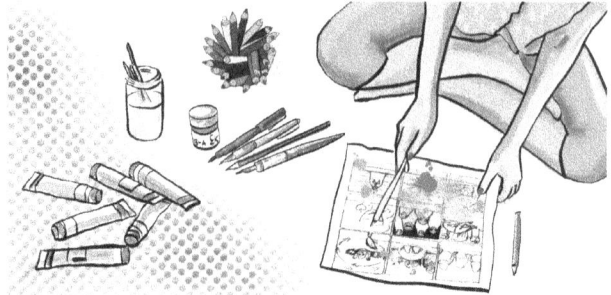

UPON IMMIGRATING TO CANADA AS A NEW MOTHER, I STARTED CHRONICLING MY IMMIGRATION JOURNEY THROUGH COMICS.

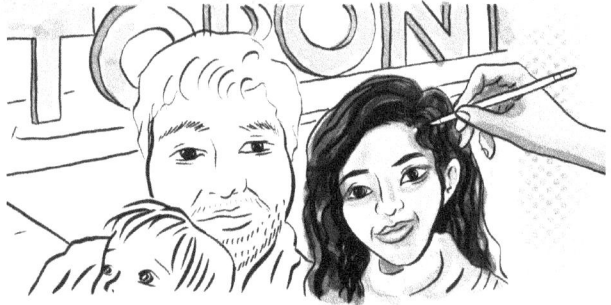

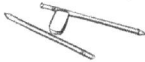

THIS MEDIUM PROVIDED ME WITH A MEANS TO DOCUMENT AND CONVEY THE GAINS AND LOSSES ASSOCIATED WITH MY NEW ROLES

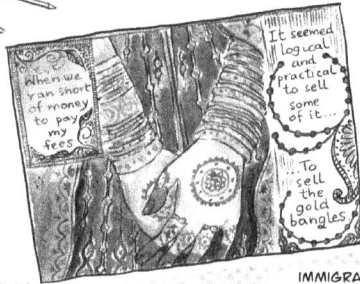

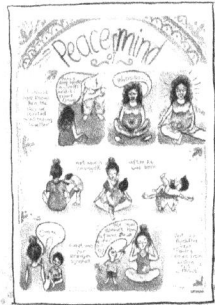

AS A STUDENT

IMMIGRANT

AND PARENT

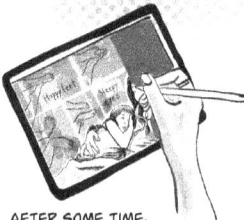

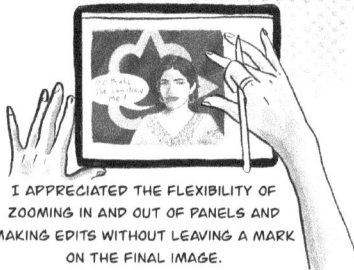

NOW, AS AN ART THERAPIST, I INTEGRATE COMICS INTO MY THERAPEUTIC APPROACH. THIS CHAPTER REFLECTS MY LEARNINGS AND EXPERIENCES.

AFTER SOME TIME, I TRANSITIONED TO CREATING DIGITAL COMICS.

I APPRECIATED THE FLEXIBILITY OF ZOOMING IN AND OUT OF PANELS AND MAKING EDITS WITHOUT LEAVING A MARK ON THE FINAL IMAGE.

accounts of mental illness that go beyond the limits of spoken language, such as the fragmented flashbacks associated with traumatic experiences (Hershler et al., 2021; Thaller, 2017).

People who read comics interpret them by responding to the tensions between image and text, sequence and surface, and time and space through macro-reading and micro-reading processes (del Rey Cabero, 2019). To construct meaning when reading comics, readers position themselves in the role of co-author of the text (Botzakis et al., 2017). This encourages individuals to approach the text with empathy, potentially leading to a profound, emotionally resonant experience.

Phenomenological encounters with comics in art therapy invite client engagement with aspects of the self, such as perceptions, experiences, beliefs, or emotions (McCreight, 2018; Mulholland, 2004). For example, Hershler et al. (2021) created a comics-based resource and clinician reference guide that highlights salient features of key concepts in trauma treatment. This illustrated toolkit incorporates metaphor rich visuals and worksheets to deliver psychoeducation on the impact of trauma. I have used this resource with clients, and some have especially identified with a comic titled *Parallel Lives*. The comic depicts a human figure walking on a pier, with text above that reads "here and now." The figure stumbles on an object labeled "something happens (trigger)" and slips into the water below the pier. As seaweed wraps around its leg the figure becomes submerged in the "there and then," eventually curled up in a ball with its head down, trapped and entangled. With concerted effort, the figure bursts through its restraints and climbs out of the water, gasping for breath. My clients have conveyed that this symbolism accurately reflects their experience of involuntarily recalling traumatic memories and losing present moment awareness. A client's emotional resonance with this comic oftentimes leads to psychoeducational discourse and increased understanding of the neurobiological impact of trauma on the body.

In another psychoeducational resource, Haines and Standing (2015) employ inventive imagery and simple descriptions to communicate experiences of dissociation, fight and flight responses, and the organization of traumatic experiences as visual images and physical sensations. Resources like these help clients demystify perplexing implicit, embodied impulses and somatosensory memories of past traumatic events.

Julia Dachez's (2020) and Rees Finlay's (2019) accounts of being diagnosed with autism in adulthood depict daily experiences of navigating a sensorially saturated and vitality depleting world with people who often misunderstand and marginalize them. These stories present autism as a complex and multifaceted identity rather than a rigid set of symptoms, challenging stereotypes and promoting counter-narratives to medical models of disability (Scavarda & Moretti, 2024; Walker, 2021).

Comics and graphic novels, such as the ones described above, create opportunities for multilinear ways of engaging with novel or complex ideas (del Rey Cabero, 2019). A bibliotherapeutic approach, in conjunction with artmaking in response to comic literature, is one way art therapists can guide clients into engaging relationally with thematic concepts of identity or biopsychosocial models of wellness (McCreight, 2018).

Although artworks created in art therapy usually focus on a single image at a time, the construction of sequential artworks has proven to be equally, if not more, effective for working through problems (Phang, 2023). When clients create sequential art, the development and manipulation of characters and the exploration of narrative possibilities and outcomes allow for a sense of control and agency. Comics offer a structure whereby the interaction of characters dialoguing in metaphorical settings can support the development of affect consciousness, multiple points of view, psychological awareness, empathy, and mindfulness (Havsteen-Franklin, 2016). Clients' use of language and metaphor within the comic frame is a bridge through which what is yet unknown to the individual can become familiar (Carpendale, 2009). The creation of fictional or fantastical settings and storylines, archetypal figures, and dramatic action is an opportunity to conceptualize themes and tropes as self-symbols and allegories for intrapsychic conflicts (Mulholland, 2004). By assembling comic narratives, individuals can communicate, reframe, and recontextualize negative thinking processes, identify internal resources, and explicate coping methods that support emotional regulation (Fernandez & Lina, 2020; Fishman, 2015; Johansson & Hannula, 2014; Shilling, 2013). Easily incorporated into therapeutic frameworks such as Cognitive Behavioral Therapy, Internal Family Systems, Narrative Therapy, and Mentalization, comics externalize and organize cognition, sensation, and affect (Fernandez & Lina, 2020; Gallardo, 2011; Khan, 2021b; Mardou Draws, n.d.; Mulholland, 2004; Phang, 2023; Song et al., 2022).

Composing sequential narratives

Comics can accommodate a diverse range of drawing skills, from stick figures to hyper-realistic representations, for purposes of fictional or personal storytelling (Shwed, 2016). When creating a comic's story space, the creator is faced with decisions regarding the composition, shape, and size of the panels, framing, borders, gutter space, word balloons, captions, and other aspects of the comic that inform the style and subject of the work (Grant, 2019; Shwed, 2016).

Art therapists can facilitate clients' comic compositions by providing a range of paper sizes and art materials, closely observing clients' preferences as well as the steps they take toward assembling their visual narrative. Additionally, therapists can offer comic page templates, graphic elements such as magazine cut-outs and printouts of shapes, settings, characters, and dialogue, and story prompts to facilitate the client's internal and external creative process (Shwed, 2016). Mixed-media such as stickers, stencils, textured paper, textiles, print labels, masking tape, washi tape, yarn, cardboard, etc., can all be included in the panels of a comic, supporting abstract problem solving, ordering, and containing of affect (Hinz, 2020). Therapists can direct clients' focus to expressive elements such as emotional tone, movement, setting, presence and absence, contextual congruence, figure and ground relationships, use of space, color, size and shape, intensity, boundaries, and perspective, as well as symbolic content (Carpendale, 2009).

Clients may seek to discover, match, or represent an inner rhythm or facilitate mindfulness through the sequential patterning of the comic (Hinz, 2020). Some young clients enjoy sequencing their comics in unconventional ways, numbering panels so the reader must visually move up, down, and across the comic page. Creating their own rules for how the story is experienced may be a way to feel more in control of their narrative.

Art therapists can observe clients' somatic responses during the art-making process, noting how body movement correlates with the embodied intensity of their narratives, as captured within compact comic panels (Grant, 2019). The size and dimensions of the drawing surface and the constraints of a comic panel can influence the creative process, forcing adaptation, causing varied kinesthetic experiences, and sometimes resulting in a shift in the visual language (Grant, 2019). This psychosomatic experience is vividly described by Grant (2019):

> Conceptually the story seems enormous to me. It is like a dark liquid that fills me up, stretching my skin and making my head throb. To get the story out I feel the need to make big melodramatic gestures. My impulse is to wail and thrash. I want to spatter ink in violent streaks. But the marks of dark liquid must be released through a set of miniature movements. There is only 10 cm of lateral movement and 15 cm of vertical movement on the boards. I cannot change the proportions of my body, and neither can I change the proportions of the little cards. My whole body clenches. I make delicate traces over the pencil lines with the tip of the brush moving only my fingers and wrists.
>
> (pp. 6–7)

Storytelling with digital comics

The tactile, relational, and kinesthetic experiences of digital comics have parallels to—and differences from—traditional comics. For example, digital artmaking tools, such as illustration apps, create computer-generated representations of physical artmaking experiences. A finger or digital pen used on the screen of a digital device can simulate splattering watercolors onto a canvas, minus the sensation of wet paint on one's skin.

Evolving alongside digital technology, digital comics offer a range of possibilities through animation, sound, and interactive features, bringing stories to life. Alt-texts, text that appears when scrolling over images, and *hypercomics* (webcomics in which reader's choices influence the sequence and outcomes of events) are interactive forms of digital comics that incorporate multiple narrative structures (Goodbrey, 2013). Defined by McCloud (2009) as a medium with an *infinite canvas*, webcomics offer room for creative exploration that extends page and print formats, although most webcomics continue to follow a page-by-page structure.

When published as a series, webcomic blogs can have a positive social impact. In her webcomic, *Hyperbole and a Half*, Allie Brosh illustrated her personal experience of depression, including how it interfered with her daily activities and the self-criticisms it elicited (Misemer, 2017).

She received multiple responses from people who said it was reassuring for them to see their experiences made visible and to participate in public discussions about mental health concerns. Her comics blog built an online community of individuals who came together over a shared struggle (Misemer, 2017).

Jamerson (2017) incorporated digital comics into *Expressive Remix Group*, a multimodal expressive therapy approach for youth from Los Angeles at risk of gang involvement. Over a 13-week timeframe, Jamerson facilitated arts-based projects using traditional art media in combination with digital technologies. He drew upon remixing as a metaphor for clients' integration of multiple forms of narrative—such as poetry, song lyrics, and stories—through digital technology. The clients incorporated digital storytelling, mask making, animation, comics, magazine covers, movie posters, and the creation of a virtual world, culminating in a "creative showcase theatre" (p. 279) for friends and family members of participants.

The magic circle of comics

The concept of the *magic circle* illuminates the role of comics and digital applications in art therapy. Coined by game theorist Johan Huizinga (1938/1949), the magic circle refers to the space and time in which individuals engage in play or imaginative activities. Within this distinct, temporal, imaginal circle, individuals are free to explore their thoughts, emotions, and experiences without fear of judgment or consequence (Snyder, 2021). The boundaries of reality are suspended, allowing for a deeper and more meaningful exploration of the self.

Within a therapeutic context, the therapist co-creates the magic circle with their client, mirroring the client's experiences, identifying emotions, and gently supporting the client as they risk vulnerability and test new ways of coping (Snyder, 2021).

Within comics, the magic circle may include the page layout, the comic panels, the expressive and evocative potential of the art materials used, and the physical space within which the creative encounter between client, artwork, and therapist takes place. It is the liminal play space of relatedness within which a client's emotional content and fantastical imaginings can be made visible and their fears can be countered in a non-threatening manner.

Comics and the Expressive Therapies Continuum

The multimodal medium of comics can incorporate all four levels of the Expressive Therapies Continuum (ETC), a theoretical framework for understanding the types of information processing associated with various art media. Through dialogue, captions, and narration in comics, individuals can connect with the cognitive aspect of the ETC. Comics can activate the perceptual and symbolic components of the ETC through storytelling and character development. Traditional comics can evoke a sense of movement and action through illustration style, perspective, and composition. Panel arrangement and visual cues, such as motion lines and gestures, can convey a dynamic sense of movement. However, the kinesthetic involvement of the comic creator may be impacted by the type of art materials used. Digital comics can combine audio and visual elements for enhanced sensory engagement. As individuals engage in comic creation through visual storytelling, involvement in one art form can often catalyze creativity in others (Hinz, 2020). For instance, drawing can synergize with written expression and increase the potential for experiencing creative flow.

Comics in individual and group art therapy

Building a comic together with a client, jointly contemplating how best to represent each part of the narrative, offers opportunities for reflexive dialogue on what matters most to the client. Retelling their story in the presence of an empathic witness can empower clients to deconstruct problems and reconstruct alternative worldviews.

In my private practice, I have introduced comic art-based exercises for individual and group art therapy. Therapeutic goals have included establishing and strengthening the therapeutic alliance, emotional expression and regulation, exploration of self-image and identity, interpersonal relating, mentalization, revisiting past events from a strengths-based perspective, and increasing self-understanding and mindfulness (Khan, 2021b). Approaches to address some of these goals are discussed below.

Co-regulating with the collaborative comic jam

As I establish a therapeutic alliance in the initial two to three art therapy sessions, I often introduce *comic jam* (Bennett, 2022) exercises to
foster and augment co-regulation and client attunement. A comic jam
is a collaborative art exercise in which individuals take turns drawing
panels or pages for a single comic. I usually start by marking out panels on a large sheet of paper or printing a five- to seven-panel comic
template. I offer markers, sharpies, drawing pencils, and a black Pentel
Brush pen to clients, inviting them to draw the first panel. However, at
this early stage in our relationship, they often defer to me to begin the
comic. Taking into consideration the client's affect, level of comfort,
and therapeutic goals, I commence by drawing a prompt to initiate dialogue within the comic on the client's hopes and fears for therapy, their
perceived level of safety, and their relational fears or needs. Each panel
offers a bordered container for the client to name and identify their
needs in the present moment and be met with reciprocal and atten-
tive presence. This comic exchange explicates our developing relational
dynamics, fosters empathy and rapport, and enhances our felt sense of
each other. The comic jam exercise can continue for a few sessions and
be revisited at any time, when there is a need to repair ruptures in the
relationship, address power dynamics, or practice co-regulation and
relationship-building skills. It offers therapeutic containment and an
experience of accompaniment for clients attempting to unearth difficult
or distressing content.

Within groups, comic jams offer a playful check-in activity at the beginning of a session, as a means for participants to introduce themselves and
prepare for collective artmaking. The exercise lends itself to relationship
building, establishing group cohesion, practicing appropriate boundaries,
and externalizing group dynamics. Online artmaking tools offer collaborative platforms for drawing comics onscreen.

Chronicling communal experiences with a textile story comic

The comics medium offers many mixed-media possibilities, including
fiber art. Groensteen (as cited in Nordenstam & Wictorin, 2022) emphasizes the continually changing medium of comics throughout its history,

identifying the popular format as the most recent one. Historically, story cloths or tapestries were created to tell collective stories (Miskin as cited in Nordenstam & Wictorin, 2022). Introducing fiber arts into comic-arts-based storytelling exercises can provide a kinesthetic and mindful means to process trauma (Hinz, 2020). Because textiles are familiar and intimate, they hold memories and experiences that are both personal and universal (Garlock, 2021; Homer, 2021).

In 2020, amid the global lockdowns prompted by the COVID-19 pandemic, I provided individual and group mental health support through telephonic and virtual conferencing. Working as a mental health professional during this time of collective trauma, I shared with my clients the experience of facing an invisible and unpredictable threat. Chronic, prolonged stress and pervasive instability weighed heavily upon many people's mental and physiological well-being.

To counter this debilitating psychological crisis, I initiated the creation of a textile story comic to document the year from January to December 2020, including both my own and my clients' encounters with the pandemic (Khan, 2021a). We all were social distancing, and yet we connected virtually from the most intimate of places, our homes. Clients shared their stories with me through audio and video recordings and photographs, which I integrated onto 12 sequential panels representing the months of the year. Layers of stitched textiles in combination with written text reflected the intermingling of individual experiences and the convergence of professional, social, and personal lives. Once completed, it allowed us to step back and focus on our individual and collective strengths, connecting us to our histories and to each other.

The word to image story and comic conversations

In addition to group collaborations, I have supported clients in crafting individual comic narratives. Topics have included school trips, conflicts with teachers, illness, body neutrality, interpersonal relationships, self-concept and identity, existentialism, immigration, video games, and relationships with technology. I sometimes invite clients to author a seven-sentence story about an event or conflict they would like to address. This provides an opportunity for them to draft a narrative adopting logical thought processes.

Next, they illustrate the written text in comic format. The transformation of words into sequential images requires analytical, symbolic, perceptual, affective, and creative thought processes that together can result in deeper emotional processing and therapeutic insights (Hinz, 2020; Khan, 2021b). For example, when I worked with a socially marginalized adolescent client, information not included in their initial word-based telling of their story emerged vividly in their comic. Through illustrating experiences of discrimination, bullying, and rejection in settings like a school and a public bus, the client situated their personal experience within a wider, social context. As a result, they gained heightened awareness of intersectional factors and worked toward reclaiming personal empowerment.

Introducing theory of mind (Brunet et al., 2003), mentalization, and/or intersectional thought processes can be facilitated by inviting clients to create several comics on the same event from differing perspectives. Clients can also visually represent social interactions and use comics to practice difficult conversations or improve communication skills (Gallardo, 2011).

Digital comic integrations

Digital comic creation requires some degree of comfort using digital technologies. In my experience, clients who express interest in creating digital comics in therapy either have prior experience with digital artmaking or are intrigued by the possibility of creating complex imagery with the ease artmaking apps or artificial intelligence (AI) offer. Digital comic creation can incorporate photographs, scans, and tracings. Clients can easily vary the size and dimensions of the panels and composition, use AI integrations to assist with illustrating the panels, and ensure continuity throughout the comic narrative.

Comic creation in VR invites the possibility of "walking through" the panels of a comic. Clients can create multiple artistic panels within limitless virtual space, housed within a background of their choice (e.g., floating in space, resting underwater, etc.). The comic can be viewed and experienced through immersion in and through the artwork, offering different perspectives and multidirectional ways of engaging with the content.

AN ART THERAPY WORKSHOP FOR NEURODIVERGENT ADULTS AT A SUPPORTED INDEPENDENT LIVING PROGRAM INVITED MENTALIZATION BASED APPROACHES TO INITIATING FRIENDSHIPS.

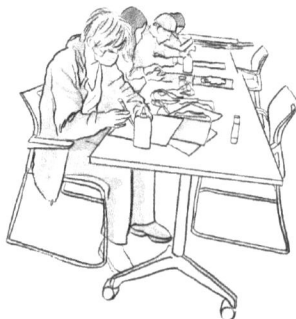

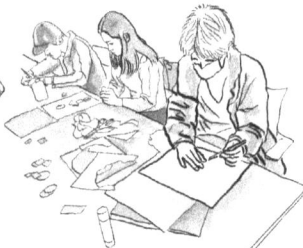

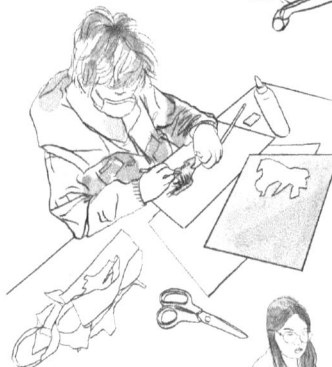

PARTICIPANTS DEVELOPED CHARACTER SKETCHES OF A PROTAGONIST AND A POTENTIAL FRIEND AS THEY DISCUSSED THEIR CHARACTERS' BACK STORIES AND INTERESTS WITHIN THE GROUP SETTING.

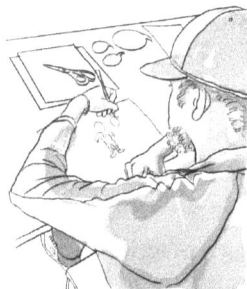

A SPORTY CHARACTER NAMED 'SWAGGY',

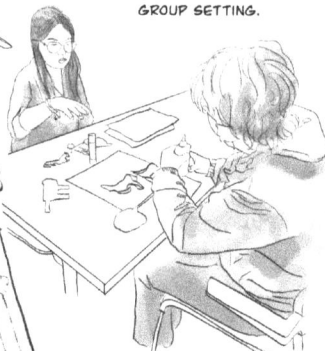

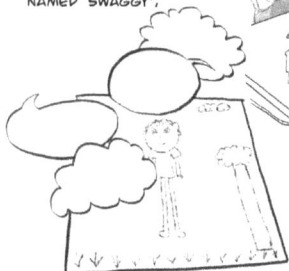

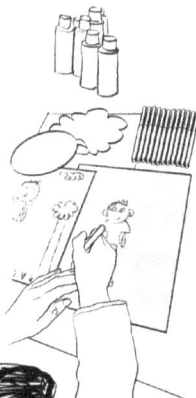

A BLACK HORSE WHO LIKES TO HEADBUTT,

A BABY WHALE WHO LIVES IN A POD WITH HIS MOTHER,

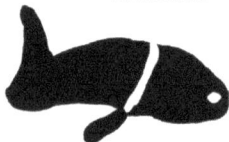

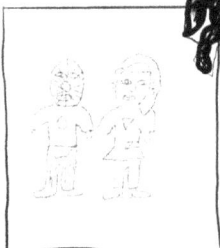

AND A 49-YEAR-OLD SPIDERMAN WERE IDEATED AND REPRESENTED ON 3 X 3 SQUARE PIECES OF CRAFT PAPER.

ART MATERIALS INCLUDED INDIVIDUAL 1 FT. X 4 FT. X 5.2 MM PIECES OF PLYWOOD, ACRYLIC PAINT, CRAFT PAPER, MARKERS, GLUE, SCISSORS AND DRAWING MATERIALS.

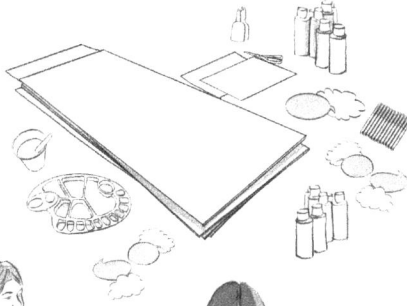

PAPER CUT OUTS OF SPEECH BUBBLES AND THOUGHT BALLOONS CREATED OPPORTUNITIES FOR PARTICIPANTS TO ARTICULATE THOUGHTS AND FEELINGS ACCOMPANYING INITIAL SOCIAL INTERACTIONS.

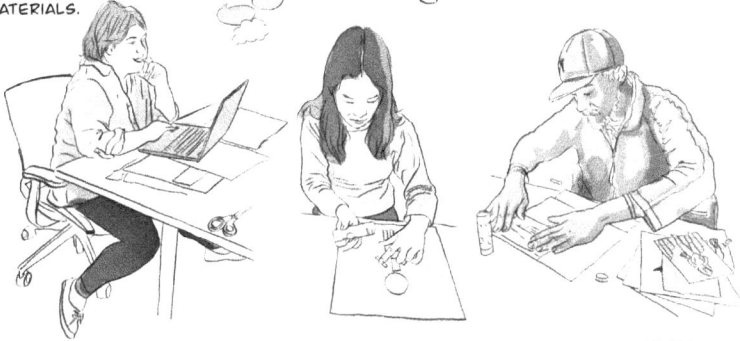

THE FINAL COMICS ON PLYWOOD PANELS FEATURED A COFFEE SHOP ENCOUNTER BETWEEN SPIDERMAN & WONDER WOMAN, SWAGGY'S INITIAL OUTINGS WITH A NEIGHBOUR, BAILEY THE HORSE'S EXPERIENCES ON A FARM, AND A LOST BABY WHALE'S RESCUE BY A HAMMERHEAD SHARK.

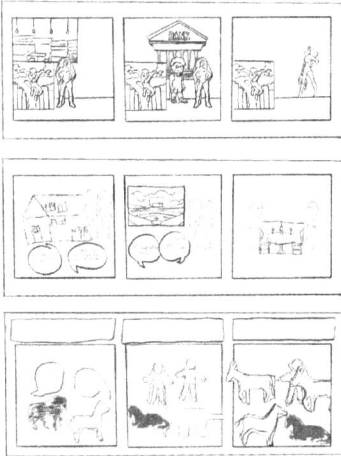

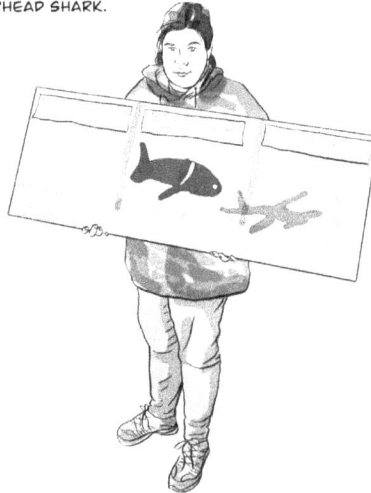

CONCEPTUALIZING THE COMIC CHARACTERS AND NARRATIVES INVITED PARTICIPANTS TO EXPLORE PERSONAL SYMBOLS AND METAPHORS. SEQUENCING THEM THROUGH WORDS AND IMAGES OFFERED A STRUCTURE TO VISUALLY REPRESENT AND PRACTISE SOCIAL INTERACTIONS. ACCOMPANYING DISCUSSIONS WITHIN A GROUP SETTING CREATED OPPORTUNITIES FOR EXPERIENCING UNIVERSALITY WHILE ALSO STRENGTHENING PEER RELATIONSHIPS.

Conclusion

Comics serve as portals into the transitional magic circle, inviting clients and therapists to co-author narratives and test new ways of coping, fostering deep connections and insight. In the context of art therapy, comics support a phenomenological encounter with the self. Through illustrating comic narratives, individuals can navigate complex themes such as identity and trauma. In group settings, comics become vehicles for communal storytelling that supports universality and allows group members to navigate the psychological and intersectional complexities of their lived experiences. Digital technologies, including virtual reality and AI, expand the boundaries of the magic circle, offering immersive and interactive experiences that blur the lines between reality and imagination. By channeling the potential of multimodal sequential storytelling, therapists can guide clients in expressive narrative processes that lead to greater internal and external well-being within their social systems and lived environments.

References

Bennett, M. (2022, July 15). *How to comics jam!* www.MarekBennett.com. https://marekbennett.com/2022/07/15/comicsjam/

Botzakis, S., Savitz, R., & Low, D. E. (2017). Adolescents reading graphic novels and comics: What we know from research. In K. A. Hinchman & D. Appleman (Eds.), *Adolescent literacies: A handbook of practice-based research* (pp. 310–322). Guilford Press.

Brunet, E., Sarfati, Y., Hardy-Baylé, M.-C., & Decety, J. (2003). Abnormalities of brain function during a nonverbal theory of mind task in schizophrenia. *Neuropsychologia, 41*(12), 1574–1582. https://doi.org/10.1016/s0028-3932(03)00119-2

Carpendale, M. (2009). *Essence and praxis in the art therapy studio.* Trafford On Demand Pub.

Czerwiec, M. K., Williams, I., Squier, S. M., Green, M. J., Myers, K. R., & Smith, S. T. (2015). *Graphic medicine manifesto.* Penn State Press.

Dachez, J., Caroline, M., Vaslet, F., & Gauvin, E. (2020). *Invisible differences: A story of asperger's, adulting, and living a life in full color.* Oni-Lion Forge Publishing.

del Rey Cabero, E. (2019). Beyond linearity: Holistic, multidirectional, multilinear and translinear reading in comics. *The Comics Grid: Journal of Comics Scholarship, 9*(1), 1–21. https://doi.org/10.16995/cg.137

Fernandez, K. T., & Lina, S. G. (2020). Draw me your thoughts: The use of comic strips as a cognitive behavioral therapy intervention. *Journal of Creativity in Mentalc Health, 15*(1), 17–29. https://doi.org/10.1080/15401383.2019.1638861

Finlay, R. (2019). *Reaffirmation: Coming to terms with an autism diagnosis.* Damn Dirty Comics.

Fishman, A. (2015, June 6). *Radiation gave me superpowers: Using autobiographical comics to relieve cancer-related anxiety in groups* [Paper presentation]. Symposium of

International Association for Social Work with Groups, University of North Carolina at Chapel Hill, United States.

Gallardo, L. (2011). Use of comic strip conversations: Therapeutic interventions producing positive outcomes for partially included children who have autism spectrum disorders. *Perspectives on School-Based Issues, 12*(3), 101–107. https://doi.org/10.1044/sbi12.3.101

Garlock, L. R. (2021). Making sense of the senseless through story cloths. In L. Leone (Ed.), *Craft in art therapy: Diverse approaches to the transformative power of craft materials and methods* (pp. 190–203). Routledge.

Goodbrey, D. M. (2013). From comic to hypercomic. In J. C. Evans & T. Giddens (Eds.), *Cultural excavation and formal expression in the graphic novel* (pp. 291–302). Inter-Disciplinary Press.

Grant, P. (2019). The board and the body: Material constraints and style in graphic narrative. *The Comics Grid: Journal of Comics Scholarship, 9*(1), 1–18. https://doi.org/10.16995/cg.145

Green, M. J., & Myers, K. R. (2010). Graphic medicine: Use of comics in medical education and patient care. *The British Medical Journal, 340*, 574–577. https://doi.org/10.1136/bmj.c863

Haines, S., & Standing, S. (2015). *Trauma is really strange*. Singing Dragon.

Havsteen-Franklin, D. (2016). Mentalization-based art psychotherapy. In J. Rubin (Ed.), *Approaches to art therapy: Theory and technique* (pp. 126–138). Routledge.

Hershler, A., Hughes, L., Nguyen, P., & Wall, S. (2021). *Looking at trauma: A tool kit for clinicians*. Penn State University Press.

Hinz, L. D. (2020). *Expressive therapies continuum: A framework for using art in therapy*. Routledge.

Homer, E. S. (2021). Embroidering pieces of place. In L. Leone (Ed.), *Craft in art therapy: Diverse approaches to the transformative power of craft materials and methods* (pp. 99–107). Routledge.

Huizinga, J. (1949). *Homo ludens: A study of the play-element in culture*. Routledge & Kegan Paul [Original work published 1938].

Huxtable, A. E., Bordonaro, G. P. W., & Schamke, L. (2022). *A graphic guide to art therapy*. Jessica Kingsley Publishers.

Jacobs, D. (2007). More than words: Comics as a means of teaching multiple literacies. *English Journal, 96*(3), 19–25. https://doi.org/10.2307/30047289

Jamerson, J. (2017). Expressive remix therapy: Using digital media art as a therapeutic intervention with transition-age youth. In S. L. Brooke (Ed.), *Combining the creative therapies with technology: Using social media and online counseling to treat clients* (pp. 74–84). Charles C Thomas Publisher.

Johansson, J., & Hannula, M. S. (2014). How do Finnish children express care and justice in comic strips and written narratives? *Journal of Moral Education, 43*, 516–531. https://doi.org/10.1080/03057240.2014.900481

Khan, R. (2021a, August 10). *Collective trauma and temporal experiences during COVID-19 pandemic* [Video]. YouTube. https://www.youtube.com/watch?v=pn9WROdAY-4

Khan, R. (2021b). Comics in online art therapy with Pakistani adolescents. *Canadian Journal of Art Therapy, 34*(1), 33–44. https://doi.org/10.1080/26907240.2021.1914988

Lucas-Falk, K. (2010). Comic books, connection, and the artist identity. In C. H. Moon (Ed.), *Materials and media in art therapy: Critical understandings of diverse artistic vocabularies* (pp. 231–255). Routledge.

Mardou Draws. (n.d). *Therapy session comics*. https://ifscomics.com/therapy-session-comics/

McCloud, S. (1994). *Understanding comics: The invisible art*. Tundra Publishing.

McCloud, S. (2009, February) *Webcomics*. Scottmccloud.com. https://www.scottmccloud.com/1-webcomics/index.html

McCreight, D. (2018, February 1). Creating comics with clients. *Counseling Today, 60*(8), 36–41. https://ctarchive.counseling.org/2018/02/creating-comics-clients/

Misemer, L. (2017, June 17). Webcomics building communities: Depression and visibility in hyperbole and a half [Conference session]. Graphic Medicine Conference, Seattle, WA. https://www.graphicmedicine.org/ wp-content/uploads/2017/05/Full-Conference-Program-1.pdf

Moretti, V. (2023). *Understanding comics–based research: A practical guide for social scientists.* Emerald Publishing Limited.

Mulholland, M. J. (2004). Comics as art therapy. *Art Therapy, 21*(1), 42–43. https://doi.org/10.1080/07421656.2004.10129317

Nordenstam, A., & Wictorin, M. W. (2022). Comics craftivism: Embroidery in contemporary Swedish feminist comics. *Journal of Graphic Novels and Comics, 13*(2), 174–192. https://doi.org/10.1080/21504857.2020.1870152

Phang, C. (2023). Individual versus sequential: The potential of comic creation in art therapy. *International Journal of Art Therapy, 29*, 1–11. https://doi.org/10.1080/17454832.2023.2261537

Rifkind, C., Christopher, B., & Alice, R. L. (Illustrator). (2019). How comics work [Brochure]. Department of English, University of Winnipeg. https://www.uwinnipeg.ca/1b19/docs/how-comics-work-web-cc-by-nc-nd.pdf

Scavarda, A., & Moretti, V. (2024). Health got graphic! The role of Graphic Medicine in unpacking autism. *Disability & Society, 40*, 1–23. https://doi.org/10.1080/09687599.2023.2289361

Shilling, R. D. (2013). *Therapeutic storytelling authoring tools for post-traumatic stress.* DARPA SBIR 11.2 Topic 003. https://amgolike.files.wordpress.com/2015/03/graphicnovelarttherapyfinal.pdf

Shwed, A. (2016). Crisis averted in infinite lives: Utilizing comics as clinical art therapy. *Intima: A Journal of Narrative Medicine.* https://static1.squarespace.com/static/54bc1287e4b09cb81d8d8439/t/57ee9caf46c3c43f7265ca34/1475255473688/Crisis+Averted+FA16+FINAL.pdf

Snyder, K. (2021). The digital art therapy frame: Creating a 'magic circle' in teletherapy. *International Journal of Art Therapy, 26*(3), 104–110. https://doi.org/10.1080/17454832.2020.1871389

Song, J. E., Ngo, N. T., Vigneron, J. G., Lee, A., Sust, S., Martin, A., & Yuen, E. Y. (2022). Chatogether: A novel digital program to promote Asian American Pacific Islander Mental Health in response to the COVID-19 pandemic. *Child and Adolescent Psychiatry and Mental Health, 16*(1). https://doi.org/10.1186/s13034-022-00508-4

Speigel, A. N., McQuillan, J., Halpin, P., Matuk, C., & Diamond, J. (2013). Engaging teenagers with science through comics. *Research in Science Education, 43*(6), 2309–2326. https://doi.org/10.1007/s11165-013-9358-x

Thaller, S. (2017). Comics, adolescents, and the language of mental illness: David Heatley's "Overpeck" and Nate Powell's Swallow Me Whole. In M. A. Abate & G. A. Tarbox (Eds.), *Graphic novels for children and young adults: A collection of critical Eesays* (pp. 45–58). University Press of Mississippi. https://doi.org/10.2307/j.ctv5jxmqd.7

Walker, E. (2021, August 10). Good grief and comic relief: Why comics have the power to transform education for Neurodiverse people. *It's Nice That.* https://www.itsnicethat.com/articles/ellen-walker-muses-and-demons-illustration-opinion-100821

Wisenthal, P. (2017). The power of digital-comic therapy in schools. *The Atlantic.* https://www.theatlantic.com/education/archive/2017/05/the-power-of-digital-comic-therapy/526911/

13

THE IMMERSIVE WORLDS OF THERAPEUTIC GAMING AND SCANOGRAPHY FOR ART THERAPY

Christina Marrero and Natalie Rae Carlton

Apps, screens, hardware, and software used as art therapy media influence clients' interpersonal and sensory experiences and require thoughtful consideration. As digital media scholars and educators, we discuss in this chapter several media qualities and rationales associated with using virtual reality (VR) platforms for therapeutic gaming and Scanography. Our intention for describing older, accessible media, such as scanners and copiers, alongside contemporary, resource-heavy technology, such as simulated VR environments and gaming, is to compare the interpersonal and group benefits, sensory experiences, and challenges of working with each.

Social positioning and life experiences are critical to our worldviews and biases related to technology. Natalie identifies as cisgender, neurodivergent, queer, able-bodied, and a U.S. Military *brat* (homes in multiple locations). Natalie is White with a mixed European ethnic ancestry, has attained middle-class status, holds a doctorate, and is employed in higher education. Within queer and counter-culture movements, Natalie has created music and artworks with analog and digital media and has been assisted by AI grammar and spell-check tools. Due to these influences, Natalie recognizes the importance of active participation in digital literacy, including critically evaluating media effects and challenging the cultural biases and societal control associated with

DOI: 10.4324/9781032720166-15

online mechanisms. Christina is a cisgender, queer, biracial (Black and mixed European heritage), *geriatric millennial* (comfortable with both analog and digital forms of communication) from Philadelphia. She is neurodivergent and a lifelong gamer belonging to a committed online gaming community. For Christina, gaming has offered opportunities to understand her identity beyond the constraints of a religiously conservative community.

Therapeutic digital gaming

Whether digital or not, a game can be understood as an intentionally structured experience with rules, objectives, interactive components, and players. The games used in therapeutic settings may include tabletop, video, board, and playground-style games. Games can be applied within various psychotherapeutic approaches to promote desired therapeutic outcomes (Bean, 2018; Franco, 2016; Rice, 2023).

A video game "requires human interaction with a user interface or program generating visual feedback" (Bean, 2018, p. 10). Gaming happens on several platforms, including consoles, personal computers (PCs), VR headsets, and mobile devices. Video gaming on any of these interfaces and programs offers potential psychological benefits beyond amusement. Reer and Quandt (2020) asserted that video games favorably impact people's well-being in three domains: promoting positive affective states, providing the opportunity to fulfill psychological needs, and increasing appreciation of meaningful experiences. Austin (2010) connected the experience of engaging with video games to Winnicott's theories of mirroring and a sense of self. Therapists can leverage the video game's innate mirroring characteristics to engage deeply felt struggles with identity, trauma, and attachment.

Those who hold marginalized identities or live with stigmatized mental health conditions may find solace in video game representation. Avatars in video games can encourage a deep exploration of personal identity and aid in facing uncomfortable facets of the self (Bean, 2018; Rice, 2023; Sawyer, 2020). In role-playing games, creating a unique avatar allows players to have a more flexible experience of social identity than in daily life (Sawyer, 2020). For example, Baldur's Gate 3 (2023) uses the Dungeons and Dragons character creation process to allow players to choose unique backgrounds, skill sets, racial, sexual, and gender identities, and moral alignments.

Video game players may benefit from using a predesigned avatar with a storyline that resembles their own. For example, Senua from the game Hellblade: Senua's Sacrifice (2017) has been lauded as a successful representation of the challenges of living with psychosis (Ferchaud et al., 2020). In the game, the player engages in psychotic symptoms to solve puzzles, survive horrific circumstances, and rescue a lost loved one. The psychosis, inclusive of both visual and auditory hallucinations, is simultaneously terrifying and essential. Thus, the game avoids romanticizing mental health struggles while increasing awareness and acceptance.

The video game Omori (2020) presents the story of a boy living in a dissociative world due to a traumatic experience he cannot recall. As the game progresses, the main character becomes increasingly aware of precipitating events. To progress, the player must make decisions that affect the character's interpretation of the events. A client and I [Christina] played this game together to encourage the expression of suppressed trauma-related content. Toward the end of the game, the client had made significant strides toward developing self-empathy and self-compassion. Additionally, the client could tolerate disclosing anger about their history without disproportionate shame.

Video games such as Dys4ia (Anthropy, 2012), Unpacking (2021), and Venba (2023) have the player uncover the narrative of a person with a marginalized identity (transgender, bisexual, and immigrant identities, respectively). For players who embody marginalized identities, games like these provide opportunities to experience validation or success through "symbolic enactment" (Rusch & Phelps, 2020, p. 6). In all these games, the effect of engagement with objects or game mechanics mirrors the experiences of people holding marginalized identities. In general, games can foster increased empathy or acceptance of previously unacknowledged aspects of the self.

Virtual reality and art therapy

A video game is, by its nature, a VR. The player becomes psychologically immersed in another dynamic world with its own rules and reactions. In VR, players no longer see their physical surroundings. The immersive qualities of VR have been used to provide specific psychotherapeutic interventions, such as exposure therapy for treating anxiety, PTSD, and phobias (Carl et al., 2019; Eshuis et al., 2021). VR's use for the assessment of psychotic symptoms has also been explored, with promising applications as a psychosocial intervention (Chan et al., 2023).

Several case studies have been published by art therapists that illustrate specific uses of VR (Bodenbender, 2022; Liu & Chang, 2018; Zeevi, 2021). A pilot study by Kaimal et al. (2020) determined VR tools encourage imagination and physical play. For embodied levels of engagement, the experience of haptic media feedback has significant sensory variables unique to VR. While immersed in the virtual environment, tactile feedback comes from unseen objects, such as the floor, hand controllers, air movement in the room, sensations inside the player's body, etc. Hacmun et al. (2018) identified freedom from physical limitations and the ability to build unreal environments as therapeutic advantages when creating art in VR.

Liu and Chang (2018) noted the tendency of art therapists to compare VR art materials to physical ones, possibly to make sense of the perceived disconnection between felt sensations and their visual field. In VR, haptic feedback does not happen simply due to immersion in the technology; there are literal and imagined bodily sensations designed into the experience. Haptic technology, such as vibrations and pressure, is deliberately added to enhance a sense of touch within the virtual artmaking environment. How and when the haptic feedback occurs may be challenging to understand for someone unfamiliar with VR or outside the experience.

Immersion comes with quirks that can add unexpected discoveries and humor or provoke anxiety. For example, when setting up the Quest software, the player focuses on a pair of disembodied, cartoonish hands. If VR controls are held incorrectly, the player will observe their hands as unnaturally twisted. Fortunately, newer headsets offer a mixed-reality option. When this setting is enabled, both the software in the headset and the physical world can be seen. Art therapists can limit the client's inadvertently walking into furniture or other people by using this setting in initial VR sessions.

To date, the therapist remains outside the client's creative process in VR unless a second headset is used or the content visible to the player

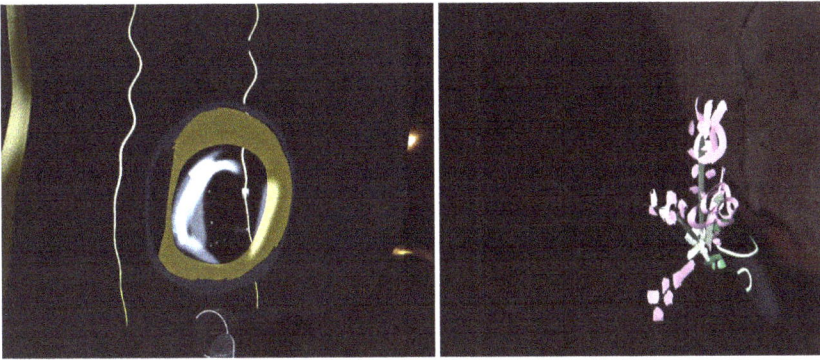

Figure 13.1 Nighttime mixed-reality painting in Open Brush, Christine Marrero

is streamed onto another device (called *casting*), enabling the therapist to see what the player is doing. Though not a perfect replication of the player's experience, casting provides enough information for the therapist to make informed therapeutic decisions. In VR, the art therapist participates by observing, choosing how directive to be, assisting the client with selecting content and materials, and potentially joining in the creative process if software and hardware allow.

An example of an art-based game using Open Brush

Virtual reality preparation

Despite its association with games and play, VR can feel strange. Art therapists are advised to have a short conversation with clients about their familiarity with the medium so that tutorials can be integrated into sessions. While in the virtual landscape, a person's proprioception is tethered to the avatar rather than their physical self. Ways to approach clients' dissonance while moving in and out of the virtual space should be discussed. Users can be allowed to begin by sitting or standing (Kaimal et al., 2020) and encouraged to schedule breaks to maintain a feeling of being grounded. Also, the mixed-reality option on some headsets might help mitigate feelings of isolation or anxiety.

Open Brush instructions

To introduce the art program *Open Brush* (2021) to a small group of clients, I (Christina) cast my headset's screen on the television and provide a short tutorial on the software. Open Brush is an art-based game in which one player is the artist, and the other players in the room are the instructors. Each client-instructor takes a turn giving directions to the client-artist. Directions include spatial cues (above, behind, below), color indicators, and shape descriptions. The artist does their best to represent the image described by the instructors in a 3-dimensional artistic environment while their creative process is cast on a television screen. Through this game, participants have opportunities to engage their theory of mind, communication skills, and empathy.

Gameplay

At first, participants may be hesitant. After each client-instructor has given one direction and the client-artist has successfully interpreted the directions, the game often moves more quickly. The artist's approach can be flexible as they move around the virtual space. They can crouch, extend, pinch, and open their arms to make the desired marks. Their movements reflect the embodied experiences frequently described in the VR art therapy literature (Bodenbender, 2022; Hacmun et al., 2018; Kaimal et al., 2020; Liu & Chang, 2018). As client-instructors watch the artwork appear on the television, they can experience moving toward and away from the horizon line, and witness objects spun upside down as the artist works to add or remove colors and other features. VR supports artmaking that uses large strokes to build dynamic, 3D environments made of bold, layered swaths of color, all without making a mess in the art space.

Aftercare

During verbal reflection on the VR experience, client-artists often say they did not feel anxious creating in front of others because they could not see the other participants' faces. The client-artist may be tired after a game, as VR artmaking can be physically energetic. Aftercare might be necessary because VR can affect ocular perception, balance, and proprioception in people with certain neurological conditions. Assessments, such as the Virtual Reality Sickness Questionnaire (Kim et al., 2018), can be administered after VR sessions to analyze the severity of adverse reactions and plan future VR interfaces.

Clinical applications in the literature

Hacmun et al. (2018) highlighted three clinically significant potentials in VR artmaking. The first is the engagement of a user's sense of presence. Presence, or one's understanding of self in the environment, is tied to visual and sensory cues. VR allows for the manipulation of these cues by the user and by programmed software. The artist's interpretation of their scale and position changes in reference to the placement and size of their artwork. The ability to attune to and fine-tune one's presence could make VR a valuable way to address disruptions in self-body relationships.

VR's second clinically significant feature is encouraging client perspective-taking (Hacmun et al., 2018) or promoting thought-process flexibility. For example, VR users can approach their artwork from different angles. They can also access *as-if* and *unreal* materials. Through casting, the artwork is visible from first- or third-person perspectives. Examination of this highly flexible experience in the therapy setting could be used to address psychological rigidity.

VR's third clinically significant potential is engagement within a playful and immersive holding environment (Hacmun et al., 2018). The holding environment concept helps therapists understand and meet clients' emotional and psychological safety needs (Bahn, 2022). In art therapy, this is typically the co-creative space occupied by therapist and client where reflective experiences can occur. Mixed-reality technology offers further potential for artistic engagement within the holding environment. VR artists can now see their surroundings, use VR art to create artwork that incorporates their environment, and save the combined image. They can repeatedly retrieve the artwork and witness their artistic impact on the holding environment of the therapy room. Co-creating and sustaining the holding environment might offer clients an increased sense of agency in the therapy relationship.

Literature on the therapeutic uses of VR contains advice against using it as a stand-alone treatment and recommends that therapists exercise clinical judgment and collaborate with other providers when using VR with vulnerable clients. For example, Chan et al.'s (2023) meta-analysis of the relevant literature determined that VR interventions may be effective at alleviating specific psychotic experiences, such as paranoid delusions. However, these researchers noted that VR interventions were consistently delivered in conjunction with cognitive-behavioral interventions.

Scanography

Scanography is a media process by which digital imagery is created using scanning functions, including those available in most current copier machines. Flatbed scanners can be 2-D or 3-D in their design and work by capturing light reflected off an object or surface and converting it into digital data. Scanography is also called Xerox art or scanner photography.

Visual artists began using scanners in the early 1980s, coinciding with increased availability and affordability of the devices. Artists may be drawn to the ability of scanners to capture high-resolution, intricately detailed images of objects, offering unique perspectives and aesthetic qualities. Over the years, scanography has evolved and become an established art form with distinct media characteristics and creative expressions.

Scanography has been used to explore the natural environment and human-made objects and to express the self in both embodied and psychological forms. Gerbeza (2023) described using medical scans to reclaim and reimagine their medical narratives, resulting in a visual work titled *Painscapes*. The series documented Gerbeza's "experiential knowledge of pain rather than imposing a traditional medical lens of pain" (p. 104). British art therapist Murray Hamilton (2016) produced a short video titled *Scanography and Art Therapy*, which details methods for introducing clients to scanning a range of objects in expressive ways.

Gerbeza (2023) and Hamilton (2016) discussed the benefits of embodied physicality when using a scanner. These include explorations of one's interior self through visual symbols and metaphors. Gerbeza (2023) engaged in building images through multiple manipulations, such as adding, subtracting, and adjusting objects, as well as playing with light and composition. This dual technological and haptic image-building activity requires patience and time. While simple scans can be made quickly and result in immediate gratification, other images require multiple attempts at curating and refining the scans to reach the desired visual impact.

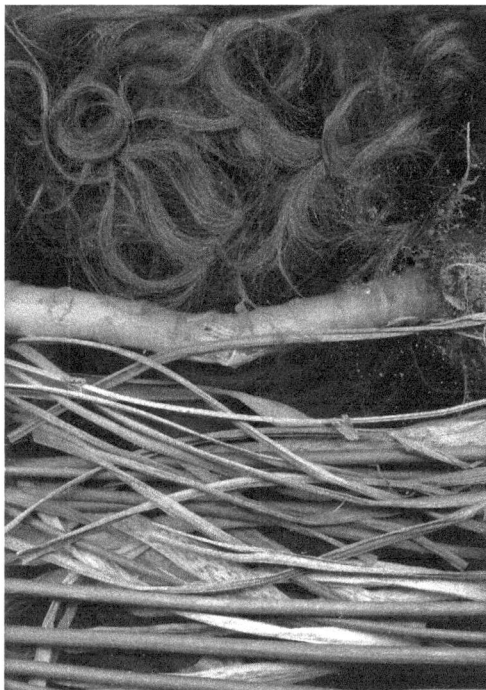

Figure 13.2 Garden Movement, scanography image, Natalie Carlton.

The human body and physical gestures are the scanography subjects of artists such as Mary-Josephine Fulton (Staebler, 2024). In contrast, Mariëtte Kotzé's work (StateoftheART, 2019) consists of ink-wash paintings made directly on the scanner bed and refined through photographic edits and additional digital processes. These artists and many others have elevated scanography to a fine art form, partly due to capturing subtle details, imbuing objects with a sense of intimacy, and conveying reverence for nature's materials. Artists' works have also highlighted the scanner's transformative power by revealing the hidden beauty in overlooked and everyday objects, such as how Jillian Mayer (Mallett, 2018) incorporated projections of scanned images into performance art using repurposed TSA security X-rays.

Experimenting with scanography techniques

Scanography can challenge traditional notions of photography and photocopying, expand the tools possible for artistic expression, and depict intersections of reality and imagination. Scanning, like print-making, is an image created and potentially replicated. Moreover, scanned images can have unexpected dimensional qualities as objects placed directly on the glass appear in the foreground and objects in subsequent layers show up as background. This is because the light source in the scanner travels under the objects and then is reflected on the sensor so that the images become *mirrored* or directionally captured from the glass surface up.

My (Natalie's) use of scanography in art therapy has included open exploration directives and step-by-step instructions to support experimentation with various objects, scanner settings, approaches, and artistic expressions. I have encouraged using scanners to capture natural objects' raw beauty and create representational to abstract forms and textures. To achieve differing depths and degrees of focus, clients can place, press down, stack, or hold the objects, fabric, other textured materials, or body parts they are scanning on or above the scanner bed. These or other elements can be moved across the image-capturing area at varied speeds to create differing light, shadow, or movement combinations. These effects are the basis of photography, using light and time to achieve desired effects.

Scanography as a therapeutic medium

Employing flatbed scanners as a therapeutic medium is an emerging, innovative approach promising to promote mindfulness, self-exploration, and emotional expression (Gerbeza, 2023; Hamilton, 2016). The resulting digital images can be physically and digitally manipulated and used as springboards for various therapeutic activities.

As with the therapeutic use of digital photography and video, scanned images can facilitate the contemplation of physical objects and their representation in digital forms (Ehinger, 2009; Mosinski, 2010). Moreover, the inherent qualities of scanography highlight the "mastery, collaboration, and control offered in the media process" (Carlton, 2014, p. 47). Scanography techniques can invite individuals to mindfully notice intricate details, patterns, and textures in their images that might otherwise go unnoticed, leading to insights about the self, relationships, and the material world.

Scanography can offer emotional expression and processing through its unique aesthetic qualities, including fragmented images of reality, blurred lines, lost details, abstract forms, and the play of light and shadow. A sense of fragmented reality can be conveyed through breaking down the imagery into strips or sections, creating a sense of disruption or distortion. Ensuing discussion can address feelings or realities, whether related to anxiety, confusion, or fractured memory, thoughts, or sensations. By using editing apps to create collages of multiple scans or by using a scanned image as the inspiration for added mark making or color, individuals can express and explore their emotional experiences. This can assist participants in discovering deeper emotions or self and relational states that are difficult to express literally.

Additional aesthetic qualities of scans include blurred details and softening of sharp edges to evoke a dream state, memory, or nostalgia. Gerbeza (2023) noted how scanning could be a complex sensory experience that heightens awareness of touch, sight, and even sound as one interacts with the scanner and the scanned objects. This heightened sensory awareness can promote mindfulness and a deeper connection to one's body, sensory systems, and environment (Vuorinen, 2024).

Scanner imagery can create dramatic visual contrasts between light and shadow, emphasizing certain features of objects while obscuring others. These effects can highlight emotions, express literal or metaphorical abstractions, or create mysterious or ominous imagery (Hamilton, 2016). Single or serial scanned images can prompt storytelling and narrative exploration and be co-created in sessions. Individuals and groups can create poems inspired by the images, using them as metaphors for personal experiences, relationships, or emotions. The technological processes of digital scanners can facilitate reflection, group exploration of narratives, and skill-building (Austin, 2010; Mosinski, 2010). Collaborative artmaking with a scanner can enable individuals to create large-scale or sequential imagery to foster connection, communication, and collective exploration of critical issues.

Conclusion

Scanography and therapeutic gaming offer playful and immersive sensory experiences, potential interpersonal benefits, and challenges for therapists to consider when using them with clients. One critical comparison between scanography and therapeutic gaming is how their tools affect the user's perception. How we interact with the haptic tools of digital media processes affects how we interpret or perceive those interactions. For example, a VR headset can persuade the brain to think we are moving and interacting within "real enough" environments by granting felt and seen forms to our actions. Similar immersive qualities are possible in scanography when unexpected or overlooked textures, shapes, and colors engage sensory experiences in disorienting or hyper-realistic ways.

Primary challenges inherent in therapeutic VR gaming and scanography are related to expense and accessibility, as well as to the patience, creativity, and experimentation required to align them with therapeutic intentions and desired outcomes. There can also be barriers related to negative sensory experiences, such as how VR can generate feelings of nausea, dizziness, and other unpleasant effects. VR also raises ethical concerns regarding how blurring the line between reality and virtuality may have adverse effects on some clients. Moreover, there must be intentional planning about how digital imagery and artwork data are collected, stored, and shared to ensure clients' privacy and confidentiality.

Scanography and therapeutic gaming can strengthen relationships and social connections. They can spark new learning and new conversations through exploration of media effects and skill-building processes, encourage playful collaborations and co-creations between participants, foster empathy and observation, and promote shared experiences. By manipulating 'as-if' environments, clients and innovative therapists can extend digital media creativity to encourage communication, identity development, and problem solving.

References

Anthropy, A. (2012). Dys4ia (PC version) [Video game]. Self-published.
Austin, B. (2010). Animated therapy: 3D computer animation & video games in art therapy with adolescents. In C. H. Moon (Ed.), *Materials & media in art therapy: Critical understandings of diverse artistic vocabularies* (pp. 199–213). Routledge.
Bahn, G. H. (2022). Understanding of holding environment through the trajectory of Donald Woods Winnicott. *Journal of the Korean Academy of Child and Adolescent Psychiatry, 33*(4), 84–90. https://doi.org/10.5765/jkacap.220022
Baldur's Gate 3 (PC Version) [Video game]. 2023. Larian Studios.

Bean, A. M. (2018). *Working with video gamers and games in therapy: A clinician's guide.* Routledge.

Bodenbender, C. (2022). Art therapy with virtual reality. In M. Winkel (Ed.), *Virtual art therapy: Research and practice* (pp. 195–207). Routledge.

Carl, E., Stein, A. T., Levihn-Coon, A., Pogue, J. R., Rothbaum, B., Emmelkamp, P., Asmundson, G. J. G., Carlbring, P., & Powers, M. B. (2019). Virtual reality exposure therapy for anxiety and related disorders: A meta-analysis of randomized controlled trials. *Journal of Anxiety Disorders, 61,* 27–36. https://doi.org/10.1016/j.janxdis.2018.08.003

Carlton, N. R. (2014). *Digital media use in art therapy* [Unpublished Master's Thesis]. Lesley University.

Chan, K. C., Hui, C. L., Suen, Y. N., Lee, E. H., Chang, W. C., Chan, S. K., & Chen, E. Y. (2023). Application of immersive virtual reality for assessment and intervention in psychosis: A systematic review. *Brain Sciences, 13,* 471–497. https://doi.org/10.3390/brainsci13030471

Ehinger, J. F. (2009). *Exploring dreamspace through video art with at-risk youth* [Unpublished Master's Thesis]. Pratt Institute.

Eshuis, L. V., van Gelderen, M. J., van Zuiden, M., Nijdam, M. J., Vermetten, E., Olff, M., & Bakker, A. (2021). Efficacy of immersive PTSD treatments: A systematic review of virtual and augmented reality exposure therapy and a meta-analysis of virtual reality exposure therapy. *Journal of Psychiatric Research, 143,* 516–527. https://doi.org/10.1016/j.jpsychires.2020.11.030

Ferchaud, A., Seibert, J., Sellers, N., & Escobar-Salazar, N. (2020). Reducing mental health stigma through identification with video game avatars with mental illness. *Frontiers in Psychology, 11,* 1–10. https://doi.org/10.3389/fpsyg.2020.02240

Franco, G. E. (2016, October 24). Videogames as a therapeutic tool in the context of narrative therapy. *Frontiers in Psychology, 7.* https://doi.org/10.3389/fpsyg.2016.01657

Gerbeza, T. (2023). Narratives of repair and the re-articulation of the pained self: A study in painscapes. In C. Riegel & K. M. Robinson (Eds.), *Health humanities in application* (pp. 103–122). Palgrave Macmillan. https://doi.org/10.1007/978-3-031-08360-0_5

Hacmun, I., Regev, D., & Salomon, R. (2018). The principles of art therapy in virtual reality. *Frontiers in Psychology, 9,* 1–7. https://doi.org/10.3389/fpsyg.2018.02082

Hamilton, M. (2016, February 23). Scanography and art therapy [Video]. https://www.youtube.com/watch?v=WwhTmI_8y6U

Hellblade: Senua's Sacrifice (Playstation 4 version) [Video game]. 2017. Ninja Theory.

Kaimal, G., Carroll-Haskins, K., Berberain, M., Dougherty, A., Carlton, N., & Ramakrishnan, A. (2020). Virtual reality in art therapy: A pilot qualitative study of the novel medium and implications for practice. *Art Therapy: Journal of the American Art Therapy Association, 37*(1), 16–24. https://doi.org/10.1080/07421656.2019.1659662

Kim, H. K., Park, J., Choi, Y., & Choe, M. (2018). Virtual reality sickness questionnaire (VRSQ): Motion sickness measurement index in a virtual reality environment. *Applied Ergonomics, 69,* 66–73. https://doi.org/10.1016/j.apergo.2017.12.016

Liu, Y., & Chang, C. (2018). The application of virtual reality technology in art therapy: A case of Tilt Brush, *1st IEEE International Conference on Knowledge Innovation and Invention,* Jeju, South Korea, 47–50. https://www.doi.org/10.1109/ICKII.2018.8569081

Mallett, W. (2018, November 20). Julian Mayer makes pretty art from airport scanners. *Vulture.* https://www.vulture.com/2018/11/jillian-mayer-makes-art-from-airport-scanners.html

Mosinski, B. B. (2010). Video art and activism: Applications in art therapy. In C. H. Moon (Ed.), *Materials & media in art therapy* (pp. 257–270). Routledge.

Omori (PC version) [Video game]. 2020. Omocat.

Open Brush (PC Version) [Video Game]. 2021. Icosa Foundation.

Reer, F., & Quandt, T. (2020). Digital games and well-being: An overview. In R. Kowert (Ed.), *Video games and well-being: Press start* (pp. 1–21). Palgrave Macmillan. https://doi.org/10.1007/978-3-030-32770-5_1

Rice, R. (2023). *Video games in psychotherapy*. Routledge.

Rusch, D. C., & Phelps, A. M. (2020). Existential transformation game design: Harnessing the "psychomagic" of symbolic enactment. *Frontiers in Psychology, 11*, 1–16. https://doi.org/10.3389/fpsyg.2020.571522

Sawyer, S. (2020). Oh me, oh my!: Identity development through video games. In R. Kowert (Ed.), *Video games and well-being: Press start* (pp. 49–64). Palgrave Macmillan.

Staebler, C. (2024, January 30). Scanography - the Art of Scanning. https://www.scanography.org/index.html

StateoftheART Gallery. (2019, August 21). In the studio with Mariëtte Kotzé [Video]. https://www.youtube.com/watch?v=RzDLEhe0Brs

Unpacking (PC Version) [Video game]. 2021. Humble Games.

Venba (PC Version) [Video game]. 2023. Visai Games.

Vuorinen, J. (2024). Scanography: Photographic art between the realms of sight and touch. *Journal of Aesthetics & Culture, 16*(1). https://doi.org/10.1080/20004214.2024.2427404

Zeevi, L. S. (2021, Febraury 4). Making art therapy virtual: Integrating virtual reality into art therapy with adolescents. *Frontiers in Psychology, 12*, 1–10. https://doi.org/10.3389/fpsyg.2021.584943

14

THE KITCHEN AS METAPHOR

SHAPING TOGETHERNESS AND THERAPEUTIC MAKERSPACES IN MARGINALIZED COMMUNITIES

Rochele Royster

The kitchen exemplifies homemade community care. It provides a sense of place that transcends physical boundaries, yet fosters stability through daily rituals and embodied practices. Rooted in materiality and process, the kitchen serves as a site for cultivating identity and belonging. Like the kitchen, therapeutic makerspaces emphasize *togetherness* and *making* as means for cultivating wellness among individuals and communities. Heidegger (as cited in Zigon & Throop, 2021) posits that the essence of humanity lies in being with others, challenging the notion of the individual as a solitary entity.

This chapter considers the topic of togetherness as essential to wellness and community spaces through personal narratives and reflections on creative practices, contemplating the multifaceted role of the kitchen as a metaphor for shaping experiences of space, identity, togetherness, and liberation.

My approach to art therapy praxis is rooted in my identity as a Black woman raised in the rural south of the United States and has evolved through my experiences as a mother, daughter, sister, and wife, intertwined with my professional roles as educator, art therapist, and community psychologist. In my early career as an art therapist, I considered what art therapy should and could look like in the Black and Brown communities where I lived and worked. I looked to places like kitchens,

DOI: 10.4324/9781032720166-16

classrooms, community gardens, and art studios for communal wisdom, which led me to curating inclusive, activist spaces informed by the Black and Indigenous cultural stewards encountered in my life along the way.

The kitchen as metaphor for therapeutic makerspaces

The materiality of the kitchen shapes our embodied experience of space and communal creation, influencing the construction of identity (Oglesby, 2021–2022). Kitchens, which are some of the most frequented spaces in people's lives, hold deeply rooted memories. I recall childhood scenes from my grandmother's busy kitchen, where pots simmered and overflowed. The steam danced around, obscuring the windows, enveloping the space in warmth. I remember the sight of women in curlers, multitasking, tending to ovens and safeguarding platters of fried chicken, gumbo, and roasted potatoes. I was often entrusted with tasks—snapping beans or peeling potatoes—while seated at the table, quietly absorbing the lively scene unfolding around me.

On countless occasions, I have found myself in the kitchens of friends and family members, their tables becoming sacred stages where the narratives of life materialize. The kitchen is often the epicenter of safety, belonging, and cultural identity. It is also a space that bears witness to the full spectrum of human emotion—sorrow, anger, rage, and joy. For this reason, the kitchen can transform into a critical, challenging, or even unsafe location where conversations are marked by tense, loud, or trembling voices.

Even kitchens centered in care can be confining. At the home of my babysitter, an old plantation house, a smaller building adjacent to the main house stood as a reminder of the past. Here, in the original kitchen, a large open fireplace served as the focal point—a place where enslaved women toiled tirelessly, preparing meals. Such kitchens often doubled as dwellings, with women sleeping on the kitchen's floor so they could tend the fire throughout the night. While the kitchen provided sustenance, it did so sparingly, with the cooking done predominantly for the enslavers' benefit rather than for the enslaved. This history reverberates in memories of my grandmother's catering business and her safeguarding plates of food from hungry hands in her bustling kitchen—a lingering testament to prioritizing the needs of others over her own needs or those of her family.

In the kitchens of my childhood, I found solace, connection, and an enduring sense of care—a legacy that continues to shape my life and art therapy practice to this day. I also learned to navigate controversy, master the art of de-escalating or encouraging conversations as needed, and managing diverse tasks and personalities simultaneously. These kitchens offer lessons for art therapy community spaces, which can be both nurturing and challenging. When problems arise, art therapists must be skillful navigators, present and intentional in moving through change and conflict.

Material and immaterial aspects of therapeutic makerspaces

If community is the product, what elements are essential, what *stuff* is needed for it to materialize? What components are woven, pasted, or hammered together to construct freedom spaces and sustainable community care? Here I consider *materials* both intangible and tangible, applying them to the context of community care.

Within therapeutic makerspaces, just as in kitchens, physical materials encompass the tools and tangible objects used in creative making practices. These objects are what artists and art therapists typically think of as *materials*. However, the intangible aspects of both kitchens and art studios—such as beliefs, values, norms, stories, rituals, and customs—are at least as important to co-creating community care and liberation.

By prioritizing the tangible/intangible gestalt of makerspaces, participants are able to perceive, articulate, and give form to shared community experiences, resulting in a space where togetherness is palpable and meaningful (Timm-Bottos, 2017). Abstract concepts can materialize into both tangible art products and social outcomes when a makerspace is aimed at fostering autonomy, self-actualization, belongingness, and social empowerment (Robertson & Vinebaum, 2016). Below I consider just three of the many intangible materials that are often at play in makerspaces serving marginalized communities: togetherness, blackness, and storytelling.

Togetherness as material

Social Exchange Theory proposes that relationships are transactions guided by reciprocity. Togetherness is achieved when the benefits of social interaction outweigh the drawbacks, fostering mutually fulfilling relationships (Miller & Bermudez, 2004). Cultural differences play a significant role in how costs and rewards are perceived, with collectivist cultures valuing group obligations, and in-group needs while individualistic cultures value personal identity, rights, and desires (Ting-Toomey, 1994).

In the kitchen, togetherness is expressed through shared experiences of cooking, eating, and conversation. In a therapeutic makerspace, togetherness is similarly expressed through conversation, making, and nurturance, but the tangible result of making practices is typically art rather than food. Intentional togetherness in doing and making cultivates both autonomy and connection. In the studio space, there is an interplay between the individual and the collective as relationships with others facilitate the discovery and understanding of oneself (Zigon & Throop, 2021). Artmaking can also offer a means for seeing beyond oneself, fostering socio-cultural-political awareness, and forging connections and empathy with others.

Engaging in collective activities becomes a process of meaning-making whereby individuals connect with one another and their surroundings through stories, art, advocacy, and activism. Within this context, meaning is not static but fluid. It is subject to exploration, interpretation, negotiation, and continuous reshaping, ultimately leading to possibilities for change, growth, and healing.

During my time teaching in the Chicago Public Schools system, amid the backdrop of gun violence directed against Black and Brown bodies, the small classroom I shared with students became the site of an impromptu art collective. Using fabric, yarn, feathers, and found objects, the students and I sought solace, reflection, and mutual support during tumultuous times. I witnessed the innate ability of students to foster communities of care as they ventured beyond the school to organize artmaking circles in their homes and churches. Through their collective efforts, they created pathways for self-care and community healing. Students meticulously wrapped and bound pieces of fabric with yarn, crafting dolls that embodied their loss and grief. These dolls, adorned with feathers, beads, and various found objects, served as powerful catalysts for conversation and mutual care among the students. Through their collaborative efforts in both making and exhibiting the dolls, the students drew attention to the pervasive issue of gun violence and highlighted the urgent need for societal awareness and action (Royster, 2021).

Blackness as material

In the context of therapeutic makerspaces, frameworks such as Critical Race Theory (CRT) and Postcolonialism help to conceptualize blackness as material within liberatory spaces. Examining power, privilege, systemic oppression, and the intersectional identities that shape inclusive spaces gives credence to the idea that making spaces inclusive of Black people, especially Black women and girls, makes spaces inclusive for ALL people. By prioritizing accessibility for marginalized groups, we remove barriers that might also hinder those with greater privilege, ultimately fostering a more equitable and welcoming space for all participants.

Critical Race Theory examines how race intersects with systems of power and privilege to perpetuate inequality and oppression, scrutinizing how racism has shaped social structures and institutions (Crenshaw, 2019). I recall my experience of attending K-12 schooling where I had only one Black teacher, and how the environment created by that teacher felt different to me. Because she understood our intersectional identities, she protected and empowered me in the face of anti-Black racism. Likewise, the meaningful involvement of art therapists of color is crucial for creating inclusive makerspaces. When individuals encounter predominantly White people in positions of power and authority, harmful colonial power structures are reinforced.

"I remember the very day I became colored. I was not Zora of Orange County anymore, I was a little colored girl" (Hurston, 1928). This quote captures Hurston's acknowledgment of her blackness upon leaving the familiar confines of her all-Black hometown for a predominantly White community. She realized how her blackness was used to try to limit her, but also how that made her different and dynamic. She applied the word *colored* as both noun and verb, defining and conceptualizing her Black identity as it was being constructed through encounters with White people within various social contexts. Geller (2012) posits that blackness is not inherent but rather a product of societal constructs. Yet, blackness also holds great significance. Black identity is shaped, through naming, by external forces such as the community, media, and state, but it is also created, supported, and nurtured in safe, communal, Black liberatory spaces, like Hurston's Black run hometown of Eatonville, Florida.

Like Hurston, I too have vivid memories of coming to understand my blackness. My elders shared stories about navigating spaces of whiteness outside the safe confines of home and entering a world where blackness might be seen as a problem, a threat, or ignored altogether. I was instructed on how to conduct myself in such spaces—how to shrink myself to fit in when needed—but also coached on how to shine in my blackness and to know that love, safety, and culture could be found and nurtured in our kitchens, homes, and community spaces. External pressures dictated our behaviors, stifled our freedom of expression, and shaped our identities and the image we presented to the world. But who was I beyond these constricted notions? Within Black-inclusive spaces, I was able to explore and discover my true self, free from the confines of internalized racist stereotypes that had been imposed on my Black body.

Black individuals who are empowered with the agency to shape their own narratives, including the origins and significance of their blackness, are able to reclaim autonomy over their body, identity, and stories, and to challenge stereotypes. The forming of authentic narratives is important not only for those identifying as Black, but also for individuals of varying racial backgrounds. Engaging in discussions about blackness prompts people—whether White or persons of color—to confront their own racial identities and to critically evaluate and deconstruct internalized, socially reinforced anti-Black biases and stereotypes.

Throughout U.S. history, Black communities have been compelled to repair the wounds inflicted by systemic injustice, which has required investment in innovative mutual aid and community care networks. Ancestral strategies of community care and collective knowledge production defy individualistic notions of self-care and patriarchal capitalist frameworks of wellness (Gipson, 2019).

My great-grandmother was a skilled quilter, weaving practicality and self-expression into her craft. Using old clothes and bleached animal feed bags, she created geometric wonders that were not just functional, but also artistic expressions of comfort and care. In the summertime, quilting became a communal affair, with neighboring women joining in to quilt the top to the backing, sandwiching the filling in between. This community of care traveled house to house to help complete quilts that were stitched by various women during the winter months. During these gatherings, which often took place in the kitchen, women would talk, laugh, give advice, craft, and make connections. Conversations were often about politics, civic engagement, gender bias, gender roles, community organizing, and relationships. A smorgasbord of snacks and potluck dishes prepared in advance was readily available. The gathering evoked a sense of belonging. It was a place to be seen and heard, to craft, to find oneself through relationships with others. I often look to these memories for inspiration when creating and holding space for others.

Storytelling as material

Stories are found in songs, weavings, quilts, dances, and the meals we cook and share. Stories are so ingrained in us that we create them even in our sleep. Narrative Therapy is based on the idea that stories help individuals understand their lives, shape their identities, and convey their beliefs to others (Kerr, 2008).

However, stories possess dual capabilities; they can perpetuate harm and uphold power inequities, or they can function as resistance through providing counter-narratives. Operating within the realm of relationships, stories can build trust, challenge power dynamics, and offer diverse perspectives (Hardy, 2022). It is important to consider the impact of stories, and to question why some stories are told, and others are not. Collective storytelling can reveal underlying assumptions about Black and Brown identities and challenge colonial interpretations. However, stories can also be appropriated, misused, and cause harm.

When I first moved to Chicago, I resided at a hostel/dormitory situated on the periphery of the University of Chicago. Although technically part of the South Side, the University campus is isolated within the Hyde Park neighborhood. I frequently heard cautionary tales about areas of the city to avoid. The narrative was clear: the South Side of Chicago, predominantly consisting of Black communities, was dangerous, and venturing there alone posed grave risks. One evening, on my journey back from downtown to my dormitory, I unintentionally fell asleep on the train and awoke to find myself in the very place I had been warned against. Stepping off the train, I realized I would have to wait at least an hour for the next train in this unfamiliar, dimly lit neighborhood. As I sat on a bench on the train platform, a young Black man approached me with a brown paper bag in hand. He sat down beside me and looked me over. Uncertain about what to expect, I recalled the cautionary tales from my housemates. "You want half my sub, Slim?" The young man offered me half of his sandwich, noting that I looked hungry. In that moment, I experienced a whirlwind of emotions—embarrassment, shame, and relief flooded over me. "I'm okay," I responded. But I was distressed to realize I had internalized false narratives about the South Side, about Black men, and about vulnerability and womanhood. Even as a Black woman with positive examples of Black men in my life, when put in a vulnerable situation my immediate impulse was to rely on the story that blackness is unsafe and dangerous. I have found that telling this story to people learning to unpack their racism opens space for them to be brave and vulnerable. Collaborative storytelling offers the potential for trust building and mutual transparency (Hardy, 2022).

As a young girl, stories unfolded through both tangible and intangible elements of the kitchen—the aroma of spices, the preparation of foods, gender roles, and the rituals and work of daily life. A similar phenomenon happens in the art studio. Stories unfold through the rituals associated with preparing the space, the sensory experiences of engaging with materials, the conversations that take place, and the daily risks associated with trust and transparency. In the art studio, like in the kitchen, participants can engage deeply with each other's stories, working and making together as fellow explorers of meaning and co-producers of knowledge.

Potential of therapeutic makerspaces

The reimagined kitchen is a studio space adorned with paint palettes and shelves full of jars, echoing the essence of a bustling kitchen. Here, people gather around a table reminiscent of the kitchen table, seeking nourishment through communal creativity. Individuals converge, bringing their stories, experiences, and expertise, fostering a culture of shared learning and growth. In this studio environment, art materials serve as conduits for expression, transforming thoughts, emotions, and memories into tangible artifacts. Ideas take shape, solidifying into images that are both malleable and concrete.

Collaborative artmaking mirrors the give-and-take inherent in kitchens. Instead of "Can you pass me that knife?" or "Do you think this needs more garlic?", queries such as "Do you have the blue paint?" or "Can you hold this?" punctuate the space. Participants engage in a dance of leaning in and leaning back, actively holding space for one another while navigating their own creative making.

Within art therapy open studio spaces, community emerges organically, built upon a foundation of mutual respect and evolving at "the speed of trust" (Brown, 2017, p. 27). When establishing art therapy studios, it is important to consider the historical and present-day culture of care in the community. How have people come together to support and care for one another over time (Moon, 2023)? What are the mutual aid and care systems already in place?

The sense of belonging cultivated within the community becomes a magnet, often drawing individuals back repeatedly. Ideally, a therapeutic makerspace is characterized by meeting people on their own terms, centering mutual care practices, decentering power, and co-creating the practice's ethos (Moon, 2023). In such a space, people can be truly seen, heard, and accepted as their authentic selves, yet also grow, evolve, and be held accountable to their potential.

The studio serves as a laboratory where essential skills are not just honed, but lived—where listening, observing, valuing, and evaluating are embodied in every interaction. The principle of mutual aid takes precedence, emphasizing participation, solidarity, and mobilization toward social action. This stands in contrast to an experience framed as charity, which often fails to deepen participants' connections to broader issues or struggles for justice (Spade, 2020). Through its ability to create new realities, art can be an impactful means of generating meaning (Zittoun & Brinkmann, 2012) and facilitating social change.

Therapeutic makerspace practices are deeply rooted in cultural relevance, acknowledging and celebrating the diverse identities and experiences within the community. Its aims are both community-centered and community-driven, with goals and processes shaped by the needs and aspirations of the participants, and an environment where democracy, freedom, and representation can flourish. What emerges are social models—representations of relationships and power dynamics—that offer potential for real-world application and transformation (Sholette et al., 2018).

Artwork created within these spaces can serve as a means to raise awareness about shared experiences and struggles, fostering empathy and solidarity among participants. As individuals engage in the creative process, they come to recognize their own agency and dignity, empowering them to act in support of themselves and their communities. The option for public art exhibitions can provide a platform for amplifying marginalized voices and influencing decision-makers such as politicians, stakeholders, and gatekeepers, thereby driving meaningful change. Ultimately, the aim is social transformation, with the studio serving as a catalyst for positive change.

Challenges of therapeutic makerspaces

The therapeutic makerspace is a microcosm of life, replete with messy relationships and the potential for harm. Relationships in communal spaces can be riddled with difficulties, as interpersonal conflicts and unhealthy patterns of behavior complicate togetherness and interfere with mutual care and solidarity. Art therapists understand the nuances of relationships, know how to navigate power dynamics, and possess the skills to facilitate and maintain a safe space, even during challenging or potentially unsafe conversations (Moon, 2023). They are tasked with creating a safe enough environment to warrant mutual trust and courage among participants, and the potential to facilitate repair when behaviors become harmful. Being continually attuned to interpersonal and group dynamics, as well as remaining focused on accessibility and inclusivity are essential skills.

During the 1800s, when enslaved women cooked in open hearth fires, the perilous nature of kitchen work was compounded by the risk of being consumed by flames, a fate tragically common as women's long skirts were vulnerable to catching fire. Thus, while the kitchen was central to caregiving, it also served as a crucible to the dangers of captivity. To this day, ordinary spaces like kitchens and art studios hold the potential to perpetuate power inequities and structural racism. Authentic liberatory spaces must transcend performative gestures, and evidence genuine anti-oppressive action.

Considering the complexity of human relationships, art therapists must consider how to cultivate spaces of community care that are intentional, reciprocal, and sustainable. They must be vigilant about rooting out the subtle ways racism and other oppressive systems manifest, and put into place safeguards that prevent art therapy studios from becoming spaces of confinement and harm.

As an art therapist, I have often supervised White or white adjacent interns working in predominantly Black urban spaces. Repeatedly, I have found adolescent Black girls playing with the interns' hair. Though initially unsure why this troubled me, I came to understand that the interns, despite good intentions, failed to grasp the deeper implications of this interpersonal dynamic. They overlooked the complex history of racism as expressed through the unacceptability, surveillance, and policing of Black hair. They failed to recognize how anti-Blackness permeates social spaces, and how the violence of discrimination—in this case, unequal standards of beauty—becomes internalized by Black individuals. This interracial dynamic underscored the importance of examining the roots of oppression and how it is perpetuated across time through daily interactions. Only with this socio-political-historical understanding can art therapists create truly inclusive and empowering environments. I always ask myself and guide my interns to ask, "Who is this benefitting and how?"

To model liberation within these systems, art therapists must actively challenge their own and others' biases and discriminatory behavior. Importantly, this means apologizing when wrong and taking steps to correct missteps, fostering a culture of accountability and growth. Sometimes, modeling a liberatory approach means acknowledging when a situation cannot be salvaged and starting anew, understanding the necessity of letting go and embracing change. Ultimately, within a thriving makerspace people learn how to navigate these complexities together and to support one another's mutual liberation.

Conclusion

This chapter considers alternatives to traditional mental health care through adopting a community-based approach that prioritizes accessibility, inclusivity, mutual care, and cultural relevance. Attuned to social determinants of mental health, art therapists can engage in social justice critique/analysis and collaborate with others to create liberatory spaces.

Such spaces address the root causes of social issues through art, dialogue, and actionable steps toward social change.

By tapping into the cultural resources and wellness rituals embedded in daily life, such as those that take place in the home kitchen, the potential of community care can be harnessed. The shared sense of togetherness and acceptance often experienced in kitchens mirrors the relational dynamics that can be found in community studio spaces. In a functioning kitchen, each person has a designated task and contributes to a collective goal, which fosters a culture of everyone being appreciated and valued. Similarly, in a community art therapy studio, each participant is encouraged to contribute what they can in relation to time, effort, knowledge, and resources, based on an understanding that their presence and support is essential to the group's flourishing.

As art therapists and community members, it is essential to advocate for sustainable solutions to social injustice, adopt intersectional approaches to care, and support community-led initiatives. Through nurturing, activist community makerspaces, art therapy can evolve into a preventative healthcare practice, addressing individual well-being while also playing a vital role in broader social transformation and liberatory praxis.

References

Brown, A. M. (2017). *Emergent strategy: Shaping change, changing worlds.* AK Press.

Crenshaw, K. (2019). *Seeing race again: Countering colorblindness across the disciplines.* University of California Press.

Geller, P. (2012). *Making blackness, making policy.* (Publication No. 9548618) [Doctoral dissertation, Harvard University]. DASH repository. https://dash.harvard.edu/entities/publication/73120378-a57f-6bd4-e053-0100007fdf3b

Gipson, L. (2019). Envisioning Black women's consciousness in art therapy. In S. K. Talwar (Ed.), *Art therapy for social justice: Radical intersections* (pp. 96–120). Routledge.

Hardy, L. J. (2022). *Community engagement through collaborative writing: Storytelling together.* Routledge.

Hurston, Z. N. (1928, May). How it feels to be Colored me. *The World Tomorrow, 11*(5), 1–4.

Kerr, C. (2008). Narrative art therapy within a multicultural framework. In J. Hoshino & D. Cameron (Eds.), *Family art therapy* (pp. 206–232). Routledge.

Miller, M. M., & Bermudez, J. M. (2004). Intersecting gender and social exchange theory in family therapy. *Journal of Feminist Family Therapy, 16*(2), 25–42. https://doi-org.libezproxy2.syr.edu/10.1300/J086v16n02_02

Moon, C. H. (2023). The art studio as public health practice. In E. Bos & E. Huss (Eds.), *Using art for social transformation* (pp. 156–166). Routledge.

Oglesby, C. (2021–2022). The kitchen: Just a place where we make food? *Anthropology of Architecture.* https://www.anthropologyofarchitecture.com/#/new-page-47/

Robertson, K., & Vinebaum, L. (2016). Crafting Community. *Textile, 14*(1), 2–13. https://doi.org/10.1080/14759756.2016.1084794

Royster, R. (2021). Dolls4Peace memorial: Liberatory community art action and praxis. *Voices: A World Forum for Music Therapy, 21*(1). https://doi.org/10.15845/voices. v21i1.3153

Sholette, G., Bass, C., & Social Practice Queens (2018). *Art as social action: An introduction to the principles and practices of teaching social practice art.* Allworth Press.

Spade, D. (2020). *Mutual aid: Building solidarity during this crisis (and the next).* Verso.

Timm-Bottos, J. (2017). Public practice art therapy: Enabling spaces across North America. *Canadian Art Therapy Association Journal, 30*(2), 94–99. https://doi.org/10.1080/08322473.2017.1385215

Ting-Toomey, S. (1994). Managing conflict in intimate intercultural relationships. In D. D. Cahn (Ed.). *Conflict in personal relationships* (pp. 47–77). Routledge.

Zigon, J., & Throop, J. (2021). Phenomenology. In F. Stein (Ed.), *The open encyclopedia of anthropology* (n. p.). https://doi.org/10.29164/21phenomenology

Zittoun, T., & Brinkmann, S. (2012). Learning as meaning making. In N. M. Seel (Ed.), *Encyclopedia of the sciences of learning* (pp. 1809–1811). Springer. https://doi.org/10.1007/978-1-4419-1428-6_1851

15

THE NEOLIBERAL CO-OPTATION OF MINDFULNESS AND MANDALA PRACTICES

Kirthana Selvaraj

Introduction

The use of materials and media in art therapy is contextualized within the cultural, artistic, and therapeutic practices that structure the therapy session, including embodied practices integrated with artmaking and directives that guide what is made. This chapter addresses two culturally specific practices frequently integrated into art therapy, mindfulness and mandala making, and critically examines their use within Western therapy contexts. This chapter addresses the foundational roots of mindfulness, tracing its evolutionary trajectory from the ancient Yoga Sutras to its intersection with Hindu and Buddhist traditions, and culminating in its adaptation into Western therapeutic paradigms, including art therapy. It also provides an exploration of the cultural significance of mandalas and their relationship with mindfulness practices. As mindfulness and mandalas gain prominence within Western therapeutic discourse, critical inquiry into issues of cultural appropriation and ethical praxis are of paramount importance. This chapter unpacks the historical, philosophical, and ethical underpinnings of mindfulness and mandalas, with the aim of fostering a decolonial and ethically conscientious approach to their incorporation within therapeutic frameworks.

DOI: 10.4324/9781032720166-17

Tracing the roots

Exploring the genesis of mindfulness requires understanding the foundational philosophies from which it emerged—Hinduism and Buddhism. These philosophies are interwoven within the broader tapestry of the Dharmic traditions, expressing parallel philosophical inquiries despite their unique doctrines and rituals (Ranganathan, 2008). *Dharma* refers to guiding principles for moral conduct and spiritual growth (Kausthub, 2023).

The ancient *Yoga Sutras* text, attributed to the sage Patanjali, serves as a vital link in the broader philosophical frameworks of the Dharmic traditions. It delineates the principles and practices of classical yoga, elucidating the path to spiritual liberation through mastery of the mind. While Western yoga practices often spotlight physical postures (asanas) and bodily strengthening, classical yoga presents a holistic system aimed at uniting body, mind, and spirit (Ranganathan, 2008).

Within yoga philosophy, Patanjali outlines the eight limbs of yoga, each constituting a distinct facet of the postulant's journey toward spiritual enlightenment and holistic development. First, *Yamas* are pillars of ethical conduct that steer one's interactions with the world, advocating principles such as non-violence, truthfulness, and moderation. Second, the *Niyamas* are disciplines that nurture self-mastery and spiritual maturation, encompassing practices like contentment and self-reflection. The third limb, *Asana*, embodies the physical postures practiced in yoga to enhance strength, flexibility, and overall physical well-being. *Pranayama*, the fourth limb, entails breath control aimed at fostering vitality and harmonizing the body-mind continuum. *Pratyahara*, the fifth limb, invites withdrawal from external sensory stimuli, facilitating heightened self-awareness and introspection. *Dharana*, the sixth limb, revolves around concentration to cultivate mental stability and clarity. *Dhyana*, the seventh limb, signifies meditation, the practice of immersion in awareness, fostering reflective contemplation and insight. Finally, *Samadhi*, the eighth limb, symbolizes the pinnacle of yogic attainment—a state of being fully and indefinitely present, experiencing transcendent unity and liberation (Ranganathan, 2008). These eight limbs coalesce to form a cohesive framework for holistic development, integrating physical, mental, and spiritual dimensions.

A deeper exploration of mindfulness (sati) leads to Samadhi, a state of deep concentration and meditative absorption wherein the practitioner attains tranquility, clarity, and unity of consciousness (Rambachan, 2014). While sati lays the groundwork for cultivating focused attention (Kabat-Zinn, 1990/2013), Samadhi represents the zenith of meditative practice, wherein the practitioner enters states of profound absorption and unified consciousness (Ranganathan, 2008).

Integration into Western therapy

Integrating Eastern contemplative traditions into Western therapeutic methodologies marks a significant cultural and clinical evolution (Kabat-Zinn, 1990/2013). Within contemporary psychology, mindfulness is defined as a state of consciousness, attention, or even an information-processing method that prioritizes present-focused awareness (Fricker, 2007). One technique, Mindfulness-Based Stress-Reduction, integrates Eastern practices, such as mindfulness meditation, into a secular program to help individuals manage stress and improve their overall well-being. Similarly, Mindfulness-Based Cognitive Therapy combines aspects of mindfulness with cognitive therapy to treat depression (Kabat-Zinn, 1990/2013). As these interventions gain traction, it becomes crucial to acknowledge the interplay between Eastern practices and Western psychological paradigms, raise questions about cultural appropriation, and consider ways of preserving these practices' original context and meaning.

A critical examination

The Western co-opting of mindfulness practices and mandalas has several implications. First, by removing these practices from their cultural roots, there is a risk of erasing the historical and spiritual contexts that give them authenticity, depth, and meaning (Ausman, 2020; Ishikawa, 2018). This superficial engagement can undermine the true potential of these practices for personal and collective transformation (Brammer, 2010) and lead to a homogenized understanding of mindfulness that lacks cultural sensitivity and awareness (Bhabha, 2021).

Second, the commercialization of mindfulness and mandalas often reduces these practices to mere tools for personal well-being, ignoring their broader cultural significance (Badr, 2022; Bhabha, 2021). This commodification results in the exploitation of cultural symbols for profit, often without benefiting the communities from which these practices originate (Badr, 2022).

Finally, practitioners and therapists using mindfulness and mandalas in their work must recognize the complexities of cultural exchange, acknowledge the cultural origins and meanings of these symbols/practices, seek to understand their spiritual contexts, and ensure that their use does not perpetuate harm through cultural appropriation (Badr, 2022; Ishikawa, 2018; Selvaraj, 2021). Therapists must also refrain from assuming a client's familiarity with cultural symbols, recognizing that the disruptive legacy of colonization has often severed communities from their cultural roots (Putcha, 2020). Attending to the ethics of cultural exchange is complex, but vitally important.

The personal is political, the political is personal

Influenced by Eurocentric and psychoanalytic lenses, mindfulness and yoga are often viewed as politically disengaged practices (Hagan, 2021; Ranganathan, 2022). However, at the core of the Yoga Sutras lies the social and ethical principle of *ahimsa*, or non-violence, which emphasizes compassion, empathy, and respect for all beings (Prana, 2003). From thoughts and words to actions, ahimsa calls for people to be mindful of the impact they have on others and the world around them.

Within an intersectional framework, ahimsa extends beyond personal interactions to addressing systemic injustice. The Yoga Sutras highlight the importance of self-awareness, mindfulness, and inner peace as pathways to liberation from suffering. But this liberation is not limited to one's own well-being; it encompasses the collective liberation of all beings from the cycle of suffering. Thus, the practice of mindfulness is inextricably linked to broader social justice initiatives, as it encourages addressing the root causes of suffering and striving for equity and liberation for all (Ranganathan, 2022).

In therapy settings, an intersectional approach to mindfulness practice goes beyond a myopic focus on individual emotion regulation and addresses moral and existential concerns (Ranganathan, 2022). The revolutionary potential of mindfulness lies in the capacity for practitioners to serve as vehicles for societal transformation, fostering resilience, equity, and compassion amid the enduring complexities of human existence.

Epistemic injustice

Neoliberal ideologies prioritize individual success, self-regulation, and self-care, thereby neglecting systemic issues and collective healing (Selvaraj, 2021). Neoliberalism has led to the commodification of mindfulness, reducing it to a technique without acknowledging its profound psychological and social implications (Badr, 2022). The influence of neoliberal frameworks in art therapy encompasses ethical and epistemic implications (Gipson, 2017; Meade et al., 2022). In disregarding the spiritual, philosophical, and cultural contexts from which art therapy practices originate, art therapists run the risk of perpetuating forms of epistemic injustice (Fricker, 2007).

Hermeneutical injustice, a concept introduced by Fricker (2007), occurs when individuals from culturally marginalized communities are unable to fully articulate their experiences within the dominant discourse, leading to their knowledge being devalued or dismissed (Anzaldúa, 1987/2012; Medina, 2012). For example, commentators and theorists frequently interpret Eastern texts based on their own Western beliefs, thereby distorting the texts' true essence. As a result, South Asian philosophy is often compartmentalized as mysticism or religion, divorcing it from its logical and ethical dimensions. To reclaim the profound scope and comprehensive nature of Eastern philosophical traditions, it is necessary to recognize their holistic nature and develop a more nuanced understanding of their cultural contexts (Ranganathan, 2008; Sood, 2018).

The cultural significance of mandalas

It is important to consider the implications of using mandalas in art therapy. While the creation or coloring of mandalas is indeed repetitive, rhythmic, and requires a high degree of precision and attention to detail, thereby engaging the practitioner in a present moment, focused, and meditative state (Jung, 2017; Kabat-Zinn, 1990/2013), the incorporation of this practice in art therapy often overlooks the mandala's cultural and historical significance (e.g., see Curry & Kasser, 2005; Fincher, 2010; Henderson et al., 2007; Isis et al., 2024; Lorentzsen, 2019). By focusing solely on psychological benefits, there is a risk of commodifying and decontextualizing mandalas from their rich cultural heritage and diminishing the profound spiritual meanings that mandalas embody (Ishikawa, 2018; Putcha, 2020; Sood, 2018).

Originating from the Sanskrit word for *circle* and based in ancient Hindu and Buddhist traditions, mandalas serve not only as tools for individual meditation, but also as representations of the universe and spiritual guidance (Brauen & Wilson, 1997). They are deeply rooted in Yogic philosophies and symbolize the cosmic order and interconnectedness (Rangarajan, 2009).

Mindfulness and the use of mandalas are practices with profound interconnections, each enhancing the other to promote mental well-being, emotional balance, and spiritual growth (Rangarajan, 2009). While similar geometric patterns and symbolic representations exist in other cultures, such as North American First Nations Medicine Wheels, Islamic geometric art, and Celtic knotwork, the term *mandala* specifically denotes its association with Hinduism and Buddhism (Sood, 2018). These traditions imbue mandalas with deep spiritual and philosophical significance, reflecting principles of unity, harmony, and transcendence (Shearer, 2022).

In ancient Indian philosophy, mandalas symbolize interdependence between the observer and the observed, reflecting the unity of elemental forces and consciousness. *Tattvas*, fundamental cosmic principles, underline this holistic worldview, encompassing physical, mental, and spiritual dimensions (Brammer, 2010). The Sri Chakra, a prominent mandala symbol, includes diverse dimensions of existence, with its central point, the bindu, signifying both creation and dissolution. The bindu represents the union of masculine and feminine principles, embodying transformative energies essential for holistic realization. Through its intricate geometry and symbolism, the Sri Chakra elucidates the interplay of cosmic forces and individual consciousness, guiding seekers toward a deeper comprehension of unity amidst diversity (Rangarajan, 2009).

A deeper exploration of mandalas unveils a richness of meaning that extends far beyond mere stress-reduction techniques (Rangarajan, 2009). These ancient symbols embody metaphysical concepts such as impermanence, transformation, and the cyclical nature of life. Each intricate design within a mandala holds layers of significance, inviting contemplation and reflection. The concentric circles and symmetrical shapes represent the microcosm and macrocosm, illustrating the idea that the individual self is interconnected with the greater cosmic whole (Husgafvel, 2018).

At their core, mandalas symbolize the interconnectedness of all things, reflecting the unity and harmony inherent in the universe. Mandalas possess not only philosophical complexity but also spiritual significance as aids for meditation and reflection (Rangarajan, 2009). Adherents of Hinduism and Buddhism frequently use mandalas as focal points during meditation, enabling them to transcend the limitations of the self and establish a connection with the collective consciousness (Husgafvel, 2018).

Cultural appropriation

The relationship between mindfulness and mandalas is frequently discussed in terms of their psychological and therapeutic benefits, such as enhancing focused attention, reducing stress (Liu et al., 2020), or increasing personal enlightenment. However, the marketing of mindfulness and mandalas as secular tools can inadvertently perpetuate a form of cultural appropriation (Putcha, 2020).

The trend of incorporating mindfulness and mandalas into therapy reflects a broader pattern of Western imperialism in which cultural elements are extracted, commercialized, and repurposed without adequate recognition of their origins and significance (Said, 1977). The commodification of spiritual practices, including mindfulness and mandalas, reflects asymmetrical power dynamics through which Western institutions shape global narratives and practices, often at the expense of Indigenous or non-Western perspectives (Fanon, 2018; Putcha, 2020). This transformation raises significant questions about authenticity, cultural respect, and the impact of capitalist systems on spiritual and cultural practices (Kaimal & Arslanbek, 2020). Cultural insensitivity erodes the authority and autonomy of marginalized communities over their cultural heritage, perpetuating a cycle of cultural erasure and domination (Meade et al., 2022).

Cultural appropriation also strains interpersonal relationships within marginalized communities and between different cultural groups. It may lead to mistrust, resentment, and conflict as individuals grapple with issues of identity, representation, and power. It can also exacerbate feelings of cultural disconnection and displacement within marginalized communities (Starling, 2021). When sacred practices and traditions are co-opted without proper acknowledgment or respect, individuals may experience alienation from their own cultural heritage, leading to confusion of identity, a sense of loss (Ranganathan, 2022; Starling, 2021), feelings of betrayal, and spiritual distress (Kaimal & Arslanbek, 2020).

Furthermore, cultural appropriation can trigger psychological trauma or re-traumatization among marginalized communities with historical experiences of oppression. Witnessing the commodification or misrepresentation of their cultural practices can evoke painful memories of past traumas and reinforce feelings of powerlessness and marginalization (Meade et al., 2022).

Misrepresentation and appropriation also perpetuate negative stereotypes and stigmatization of marginalized communities, reducing them to caricatures or objects of curiosity. In addition, cultural appropriation can create barriers to accessing culturally relevant resources and support networks, further marginalizing affected communities and limiting their ability to engage with their cultural heritage in empowering ways (Meade et al., 2022). Thus, ensuring ethical and culturally sensitive practices in therapeutic settings is crucial to promoting healing and empowerment.

It is important here to distinguish between cultural appropriation and cultural appreciation. While it is possible for individuals from diverse cultural backgrounds to engage with and appreciate symbols or practices from other cultures, appropriation occurs when such engagement lacks understanding, respect, and acknowledgment of cultural context and significance. Art therapists who uncritically adopt symbols or practices that are not part of their own cultural history perpetuate the legacy of colonialism, reinforcing asymmetrical power relations and marginalizing the voices and experiences of people from the culture where the symbol/practice originated.

Art therapy is increasingly incorporating mindfulness and related techniques to enhance self-expression and emotion regulation (Malchiodi, 2022). The integration of Eastern methodologies, such as meditation and mandalas into art therapy often occurs without explicitly acknowledging their spiritual context or the potential risk of cultural insensitivity (e.g., Curry & Kasser, 2005; Fincher, 2010; Henderson et al., 2007; Isis et al., 2024; Lorentzsen, 2019). Mandalas are a frequently appropriated cultural symbol within art therapy, including as instruments for medical assessment or data collection (e.g., Elkis-Abuhoff et al., 2009; Parris, 2008, p. 84). While harmful intentions may not always be present, even actions based on good intentions can potentially harm clients who are deeply rooted in their cultural context (Talwar, 2010). Moreover, the misuse of mindfulness practices like meditation can be harmful to any art therapy participants, regardless of their cultural background. This potential for harm is particularly significant if therapists do not recognize and work within their cultural and educational limitations, and fail to consider the mental, emotional, psychological, and socio-cultural aspects of these practices. A little knowledge can indeed be dangerous; therapists must exercise both cultural humility and sensitivity to the diverse capacities and needs of their clients.

Ethical practices in mindfulness and mandala-based therapies

Even though empirical research supports the notion that both mindfulness and mandala practices can significantly reduce levels of stress and anxiety (Kabat-Zinn, 1990/2013; Malchiodi, 2022), it is essential to question the potential impact when these practices are used in therapeutic settings without a deep understanding of their spiritual foundations (Ishikawa, 2018; Selvaraj, 2021). In response, some arts therapists have broadly challenged cultural appropriation (Sajnani & Johnson, 2024; Talwar, 2018), and others have proposed culturally informed, sensitive, and respectful ways to include culture-specific practices (e.g., see Jhaveri, 2020).

Ishikawa (2018) offers a compelling argument for a more fundamental shift in how mindfulness is approached in educational and therapeutic settings, suggesting it should be "reoriented into its Buddhist contexts… accompanied by required lessons and trainings on Buddhist cultures, ontologies, and knowledges" (p. 108). This approach ensures that mindfulness practice is grounded in an understanding of its collective and holistic origins. Ishikawa underscores that the current individualistic, reductionist interpretations of mindfulness are a form of cultural appropriation that perpetuates oppression. They suggest that mindfulness-based programs be referred to as *attention-focusing* and *stress-reduction* strategies, rather than using terms that misconstrue mindfulness as fundamentally individualistic in nature.

Incorporating these insights into art therapy necessitates a culturally attuned approach that ensures mindfulness and mandala applications are ethically sound (Sajnani & Johnson, 2024; Talwar, 2018). To integrate Ishikawa's (2018) perspective, art therapists must first establish a solid educational foundation in the historical, spiritual, and cultural significance of mindfulness and mandalas within Buddhist and Hindu traditions. Art therapists might then introduce elements of Buddhist philosophy into meditation practices within therapy, but with cultural sensitivity and a humble acknowledgment of the limits of their knowledge.

Jhaveri's (2020) sensitive integration of traditional Indian crafts like mehndi and kolam into art therapy demonstrates the importance of deep cultural understanding. Like mandalas, kolam holds profound ritualistic and symbolic meaning in Hindu traditions. Therapists should avoid using such practices purely for aesthetic or relaxation purposes, instead guiding clients in engaging with deeper concepts like unity, protection, and the cyclical nature of life, and thereby promoting both personal growth and cultural respect.

Art therapist Michael Franklin (as cited in Jhaveri, 2020) is committed to an ethically sound use of mindfulness, viewing it as intrinsic to yoga and crucial for both the creative process and the practice of art therapy. Franklin (2001) emphasizes the integration of mindfulness across all aspects of being—body, mind, heart, and spirit—and advocates for deep, personal engagement with these practices to ensure full understanding and to develop competence in facilitating holistic healing for clients.

Both Ishikawa (2018) and Jhaveri (2020) emphasize the need for collaborative community involvement to ensure that cultural practices are used ethically. Engaging with the communities from which these traditions originate, as Jhaveri did with local women to revive kolam, ensures that traditional practices are shared in respectful, authentic ways, avoiding appropriation or distortion. Moreover, incorporating culturally specific practices in therapy can help address intergenerational trauma and foster holistic healing. Combining the principles of cultural education and community involvement, therapists might approach culturally rooted practices as pathways for both personal and collective healing.

Practitioners must also recognize the limitations of their cultural understanding and approach the use of mandalas with a sense of humility. It is essential to avoid a cursory use of any culture-specific practice in the context of therapy without a profound grasp of its cultural context (Talwar, 2010). Informed consent and collaboration with clients are crucial, especially when working with individuals from diverse cultural backgrounds (Jhaveri, 2020). Art therapists should engage in a dialogue to ensure that the use of cultural symbols or practices align with—and are respectful of—the clients' cultural beliefs and values, adapting or avoiding certain practices to demonstrate respect for individual and cultural boundaries (Talwar, 2010).

The use of accurate and respectful terminology is also important for practices that have gone through a process of extraction under the lenses of Western imperialism and epistemology, divorcing them from their traditional applications. Linguistic precision helps to maintain the cultural integrity of these practices. In addition, consulting with cultural experts or members of the Buddhist community can help ensure that the incorporation of mindfulness and mandala practices in therapy is culturally appropriate and respectful.

Finally, art therapists must commit to ongoing cross-cultural learning, remain open to feedback about cultural insensitivities or missteps, and be willing to adjust their practices accordingly. By embracing these principles, art therapists can ensure that the use of mindfulness, mandalas, and other culture-specific art forms and practices are not only beneficial for clients but also respectful of the rich cultural heritage from which the practices have emerged.

Engaging with these complex issues requires a concerted effort to elevate marginalized voices, respect cultural heritage, and challenge the hegemony of Western narratives in the global wellness industry. It is important for art therapists to deeply consider these dynamics and strive for ethical and culturally sensitive practice (Moon & Faulkner, 2024).

Conclusion

The inclusion of mindfulness and mandala practices in art therapy requires ethical considerations related to materials, media, and processes used in art therapy (Selvaraj, 2021). They may provide therapeutic tools for self-expression and emotional regulation (Ranganathan, 2008) but their adoption within Western therapeutic methodologies raises significant ethical concerns about cultural sensitivity and integrity (Putcha, 2020).

Just as therapists carefully select and utilize art materials, considering their therapeutic implications, they must approach the integration of mindfulness and mandala practices with equal thoughtfulness and ethical awareness. Moreover, therapists must navigate power dynamics within cross-cultural and therapeutic relationships (Talwar, 2010), as expressed through embodied and artmaking practices. In certain cases, it may not be appropriate for a therapist to incorporate culture-specific practices into their work at all. This kind of discernment calls for humility, ongoing education, and a strong commitment to cultural competence.

Creating an environment of critical reflection and respectful dialogue within the art therapy community is crucial for addressing these ethical concerns. By nurturing a dialectical engagement that respects diverse cultural perspectives and interrogates power, art therapy can achieve a harmonious cross-cultural synthesis, but only when art therapists ask the right questions. While the therapeutic benefits of Eastern practices can be ethically integrated into art therapy, is the original cultural significance still being preserved? And if not, whom is this practice serving?

References

Anzaldúa, G. (2012). *Borderlands: The new mestiza* (4th ed.). Aunt Lute Books (Original work published 1987).

Ausman, T. (2020). Pedagogies of enlightenment or entitlement? Hospitality, school yoga, and the trials of decolonization. *Cultural and pedagogical inquiry, 12*(2), 121–131. https://doi.org/10.18733/cpi29593

Badr, S. (2022). Re-imagining wellness in the age of neoliberalism. *New Sociology: Journal of Critical Praxis, 3.* https://doi.org/10.25071/2563-3694.66

Bhabha, H. K. (2021). Of mimicry and man: The ambivalence of colonial discourse. In A. Gupto (Ed.), *Literary theory and criticism: Recent writings from South Asia* (pp. 171–181). Routledge India.

Brammer, J. A. (2010). *Modern transnational yoga: A history of spiritual commodification* [Master's thesis, Sacred Heart University]. SHU digital commons. https://digitalcommons.sacredheart.edu/rel_theses/29

Brauen, M., & Wilson, M. (1997). The mandala: Sacred circle in Tibetan Buddhism (Excerpt) (Part 1). *The Middle Way: Journal of the Buddhist Society, 72*(3), 159–170.

Curry, N. A., & Kasser, T. (2005). Can coloring mandalas reduce anxiety? *Art Therapy, 22*(2), 81–85. https://doi.org/10.1080/07421656.2005.10129441

Elkis-Abuhoff, D., Gaydos, M., Goldblatt, R., Chen, M., & Rose, S. (2009). Mandala drawings as an assessment tool for women with breast cancer. *Arts in Psychotherapy, 36*(4), 231–238. https://doi.org/10.1016/j.aip.2009.04.004

Fanon, F. (2018). *Alienation and freedom* (S. Corcoran, Trans.). Bloomsbury Publishing.

Fincher, S. F. (2010). *Creating mandalas for insight, healing, and self-expression* (2nd ed.). Shambhala Publications.

Franklin, M. (2001). The yoga of art and the creative process: Listening to the divine. In M. Farrelly-Hansen (Ed.), *Spirituality and art therapy: Living the connection* (pp. 97–114). Jessica Kingsley Publishers.

Fricker, M. (2007). *Epistemic injustice: Power and the ethics of knowing.* Oxford academic.

Gipson, L. (2017). Challenging neoliberalism and multicultural love in art therapy. *Art Therapy, 34*(3), 112–117. https://doi.org/10.1080/07421656.2017.1353326

Hagan, C. (2021). *Practicing yoga as resistance.* Routledge.

Henderson, P., Rosen, D., & Mascaro, N. (2007). Empirical study on the healing nature of mandalas. *Psychology of Aesthetics, Creativity, and the Arts, 1*(3), 148–154. https://doi.org/10.1037/1931-3896.1.3.148

Husgafvel, V. (2018). The 'universal dharma foundation' of mindfulness-based stress reduction: Non-duality and Mahāyāna Buddhist influences in the work of Jon Kabat-Zinn. *Contemporary Buddhism, 19*(2), 275–326. https://doi.org/10.1080/14639947.2018.1572329

Ishikawa, M. (2018). Mindfulness in Western contexts perpetuates oppressive realities for minority cultures: The consequences of cultural appropriation. *Simon Fraser University Educational Review, 11*(1). https://doi.org/10.21810/sfuer.v11i1.757

Isis, P., Bokoch, R., Fowler, G., & Hass-Cohen, N. (2024). Efficacy of a single session mindfulness-based art therapy doodle intervention. *Art Therapy, 41*(1), 11–20. https://doi.org/10.1080/07421656.2023.2192168

Jhaveri, K. (2020). Healing roots of indigenous crafts: Adapting traditions of India for art therapy practice. In L. Leone (Ed.), *Craft in Art Therapy: Diverse approaches to the transformative power of craft materials and methods* (pp. 118–130). Routledge.

Jung, C. G. (2017). *Mandala symbolism: (From vol. 9i collected works)* (Trans R. F. C. Hull). Princeton University Press.

Kabat-Zinn, J. (2013). *Full catastrophe living: Using the wisdom of your body and mind to face stress, pain, and illness.* Random House (Original work published 1990).

Kaimal, G., & Arslanbek, A. (2020). Indigenous and traditional visual artistic practices: Implications for art therapy clinical practice and research. *Frontiers in psychology, 11.* https://www.ncbi.nlm.nih.gov/pmc/articles/PMC7308491/

Kausthub, S. (2023). Atha—The connection between yoga and mindfulness. *International Journal of Indian Psychology, 11*(1), 558–564. https://ijip.in/articles/atha-the-connection-between-yoga-and-mindfulness/

Liu, C., Chen, H., Liu, C. Y., Lin, R. T., & Chiou, W. K. (2020). Cooperative and individual mandala drawings have different effects on mindfulness, spirituality, and subjective well-being. *Frontiers in Psychology, 11.* https://doi.org/10.3389/fpsyg.2020.564430

Lorentzsen, K. (2019). The mandala as response art: A method for centering, containing, and exploring (Publication No. 130) [Master's Thesis, Lesley University] Digital Commons. https://digitalcommons.lesley.edu/expressive_theses/130/

Malchiodi, C. A. (2022). Frameworks for expressive arts therapy. In C. A. Malchiodi (Ed.), *Handbook of expressive arts therapy* (pp. 21–40). Guilford Press.

Meade, N. A., Branco, S. F., Burt, I., White, R. K., & Hanks, A. (2022). Cultural appropriation, appreciation, and adaption: A rejoinder to "effects of a rite of passage ceremony on veterans' well-being." *Journal of Counseling & Development, 100*(1), 96–103. https://doi.org/10.1002/jcad.12400

Medina, J. (2012). Hermeneutical injustice and polyphonic contextualism: Social silences and shared hermeneutical responsibilities. *Social epistemology, 26*(2), 201–220. https://doi.org/10.1080/02691728.2011.652214

Moon, C. H., & Faulkner, K. (2024). Intersectional care ethics in art therapy organizations. *The Arts in Psychotherapy, 89*. https://doi.org/10.1016/j.aip.2024.102165

Parris, J. M. (2008). The mandala as a visual "third space" for work with trauma survivors. *Creative Approaches to Research, 1*(2), 71–86. https://search.informit.org/doi/10.3316/informit.426521066094487

Prana, S. (2003). *Ahimsa: The practice of non-violence* [Paper presentation]. Pathways to Peace Symposium, Griffith University, Brisbane, Australia.

Putcha, R. S. (2020). Yoga and White public space. *Religions, 11*(12). https://doi.org/10.3390/rel11120669

Rambachan, A. (2014). *A Hindu theology of liberation: Not-two is not one.* State University of New York Press.

Ranganathan, S. (2008). *Patanjali's yoga sutra.* Penguin India.

Ranganathan, S. (2022). Hinduism, belief, and the colonial invention of religion: A before and after comparison. *Religions, 13*(10), 1–29. https://doi.org/10.3390/rel13100891

Rangarajan, S. (2009). The mandalic consciousness: Sri chakra as psychocosmogram. *The Trumpeter, 25*(1). https://trumpeter.athabascau.ca/index.php/trumpet/article/view/1155

Said, E. W. (1977). Orientalism. *The Georgia Review, 31*(1), 162–206. https://www.jstor.org/stable/41397448

Sajnani, N., & Johnson, D. R. (2024). *Trauma-informed drama therapy: Transforming clinics, classrooms, and communities.* Charles C. Thomas Publisher.

Selvaraj, K. (2021). Being queer and brown: A queer, decolonial, arts-based, autoethnographic enquiry into art therapy pedagogical institutions and spaces. *Journal of Creative Arts Therapy, 16*(1), 66–77. https://www.jocat-online.org/a-21-selvaraj

Shearer, M. (2022). Mantras and monetization: The commodification of yoga and culture. *Virginia Sports & Entertainment Law Journal, 21*(1), 38. https://papers.ssrn.com/sol3/papers.cfm?abstract_id=4190057

Sood, S. (2018). Cultivating a yogic theology of collective healing: A yogini's journey disrupting White supremacy, Hindu fundamentalism, and casteism. *Race and Yoga, 3*(1). https://doi.org/10.5070/R331034279

Starling, C. G. (2021). Experiences of shame, exclusion, & appropriation in mindfulness-based wellness culture [Bachelor's Honors Thesis, Portland State University]. https://doi.org/10.15760/honors.992

Talwar, S. (2010). An intersectional framework for race, class, gender, and sexuality in art therapy. *Art Therapy, 27*(1), 11–17. https://doi.org/10.1080/07421656.2010.10129567

Talwar, S. K. (Ed.). (2018). *Art therapy for social justice: Radical intersections.* Routledge.

16

PLAYING IN THE DEEP

APPLYING IMPROVISATIONAL PRINCIPLES TO THERAPY

Victoria Te You Moore and Katharine Joy Houpt

Improvisational techniques and principles have been used in psychotherapy, group psychotherapy, and psychotherapy education across numerous theoretical traditions (Bayne et al., 2021; Kindler & Gray, 2010; Lloyd-Hazlett, 2021; Phillips Sheesley et al., 2016; Schwenke et al., 2021; Todd, 2012; Wiener, 1999). While not directly commenting on improvisation, Winnicott (2005) characterized psychoanalysis as a "highly specialized form of playing in the service of communication with oneself and others" (p. 56) and stressed the importance of "formlessness" in one's dreams, analysis, and early play experiences for developing confidence and sense of self (pp. 45–46). Hamingson and Moore (2016) built upon the works of Ringstrom (2001, 2007) and Pagano (2012) in illustrating how improvisational principles and techniques can help psychoanalysts in working with enactments. This chapter's authors, Houpt and Moore, have themselves furthered the integration of improvisation (called *improv* in the United States) in clinical, educational, and professional settings in the past decade. They have written and presented on the utility of integrating improv into the fields of psychoanalysis (Hamingson & Moore, 2016), dementia care for Alzheimer's disease and related disorders (Fridley & Houpt, 2018; Houpt, 2017), 12-step recovery (Moore & Zwick, 2015), dialectical behavioral therapy (Moore & Zwick, 2016), and group psychotherapy

    DOI: 10.4324/9781032720166-18

(Moore, 2016; Moore & Hamingson, 2014). Improv has also been integral to Houpt's pedagogy as an art therapy and counseling educator.

The authors propose that the formlessness of theatrical improvisation is an art method in and of itself, created by the unconscious and imaginations of participants. What results from this play becomes an art material that can then be spontaneously shaped collectively by art therapy participants. Improvisation-trained art therapists can use improv games and unplanned long-form improv as art material and method in and of itself, and can apply principles of improv (letting go of perfectionism, accepting mistakes, following the fear, and 'yes, and') to existing art practices.

Improvisers and group therapists alike have shown that powerful, disruptive, and transformative group-level events can happen in spaces in which members feel safe and supported enough to take deep emotional risks into the unknown with one another. Drawing from their collective experience as improvisers, group therapists, and educators in the mental health and art therapy fields, the authors elucidate some unifying characteristics of transformative group phenomena that exist in theatrical improvisation, as well as highlight relevant insights beneficial to the training and development of therapists. Throughout this chapter, they also share illustrative vignettes inspired by their experiences.

Pass the clap

For the first time, as a student in an art therapy fieldwork supervision course, Ev has just shared a case from their internship site. While sharing, Ev expressed feeling vulnerable about their work and has now asked the group for feedback.

Five other art therapists-in-training look down or at their computers, eyes shifting above their masks. This is the first semester we are meeting in person after the COVID-19 lockdown. We are not accustomed to being in a room with each other instead of relating remotely through a screen. Despite my framing group supervision as a collaborative effort and encouraging the students to contribute their ideas, they do not speak.

Without explanation, I ask them to get up and form a circle. As they tentatively look around, I join them in the circle, turning to the student next to me and locking eyes. "I'm going to look at Rory and Rory is going to look at me." I lift my hands, my palms facing each other, and Rory instinctively mirrors me.

"Then we will clap our hands at the same time." We clap on cue at the word clap, as if it has been choreographed. "Then Rory is going to look at Min and Min is going to look at Rory, and they will clap their hands at the same time." They do so together, following my instructions. Then, no more words are needed. The clap is passed around the circle. Someone hesitates, throwing off the rhythm. "Don't think!" someone else side coaches. They laugh and the two students clap again, this time together. I plan to switch the direction of the clap at some point, but a student thinks of it first. Spontaneously and mischievously, the student reverses the clap route. Everyone laughs, embracing the new rule of the game, playing together. After a few minutes, we sense we are done and we all sit down, laughing. Soon, everyone bubbles over with ideas to share about Ev's clinical question.

What improv is and is not

Improv is making things up as one goes along. Theatrical improv is carried out, completely unplanned, in groups and it is ripe with group-level processes. Improv games, like the one described in the previous section, usually have a setup or structure within which unplanned exploration and processes can emerge. Improvisation happens in music, theater, dance, creative writing, and visual art. However, in this chapter the focus is on theatrical improv.

Improv is not about trying to be funny, but rather about being present with oneself and with other group members. It is also about committing to being vulnerable and real with one another, making deep interpersonal connections, taking emotional risks, and exploring the depth of those connections together (Moore & Hamingson, 2014). In improv, one expects the unexpected future while spontaneously responding to the past (Levine, 2019). Improv is about reacting with honesty (Jagodowski et al., 2015).

Improv is not psychodrama, which involves a directed and choreographed dramatization of participants' past experiences (López-González et al., 2021). As such, even though psychodrama is inspired by theatrical improvisation, it is more planned and directed. Van Der Kolk (2014) postulated that everyone has within themselves a chronological self and a moment-to-moment self. Improv helps people cultivate their moment-to-moment selves, whereas psychodrama helps people cultivate their chronological selves.

Improv, like therapy, often has a frame in which maximum freedom can operate (Levine, 2019). An improviser makes things up but is not unprepared; improvisers prepare by experiencing life (Jagodowski et al., 2015). An art therapy client needs only to have experienced life and to be willing to be open to the unknown in order to utilize improv as an art medium.

U.S. improv's origins in group social work

Theatrical improvisation has various origins throughout the world. In the United States, its roots primarily stem from the work of Viola Spolin (Szuster, 2019). Spolin first devised improvisational games as therapeutic interventions in her work with immigrant children at Chicago's Hull-House. She had trained in group social work and experimental theater with Neva Boyd, who used play to help children navigate differences and work as a group (McAndrew, 2022). Spolin later adapted these games for the training of stage actors and helped instruct members of the nation's first improvisational theater, which was established by her son Paul Sills (McAndrew, 2022). Del Close and Charna Halpern started iO Theater (2023), formerly ImprovOlympic, where improv became an art form unto itself (Halpern et al., 1994).

Improv in art therapy

In improv, the improviser IS the instrument (Asher, 2013). Art therapists introducing improv can remind clients that rather than setting up paintbrushes, clay tools, or collage materials, that their bodies and minds are the art method and material. Improvisers create a scene by discovering a *relationship* between their characters, creating an *environment* for that relationship, and allowing an *event* or situation that makes this day different from all the rest to emerge (Halpern et al., 1994).

To create an environment, an improviser may use object work, a simulation of using objects in a way that feels realistic to the viewer. For example, one might turn to their left and pick up an imaginary coffee mug from a coffee table, allowing for its suggested weight to show in the way they hold their arm. The coffee table's location is then set in the scene that the improvisers are painting. Their scene partner "yes, and's" that reality by walking around the invisible coffee table, rather than through it. Maybe later they find a magazine next to the coffee mug. The improvisers paint a scene together, just as an artist might paint that same room. In this way, improv is a visual medium (Halpern et al., 1994). Improv bridges and opens the space between physical artistic mediums and the bodies and minds of the therapist and client as medium.

Art therapists have expanded ideas about what art can mean beyond the expected visual media like drawing, painting, and ceramics (Moon, 2010). Levine stated, "in a sense, all artmaking has an improvisational element—it aims to bring something new and unforeseen into being" (Levine, 2019, p. 104). Art therapy education has been conceptualized as performance art, ranging from structured to improvised, in which "we need to learn to be comfortable with being uncomfortable" (Moon, 2012, p. 194). Art therapists have considered performance through a lens of disability studies (Talwar, 2019b; Yi, 2019). Pinna-Perez and Frank (2018) conducted performance art-based expressive arts research as psychosocial commentary on individual and collective behavior. The *Creative Dialogues Project* engaged with multiple types of creative arts media through an improvisational lens to reckon with the unknown during the start of the COVID-19 pandemic (Harvey et al., 2023).

Art therapy literature specific to theatrical improv, as this chapter focuses on, is more limited. Notably, it has been used in art therapy education. Misluk-Gervase and Ansaldo (2023) created a curriculum for art therapy students that combined applied art therapy directives with applied improvisation games to demonstrate three stages of the therapeutic process: (1) safety/attunement, (2) risk taking/acceptance, and (3) mastery/autonomy.

Improv in art

The material practices of contemporary art are virtually without bounds, and contain principles of theatrical improvisation. Christine Sun Kim (Karasawa, 2023a) plays with patterns and repetition in the relationship and language between herself as a Deaf person and an American Sign Language interpreter, just as improv scene partners look for patterns to subconsciously emerge in their dialogue and actions, accepting mistakes as gifts. The improvisers' patterns are on display on the stage, while Kim creates infographics and diagrams of patterns on paper. Miranda July's work relies on the risk inherent in human interaction and connection when "anything is possible in the moment. It is kind of like being in a dream or something, but a shared dream" (Karasawa, 2023b, 13:10). Del Close (Halpern et al., 1994) called this phenomenon in improv "group mind" (p. 87) when a group of improvisers' brains seem to meld into one as a scene unfolds and each person can see what the other sees. Alex Da Corte (Forster, 2023) gathers ephemera from American politics and pop culture to create new meaning, through installation, video, and performance, revealing psychological complexity. Art therapists too can apply improvisational principles to artmaking with clients. Inevitably, an art therapy client will make a "mistake" in a painting. What happens when they can begin to view a mistake as a gift, to *yes, and* it by turning an erroneous mark into an accepted part of the painting? And what happens when that, in turn, is applied to their view of mistakes in their own life? Art therapy clients *follow the fear* when they bravely face a blank canvas.

Watching improv in Chicago as a Chinese immigrant

First, a little background. I (Moore) am a Chinese immigrant. I like going to improv shows and sitting in the front row to be close to the action. Given the Midwestern, predominantly White context of the Chicago improv scene, what often transpires is that an improviser on stage sees me—maybe the only Asian person in the theater— and proceeds to initiate an unfortunate scene about Chinese food, Godzilla, or sushi. Except for one instance, which I share below, this type of initiation has always left me feeling othered.

In November 2019, I attended a TJ and Dave show where I sat in the front row with a Chinese American friend. We were the only visibly East Asian people in the theater. TJ Jagodowski and Dave Pasquesi begin their legendary long form shows by scanning the audience, presumably taking in the room and its vibrations, and then just begin without a verbal suggestion from the audience. They saw us and began their scene inside a Chinese restaurant. However, unlike so many similarly situated improv scenes I had suffered through before, this one felt very different. TJ and Dave did not make fun of Chinese food. Nor did they try to skirt around diversity issues or smooth them over. They did not try to put on an air of expertise about Chinese food or Chinese culture. They played doofuses who did not know much about Chinese food but who loved going to the Chinese restaurant, ordering the Lo Mein and the egg rolls, and socializing with each other and everyone else in the restaurant. Their characters went to high school with the current owner of the restaurant, who inherited it from his late father. TJ's character's comment about "I hear this place got shut down last month for health code violations" landed well because it came from a place of truth for the character, a place of affection and nosiness. The cultural differences and even common stereotypes were not denied, avoided, or sugar-coated. Rather, they were named, played through with good-natured honesty, and deeply humanized. The entire show ended up taking place in the Chinese restaurant and was a marvel to me. Instead of making the Chinese restaurant the "Other" or ignoring the difference in the room, TJ and Dave made the restaurant the flawed center of their flawed characters' lives (TJ and Dave, 2019). And I felt deeply honored by it.

Improv imbalance

The other author (Houpt) is White, and looks to examples such as the above for how to handle inevitable offers of stereotypes and assumptions in improv scenes. Even these can be turned into gifts rather than mistakes when they are subverted instead of ignored, though this largely depends on the skill of the improviser. The predominantly White, abled field of art therapy has encountered calls from art therapists of color and queer and disabled art therapists to reckon with the ways imbalanced socio-political power structures are replicated in the field (Gipson, 2017; Talwar, 2019a; Yi, 2019; Yi & Moon, 2020), and that often it is the political situations themselves that create a need for therapy (Gipson, 2017). A similar critical evaluation is needed in improv, which for much of its history "has been a straight white man's game" (Love, 2019, p. 34). Büch (2022) noted that many improv texts are solely effusive about its assets. Interviewing established Chicago improvisers, Büch asked: Why does improv tend to be a space that "continually sets up whiteness as a categorical default invisible to the white improviser?" (p. 2). In an aesthetic endeavor in which the group is expected to 'yes, and' one another and experience the phenomenon of *group mind*, White reality as the neutral default is ostracizing to anyone who lives outside of that experience

(Büch, 2022). The predominance of whiteness is disrupted by all-Black, all-Asian, and other identity-based improv groups grounded in shared experiences outside of whiteness (Love, 2019). There is a class imbalance in improv as well. Training is expensive, and improv life after training often entails expenses like paying for an improv coach and for the opportunity to audition for unpaid performances. While diversity scholarships exist, this neoliberal gesture is empty when there isn't enough outreach to have an audience big enough for the show to go on (Büch, 2022).

Letting go of perfectionism and inviting in the potential for change

Moore (2016) postulated that the thoughtful use of improvisational principles in the training of group therapists could help reduce therapists' defensiveness and develop their capacity to tolerate and work with difficult feelings. Yalom and Leszcz (2008) contend that the group therapist "who cannot be criticized openly generally is the source of scapegoating" (p. 318). In other words, if a group therapist is unable to tolerate the group's projections of ineptitude as well as their own feelings of imperfection and fallibility, then they risk generating a scapegoat in the group who will contain the therapist's and the group's feelings of incompetence. What emerges is what Rutan et al. (2014) call an *encapsulated scapegoat*, one who contains feelings the group is unprepared to tolerate or explore, and who is allowed only limited participation and expression in the group. The members, in turn, act as if the scapegoat is the only one who makes mistakes. On the other hand, if group leaders and members can integrate the projections and unwanted feelings rather than scapegoat them, they create space for potential transformation (Moore, 2016, p. 3).

This is where the improvisational principles of *yes, and…* and *no mistakes* come in. The principle of *yes, and* calls for the improviser to accept the reality that has been established by their scene partner and then *build upon it* with something of their own. The *yes, and* principle is especially crucial to an ensemble's dynamics and functioning when what needs to be *yes, and*-ed is an apparent mistake. When an ensemble acts out of perfectionism and denies such a mistake, "it scapegoats the performer who first voiced this 'mistake' and creates a split in the show between that which is acceptable and that which is not" (Moore, 2016, p. 3). On the other hand, when the ensemble can weave the mistake into the tapestry of its ongoing creation, the performers create the potential for discovery and transformation.

Mistakes are gifts

An Improvised Shakespeare *performance in 2014 illustrates the transformative power of* yes, and-ing *a performer's mistake. The show had already established that its protagonist was Princess H, played by performer A, and that this princess was looking for a prince to marry. More than halfway through the show, a performer misidentified performer B as Princess H. I (Moore) saw only a second of tension across the other ensemble members' faces before they fully embraced this new reality. There were now two Princesses H, and they were both looking for princes. Through moment-by-moment discovery, the two Princesses H eventually had an exhilarating meeting in which they found kindred spirits in one another (The Improvised Shakespeare Company, c. 2014). Imagine if the ensemble had instead tried to deny or minimize the mistake, how much more boring and less honest the ensuing show would have been!*

Lacan (as cited by Giraldo, 2016) characterizes the state of impotence as one of false solutions and immobility. Impotence can manifest in a therapy group as the therapist trying to make things happen rather than *allowing* things to happen (Moore, 2016). Impotence is often a reaction to fear and an attempt to hold onto control.

Giraldo (2016) illustrates this dynamic as a full grid with no room for movement or change. The ability to accept one's failures and mourn one's losses is what can free one up to move on from impotence and toward transformation and growth. He illustrates this state of movement as such:

X	X	X
X	X	X
X	X	X

	X	X
X		
X		X

It is in accepting and mourning the empty spaces (i.e., what's impossible) that space for movement and change is created. Adopting an improvisational mindset can help the group therapist create and maintain the potential for change in a group. Del Close, the founder of longform improvisation in the United States (Halpern et al., 1994), often told his students to "fall, and then figure out what to do on the way down" (as cited in Hamingson & Moore, 2016, p. 3). If, in moments of uncertainty and fear, the group therapist takes this courageous rather than defensive stance, what follows can be discovery and transformation.

Follow the fear

After the usual one hour of knocking on doors, negotiating with nurses and physical therapists, and carefully backing people in wheelchairs into elevators, I had gathered the art therapy group participants at the continuing care retirement community (CCRC) into a circle. Today we didn't have tables in front of us for visual artmaking, only empty space for improv. Already, Joan was eyeing me, and not so subtly nodding toward Gladys while rolling her eyes. I knew what she was intending to communicate— she had complained to me many times about participating in the same group as Gladys, who was in middle-stage dementia. Joan had founded and ran the CCRC book club and had no signs of cognitive decline. Last week Gladys had tried to drink the watercolor rinse water, and she needed increasing assistance with activities of daily living. Lately, Gladys had taken to watching Perry Mason *every night and was prone to sudden dramatic courtroom confessions when you were merely asking if she could hand you a colored pencil. Joan didn't want to be lumped in with someone like* that, *who might say or do anything at any time. Joan was dignified.*

While dementia is not a given characteristic of aging, it becomes more likely as one ages. Naturally, in a CCRC, where one plans to "age in place" and move to memory care or skilled nursing care if the need arises, many people fear the possibility of their disavowed future selves. I gave Joan a gentle nod, subtly acknowledging her emotion without granting her wish of removing Gladys from the group. I felt a moment of frustration around Joan's lack of tolerance, and the urge to control the situation rose and fell within me.

Then, I started to play. I made a sound and a movement and asked the person next to me, Margaret, to mirror it. I instructed the person next to her, Betty, to mirror Margaret's exact movement, rather than mine. Betty paused for a long while, then mirrored the movement in the way the impact of her stroke allowed. Sheila caught on, incorporating the pause, then let a sneeze escape as she waved her arm. Berna mimicked the sneeze and arm wave combination and we all laughed, not at *anyone but at the group's embrace of humanity. Berna looked at Gladys, as we all did, with bated breath. Long pause. "Alright, you got me! It was ME! Me, I tell ya! But he had it comin' to him!" A pregnant pause turned into an eruption of laughter. Suddenly, someone else chimed in from across the circle, "Gladys, how COULD you?" And another, mistaking Perry Mason for Columbo, said "Just one more thing!" Then everyone chimed in, yes-anding the courtroom drama, everyone in it together. Joan's fear and Gladys's unpredictability were both accepted. Mistakes could be made, resulting in transformation and growth, at least in that moment.*

Yes, and

The possibilities for incorporating improv in psychotherapy and art therapy are endless. Even in co-authoring this chapter, the authors relied on yes-and'ing one another. They started with uncertainty: "Do we have time for this?" "What dynamics should we choose to highlight?" "Can we still back out?" "Do I even like to write?" It wasn't until the authors let go and began to play, building off what the other had written, that a chapter began to take shape. And now, the authors invite the readers to *yes, and* this chapter by exploring the potential of improvisation and play in their own art therapy practice.

References

Asher, D. (2013). Improv Level 3. [Class] iO Chicago Training Center, Chicago, IL.

Bayne, H. B., Pufahl, J., McNiece, Z., & Ataga, J. (2021). Acting with empathy: A counseling and applied theatre collaboration. *Counselor Education & Supervision, 60*(4), 306–315. https://doi.org/10.1002/ceas.12218

Büch, M. (2022). *Whiteface: Improv comedy and anti-Blackness* (1st ed., Vol. 5). De Gruyter. https://doi.org/10.1515/9783110752748

Forster, I. (2023). *Alex Da Corte in "everyday icons"* [video]. Art in the Twenty-First Century (Season 11). https://art21.org/watch/art-in-the-twenty-first-century/s11/alex-da-corte-in-everyday-icons/

Fridley, M., & Houpt, K. (2018, September 21–23). *The Joy of Dementia: You Gotta Be Kidding!* [Conference workshop]. Performing the World Conference, Eastside Institute, New York, NY.

Gipson, L. (2017). Challenging neoliberalism and multicultural love in art therapy. *Art Therapy, 34*(3), 112–117. https://doi.org/10.1080/07421656.2017.1353326

Giraldo, M. (2016, February 22). *From the discourse of the other to the discourse with others* [Special Institute Presentation]. American Group Psychotherapy Association Annual Meeting, New York, NY.

Halpern, C., Close, D., & Johnson, K. (1994). *Truth in comedy: The manual of improvisation.* Meriwether Publishing.

Hamingson, Z., & Moore, V. T. Y. (2016, June). Acting and reenacting: Utilizing improv skills to effectively negotiate enactments. From Hamingson, Z., Moore, V. T. Y., Fenno, S., & Dworkin, N., *Play and improvisation at the relational edge* [Conference presentation panel]. International Association for Relational Psychoanalysis and Psychotherapy Conference, Rome, Italy.

Harvey, S., Wang, S., & Connor Kelly, E. (2023). A review of the Creative Dialogues Project: Using creative arts online during the COVID-19 pandemic. *Creative Arts in Education and Therapy* (Online), *9*(2), 120–142. https://doi.org/10.15212/CAET/2023/9/13

Houpt, K. (2017, September 8–10). *Improv and Dementia* [Conference presentation]. "Yes And" Mental Health Conference, Chicago, IL, iO Theater, 2023. *About Us.* https://ioimprov.com/about-us/

Jagodowski, T. J., Pasquesi, D., & Victor, P. (2015). *Improvisation at the speed of life: The TJ and Dave book.* Solo Roma Books.

Karasawa, C. (Director). (2023a). *Christine Sun Kim in "friends and strangers"* [video]. Art in the Twenty-First Century (Season 11). https://art21.org/watch/art-in-the-twenty-first-century/s11/christine-sun-kim-in-friends-strangers/

Karasawa, C. (Director). (2023b). *Miranda July in "friends and strangers"* [video]. Art in the Twenty-First Century (Season 11). https://art21.org/watch/art-in-the-twenty-first-century/s11/christine-sun-kim-in-friends-strangers/

Kindler, R., & Gray, A. (2010). Theater and therapy: How improvisation informs the analytic hour. *Psychoanalytic Inquiry*, *30*(3), 254–266. https://doi.org/10.1080/07351690903206223

Levine, S. K. (2019). *Philosophy of expressive arts therapy: Poiesis and the therapeutic imagination.* Jessica Kingsley Publishers.

Lloyd-Hazlett, J. (2021). Improv-ing clinical work with stepfamilies. *Journal of Creativity in Mental Health*, *16*(2), 231–243. https://doi.org/10.1080/15401383.2020.1762817

López-González, M. A., Morales-Landazábal, P., & Topa, G. (2021). Psychodrama group therapy for social issues: A systematic review of controlled clinical trials. *International Journal of Environmental Research and Public Health*, *18*(9), 4442. https://doi.org/10.3390/ijerph18094442

Love, M. (2019). Improv so White? *American Theatre*, *36*(3), 34–38.

McAndrew, T. M. (2022, December 19). *From Hull House to Second City: How Chicago immigrants helped change theater.* NPR Illinois. https://www.nprillinois.org/illinois/2022-12-19/from-hull-house-to-second-city-how-chicago-immigrants-helped-change-theater

Misluk-Gervase, E., & Ansaldo, J. (2023). Art therapy and applied improvisation: High impact learning strategies to enhance communication and professional identity. *Journal of Creativity in Mental Health*, *18*(4), 493–510. https://doi.org/10.1080/15401383.2021.2021118

Moon, B. L. (2012). Art therapy teaching as performance art. *Art Therapy*, *29*(4), 192–195. https://doi.org/10.1080/07421656.2012.730954

Moon, C. H. (2010). *Materials & media in art therapy: Critical understandings of diverse artistic vocabularies.* Routledge.

Moore, V. T. Y. (2016). Lessons from improvisation: Creating and holding space for change in group psychotherapy. *Newsletter of the Illinois Group Psychotherapy Society*, *2016*, *3*, 10.

Moore, V. T. Y., & Hamingson, Z. (2014). *Playing in vulnerability: Using improv principles to access, explore, and connect through vulnerable moments in groups.* [Workshop]. American Group Psychotherapy Association Annual Meeting, Boston, MA.

Moore, V. T. Y., & Zwick, K. (2015). *Playing oneself to play together: Applying improv principles to attachment and codependency in groups.* [Workshop]. American Group Psychotherapy Association Annual Meeting, San Francisco, CA.

Moore, V. T. Y., & Zwick, K. (2016). *Playing alone and together: Practicing DBT principles through improvisation.* [Workshop]. American Group Psychotherapy Association Annual Meeting, New York, NY.

Pagano, C. J. (2012). Exploring the therapist's use of self: Enactments, improvisation, and affect in psychodynamic psychotherapy. *The American Journal of Psychotherapy, 66*(3), 205–226. https://doi.org/10.1176/appi.psychotherapy.2012.66.3.205

Phillips Sheesley, A., Pfeffer, M., & Barish, B. (2016). Comedic improv therapy for the treatment of social anxiety disorder. *Journal of Creativity in Mental Health, 11*(2), 157–169. https://doi.org/10.1080/15401383.2016.1182880

Pinna-Perez, A., & Frank, R. (2018). *Sleep of reason*: Critical reflections on performance arts-based research as psycho-social commentary in expressive arts therapy praxis. *Qualitative Research in Psychology, 15*(2–3), 234–246. https://doi.org/10.1080/14780887.2018.1429908

Ringstrom, P. (2001). Cultivating the improvisational in psychoanalytic treatment. *Psychoanalytic Dialogues, 11*, 727–754.

Ringstrom, P. (2007). Scenes that write themselves: Improvisational moments in relational psychoanalysis. *Psychoanalytic Dialogues, 17*, 69–99. https://doi.org/10.1080/10481880701301303

Rutan, S. J., Stone, W. N., & Shay, J. J. (2014). *Psychodynamic group psychotherapy.* Guilford Press.

Schwenke, D., Dshemuchadse, M., Rasehorn, L., Klarhölter, D., & Scherbaum, S. (2021). Improv to improve: The impact of improvisational theater on creativity, acceptance, and psychological well-being. *Journal of Creativity in Mental Health, 16*(1), 31–48. https://doi.org/10.1080/15401383.2020.1754987

Szuster, M. (2019). Theater without a script—Improvisation and the experimental stage of the early mid-twentieth century in the United States. *Text Matters* (Łódź), *9*(9), 374–392. https://doi.org/10.18778/2083-2931.09.23

Talwar, S. (2019a). *Art therapy for social justice: Radical intersections.* Routledge.

Talwar, S. (2019b). Identity matters: Trauma and violence through art, performance, and social practice. In S. Talwar (Ed.), *Art therapy for social justice: Radical Intersections* (pp. 38–65). Routledge.

The Improvised Shakespeare Company [Performance] (c. 2014). iO Chicago, Chicago, IL.

TJ and Dave (2019). [Performance]. Old Town School of Folk Music, Chicago, IL.

Todd, S. (2012). Practicing in the uncertain: Reworking standardized clients as improv theatre. *Social Work Education, 31*(3), 302–315. https://doi.org/10.1080/02615479.2011.557427

Van Der Kolk, B. (March 3, 2014). *The body keeps the score: Integration of mind, brain, and body in the treatment of trauma.* [Special Institute presentation]. American Group Psychotherapy Association Annual Meeting, Boston, MA.

Wiener, D. J. (1999). Rehearsals for growth: Applying improvisational theater games to relationship therapy. In D. J. Wiener (Ed.), *Beyond talk therapy: Using movement and expressive techniques in clinical practice* (pp. 165–180). American Psychological Association. https://doi.org/10.1037/10326-008

Winnicott, D. W. (2005). *Playing and reality.* Routledge (Original work published 1971).

Yalom, I., & Leszcz, M. (2008). *The theory & practice of group psychotherapy.* Basic Books.

Yi, C. S. (2019). Res(crip)ting art therapy: Disability culture as a social justice intervention. In S. Talwar (Ed.), *Art therapy for social justice: Radical Intersections* (pp. 161–177). Routledge.

Yi, C. S., & Moon, C. H. (2020). Art therapy and disability studies. *Art Therapy, 37*(2), 59–61. https://doi.org/10.1080/07421656.2020.1764798

17

A BOX OF FIRED CLAY BRICKS

BUILDING HOME ON THE COMMUNITY TABLE WITH PEOPLE ON THE MOVE

Miriam Usiskin and Bobby Lloyd

This chapter focuses on a box of miniature fired clay bricks and its use within open access psychosocial group support for people on the move. Delivered by the charity *Art Refuge* on either side of the English Channel, this work responds to the psychological needs of people, both displaced and seeking asylum, where loss of home is pervasive.

Consciously and actively steering away from pathology, Art Refuge recognizes the influence of environmental, societal, and political factors that lead to people leaving home and crossing international borders. Acknowledged are the colonial histories and ongoing injustices, conflicts, oppressions, and climate emergencies that have contributed to the contexts in which millions of people around the world are on the move, with 6.1 million people being asylum seekers in 2023 (https://www.unhcr.org/refugee-statistics/).

As British passport holders, we can crisscross the English Channel between France and the UK. Our privilege carries with it a responsibility to deliver work that is contextually informed, reflexive, and congruent (Kapitan, 2015). The questioning of what materials are used, why, and if they are culturally resonant needs to be asked. Included in this chapter is an interwoven discussion of the intersectional and socio-political

 DOI: 10.4324/9781032720166-19

complexities of this work. This discussion sits alongside short extracts adapted from Art Refuge's social media posts, representing different voices of people involved in the work, with the narrative itself crisscrossing the Channel.

The Community Table

Art Refuge has developed an open access psychosocial group model called *The Community Table* to support the mental health and well-being of people who are displaced. It has evolved since 2015 out of our work on the France-UK border and the 'refugee crisis' in Europe. It has been used in various settings by a growing freelance team of art therapists, alongside artists with lived experience of displacement, in France, the UK, and further afield.

People who are displaced, alongside the community around them—humanitarian workers, interpreters, welfare officers, security guards, volunteers—are welcomed to join and make art alongside one another at the table. Collectively, this work offers a temporary community and a place to pause for a brief time (Lloyd & Usiskin, 2022).

Most people we encounter are male, of all ages but predominantly in their twenties. They have traveled mostly from north and east Africa, Asia, and across the Middle East. Separated from their families and communities, they often have limited or no psychological and financial support and face enormous challenges. Their lives, skills, experiences, roles, and reasons for leaving home are multiple, but are not given foremost attention once they are in transit and enter the asylum system.

Over the years, we have sat at these tables with men from a vast range of professions and backgrounds, including builders, architects, designers, scientists, computer programmers, and engineers. They sit alongside artists, teachers, priests, doctors, musicians, barbers, shopkeepers, sportsmen, students, writers, farmers, former soldiers, car mechanics, electricians, chefs, beekeepers, and ice-cream makers. Many speak of their studies and careers having been aborted due to poverty, war, or fleeing forced conscription. Their normal life rhythms have been suspended, along with the loss of family relationships and home.

Border politics

France

We have documented our work on the France-UK border and explored within this our use of different materials and media, including maps (Carta et al., 2023; Lloyd & Usiskin, 2020), social media (Usiskin & Lloyd, 2020), postcards, installation (Usiskin et al., 2020), kites (Kalmanowitz & Lloyd, 2016), and construction materials (Lloyd et al., 2018). The border is a longstanding crisis setting in which people who want to claim asylum in the UK find themselves needing first to navigate the political and geographic land border along with the body of water (the English Channel) that lies between the two countries. As on other European borders, people often get stuck, sometimes for months, even years.

The town of Calais in northern France, where the focus of our work has been, is a complex, messy, and often violent place for people on the move. Trafficking, exploitation, and homelessness are rife. Over the past decade, we have witnessed the active reshaping of the town and surrounding landscape, including a proliferation of hostile architecture that disrupts the environment both physically and psychologically. Numerous overt walls, fences, boundaries, barriers, and other fortifications have been built alongside increased covert surveillance, with access to public space decreasing for both people displaced and residents of the town. Over recent years, the Calais prefecture has used large rocks to block entrances to public land where individuals and families have attempted to sleep. In 2023, heavy machinery was used to move several hundred large boulders into a living site in the town center, uncannily mirroring the number of people on the move at that time.

The former makeshift camp known as *The Jungle* had an estimated population of 10,000 at its height. People built their own enclosures, structures, and encampments, often collectively with others from their own communities. This built environment not only expressed an instinctive need to create shelter, but also often echoed the architectural forms of people's cultures (Breeze, 2023). In October 2016, this camp was dismantled, and since then large camps have not been tolerated in this border setting.

In this context, our psychosocial work has taken place in The Jungle camp, living sites, a large day center, roadside psychosocial activities van, petrol station, launderette, and safe house, among other sites.

UK

The UK government's hostile environment policy has made it increasingly difficult for people seeking asylum in the UK to access safe, legal routes outside of a small number of formal resettlement schemes. People therefore reach the UK from France using irregular routes, traveling in trucks or, increasingly, in small boats. Since the withdrawal of the UK from the European Union (Brexit) in 2016, the UK government has introduced increasingly hostile, anti-migrant measures to deter people from crossing into the UK, including the Illegal Migration Act (July 2023) and Safety of Rwanda Act (April 2024). Government policies are ever changing, but deep insecurity for people on the move is consistent, elicited by their not knowing what will happen next.

Living in temporary accommodations run by the UK Home Office—hotels, ex-military camps, repurposed ships—and lack of clarity around timescales and processes has greatly impacted people's mental health. Asylum seekers are left feeling deskilled and undervalued. Existing in an ongoing state of limbo, they are prevented from working and depend on the State, voluntary sector support, and/or gig economy. These factors can lead to stress, anxiety, depression, and—for some—a loss of hope. In this context our psychosocial work has taken place in hotels, former army and air-force camps, and youth and church hall drop-in services.

Cross-Channel work and social media

The cross-Channel work takes place in indoor and outdoor spaces alongside local and international organizations and NGO's. Prevailing psycho-social-political issues include homelessness, hostility, discrimination, and violence, with campaigning and awareness-raising for safe legal routes a consistent counter-narrative to the mainstream political rhetoric. Meanwhile, a difficulty for the poorest and most marginalized is that they have no means of voicing their concerns or impacting policy debates. The use of social media forms a key element of the work of Art Refuge, acting as a platform from which images and words can be shared, and those participating can actively find voice and visibility (Usiskin et al., 2020).

Building home

Bricks as material

Bricks as a modular building material have been around for millennia. Both sun-dried and kiln-fired bricks were used 6,000 years ago in the building of the city of Uruk, Mesopotamia (Cruickshank, in Hall, 2015). Using the elements of earth, water, and fire, their color and texture is dependent on the clay from which they are made. They are sustainable, breathable, structural, and aesthetic. Because bricks are one of the most ubiquitous, strongest, and oldest of building materials, we have witnessed how immediately familiar the clay bricks are to the people who join our work. In their ordinariness, bricks manage to hold personal and cultural resonance, with many participants being builders and even brickmakers.

Bricks are a crucial material in our kit of largely pre-used and reusable materials. They are nurtured and cared for, organized, and packed back in their box, returned to again and again, and handled by many people. The desire to build and establish space has carried through our work across sites. Throughout the ever-harsher developments on either side of the Channel, during which we have observed the sleep deprivation, exhaustion, and hypervigilance of those who are displaced, there has been focused, painstaking building at The Community Table. The irony is not lost on us. Often it has been painful to watch the construction and deconstruction of miniature homes, shelters, and other buildings, while those we are working with are either homeless or in insecure temporary housing.

Manufactured in northern Europe some 50 years ago, each of our miniature red clay bricks measures 3.0 × 1.5 × 0.5 cm. While a full-scale brick is designed to be held in one hand, the dimensions of the miniature bricks are roughly the same proportions wherever they are made. The bricks encourage design, and are often used in such a way as to allow for structural loads that accommodate window and door openings and space for a roof, stairs, and room divisions.

Material politics

Denial of formal access to physical shelter in northern France exists alongside active confiscation and destruction of infrastructure, makeshift constructions, and basic possessions. This has included police smashing mobile phones, which consequently severs crucial connections. In an in-depth report about the degrading treatment of children and adults in this setting, human rights observers documented routine small-scale evictions as often as every 48 hours in Calais, and at least 90 mass evictions of encampments in northern France in 2020 and the first seven months of 2021 (Human Rights Watch, 2021).

Over the years, Art Refuge has increasingly steered clear of bringing quantities of shop bought art materials to the table, and instead is consciously concerned with reducing environmental impact and paying attention to the materials' source. The narratives, histories, and geographies of artworks made in the West are often divorced from their material origins and many generic materials (e.g., A4 white paper, pens, pencils) are mass produced and imported from other countries using cheap labor. In countering negative attitudes toward people on the move and the deliberate intent to dehumanize, we foster a culture that supports resilience. We actively strive to use materials that evoke associations to personal and cultural histories (Moon, 2010) as another way to challenge the dehumanizing cycle and cross borders. Collectively, the bricks themselves have become a cultural carrier, holding continuity across time and place, even though mortar isn't applied and rarely asked for, and the designs built are left on the table or swept away. The movement and potential of working with the bricks is a contrast to the often-static situation, hopelessness, and weight of issues.

Josie Carter, poet and member of the Art Refuge team on either side of the Channel, also volunteered in northern France in 2024. She wrote:

> The bricks cross the Channel again and again in a way that the people around the table can't. Their occupation of a cycle of re-crossing and re-use is a counterpoint to a kind of incomplete cycle that is found everywhere in Northern France coastal living sites—of donation, use, and abandonment-confiscation-destruction. Goods are given in good faith to satisfy the very real material needs of people seeking refuge, then used and discarded, or taken or destroyed by police.

People live among the debris of what has been given to them that they can no longer use: soiled clothes, broken tents, empty containers. The dynamics of the distribution of donations speaks to the ineffectiveness of the practice as a strategy to subvert the structural violence inherent in the conditions of the border. Applied repetitively and unconsciously as a sticking-plaster to cover for the impossibilities of living outside, they make the material world of the border one that reflects the disposability of its inhabitants.

In contrast to the spent debris of objects used to their exhaustion, the cyclical and periodic reappearance of the bricks seems sometimes to pierce the stuckness, repetitive rhythms, and material accretion that define Calais as an environment. The care and custodianship that go into reusing them speaks to the possibility of longevity, renewal, and sharing, as they pass through many hands and recur in many different places. Objects that are long-lasting, beautiful, and communally held are in short supply in the borderlands of Northern France. Rare too are exchanges that feel reciprocal and un-freighted by the inequalities inherent in much of the work done by NGOs with people on the move.

We see the complexities in this border setting, and that it is difficult to think clearly and reflexively. We also wonder about the unrealistic expectations and sense of disempowerment that might inadvertently be set up for people both in the here and now, and for the future as they continue their journey to the UK or elsewhere.

Home

What is prevalent on both sides of the Channel is the thinking of, longing for, and wondering about home. It could be said that the loss of home is what defines refugees (Taylor, 2013). Samer, a refugee in the UK whom we first met in Calais said, 'Home is not where you come from, it is where you feel you are safe.' Bachelard (1958/1994) links memories of home with the self: "The house we were born in is physically inscribed in us" (p. 14). With displacement and the loss of home comes what Papadopoulos

(2021) describes as "onto-ecological unsettledness" (p. 142). He suggests that this links to geography and environments where time, place, and space may literally be computed differently.

Through the bricks' sensory qualities—their tactility and aesthetics—memories, stories, and dreams emerge. Like soulful food, among the range of carefully selected materials on our tables, the bricks' texture, tone, color, and sound hold resonance. The bricks are robust but not inert. They bear the gentle marks of use over time, some softened at the edges as if washed by the sea. The individual bricks become imbued with human handling, traces of past experiences, and cultural richness held within them. Latour (2000) suggests, "things do not exist without being full of people" (p. 10). Freeman et al. (2015) suggest, "things do not exist without being full of memory" (p. 4).

The bricks make explicit the memory of home, linked with the temporal and conceptual. There are painful memories of homes lost, but also the possibility of new homes in the future. Physical engagement with the bricks helps the structures become embodied in people's minds as homes they can carry with them, along with other resources and experiences that support resilience (Lloyd et al., 2018). In the words of Abdullah, a refugee in Calais from Afghanistan who made many houses at the table: *When I try to build the rooms and everything, it is like my house. One day I will have a house like this. There are 100 things in your mind, but you forget once you start building. It is real for me, it is real. For me I am inside it.*

In both France and UK settings, people sometimes return to the table, and so there is the possibility of processing experiences over time:

> A young man from Iran who had built a series of houses last week joined us at the table again and built a new house that felt stronger than those that came before it. This time he included a garden wall, a gradual evolution from basic shelter toward a more comfortable dwelling. A young man from Afghanistan had attempted to build his family home several weeks earlier but had left abruptly. He too returned to the table today and carefully recreated the floor plan with the bricks, this time adding detail, building a strong floor, and remaining with us for some time.
>
> (Essex, England 16.02.24)

Grounding and regulation

While the physical contexts imply transience and uncertainty, and the groups take place in often busy—even chaotic—spaces, the bricks in their solidity, reliability, and durability are grounding. Building with the bricks creates a rhythm; selecting and placing in an ordered form helps regulate breathing. Once the brick courses are laid, other possibilities emerge. A structure can be built, knocked down, or returned to the box, but the material still exists. We also actively support people taking photographs on their mobile phones as a durable record they can return to and view over time.

People often play with scale, for example, with small bricks viewed in juxtaposition with the surface of large maps. Playing with scale and the repeated visual and kinesthetic movement between large and small not only introduces different perspectives but can also help integrate both cognitive and emotional processing by engaging both hemispheres of the brain (Lusebrink, 2004). It can also be a useful way to alleviate difficult feelings in the here and now, like bilateral stimulation used to support integration of difficult experiences (Tripp, 2007) and to facilitate sensory awareness and emotional regulation (Talwar, 2007).

The play between macro and micro is also a replication of wider socio-political situations. The issues around war, conflict, climate emergencies, poverty, and displacement are overwhelming. It is impossible to determine how any of this can be resolved. Working small offers the opportunity to focus in and experience something as contained and controllable, reinforced by the scale of the bricks. The work can also extend into the virtual space of social media and back to the physical table, allowing for play with perspective and scale, seeing things in different ways.

> One man built a Roman bridge out of the bricks, which he placed on top of Syria on the tablecloth map alongside a photo of the bridge he had located on his mobile phone, saying it's not far from his family home. He delighted in using the large magnifier to focus in on the bridge, and then he moved onto an elaborate construction of a larger site. He ended by mapping out a brick journey from Syria to Calais.
>
> (Calais, France, 15.11.2019)

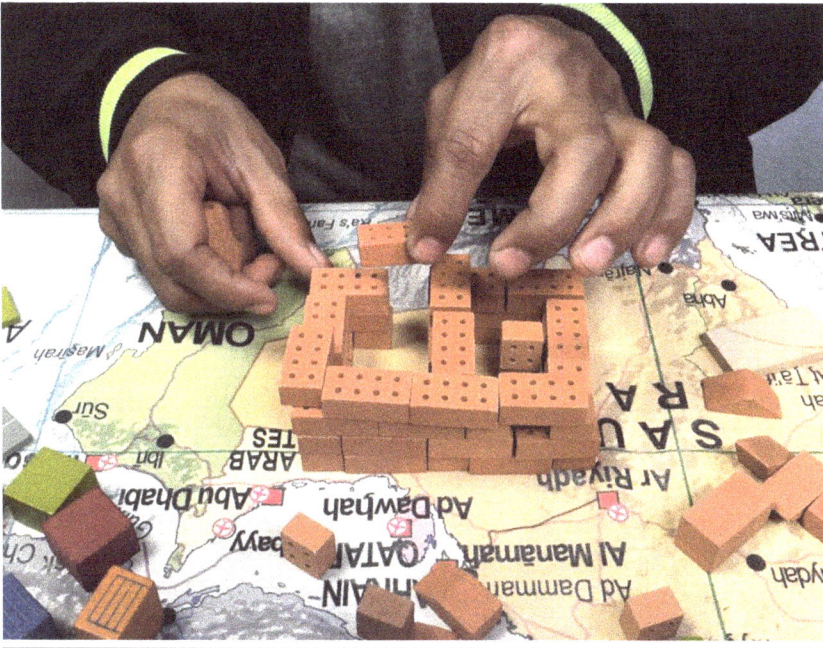

Figure 17.1 Building with the miniature bricks.

Sometimes the context makes the work's rhythm difficult to find, like an irregular heartbeat, while building with the bricks helps establish a rhythm. The sense of urgency to join the table has at times been intense, reflecting the hostile border conditions. On the first occasion we introduced the bricks in Calais, men took turns joining the table, bringing with them tension, anger, relief, and sadness.

> It was boiling hot. Some men had sunburned faces; several were dropping off to sleep in their chairs. Many appeared to be on alert, fractious, ready to snap. Men and boys, largely from Afghanistan, sat down at the table and started to build with the clay bricks. Across the two hours individuals joined the table, taking turns to sit in front of and add to the houses being carefully, expertly constructed. Poignantly, the roofs proved the hardest to build, mini roof tiles falling through the rafters. There was a queue of men wanting to have their turn. One man was meticulous about his brick courses being in line, protective of his building, not

wanting help. His friends instead gave ideas or made furniture. He told us of his lack of sleep from living over so many months in this challenging environment, and of his desire for water for the dream home he was building.

(Calais, France, 22.05.2017)

Culture, connection, and community

The modularity of the bricks can capture imagination and allow for infinite possibilities. We have observed how people place their own culture, history, traditions, ways of living, feelings, and experiences into the structures they build. Our 500 miniature bricks have been transformed into thousands of homes, buildings, shelters, and farms from across the world.

The structures are relatable, enabling a way to connect with and be supported by others around the table. Alex Holmes, letter-carver and long-term volunteer at the safe house in Calais wrote: *The bricks are so tactile, so satisfyingly solid to build with—a small house, a leaning tower, a serpentine wall. All around the table, other buildings are rising—here a*

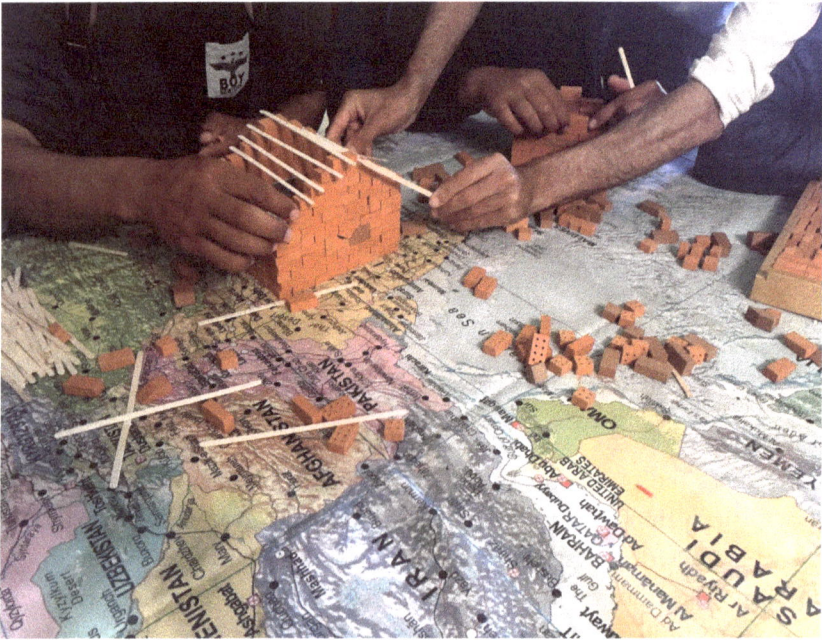

Figure 17.2 Three men build house structures using miniature bricks, Calais, France, 2017.

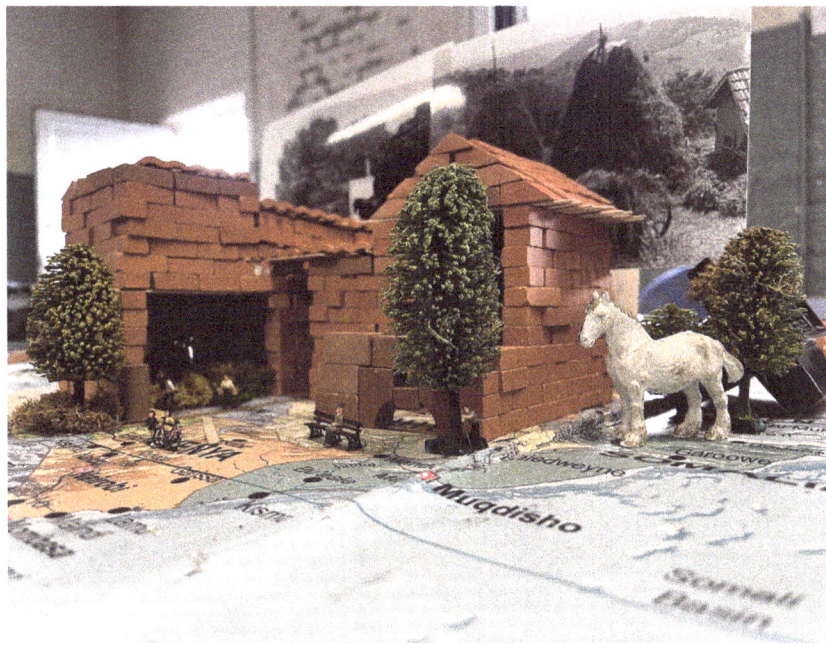

Figure 17.3 A farmhouse made out of miniature bricks, and other objects, Kent, England, 2023.

church, here an animal pen, here a round and roofed hut. Then a new idea, a railway track gradually extends across the table. The solitary constructions are now interlinked.

Aida Silvestri, interdisciplinary artist and member of The Community Table team, originally from Eritrea, wrote: *The miniature bricks hold a sentimental value in my heart and provide a comforting sense of familiarity because they remind me of my mother. When she was building her new home, there was a shortage of building bricks. Determined to find a solution, she decided to make the bricks herself with the support of friends and family. I have a vivid memory of that time, filled with laughter, songs, food, and my mother's commanding voice overseeing everything. People were gathering dirt, some were mixing the dirt with water and using their feet to create clay, while others, including my mother, were shaping the clay mixture into rectangular wooden molds.*

The bricks capture a sense of togetherness and the joy of creating something meaningful as a community. They serve as a tangible connection to my mother's strength, determination, and the fond memories I have of that time. As I work with the miniature bricks, I embrace the emotions and memories they evoke, the spirit of festivity, joy, and community that surrounded my mother's brick-making endeavor.

In another early group in Calais, the bricks brought people together around the table:

> The business at the table lent itself to a communal atmosphere where older men joined to support younger builders, developing a small construction into a large mosque complete with a shower and places to wash feet. Across the table, two builders were remembering their work together on building sites, referring to saved photos on their mobile phones of houses from their old jobs to recreate scaled down models, while a friend appointed himself as site-manager, offering advice on roof construction.
>
> (Calais 01.09.2017)

At the table are often additional boxes of miniature roof tiles and shaped bricks, alongside trees and foliage, which are used to add further texture and life to the collective dioramas that follow. They also help reflect the very practical realities for people living outside, such as the changeable weather.

> At the day center, in the fiercest heat of the day, buildings were constructed with roofs, but no windows and doors. Here was the shade so desperately needed, but there was no access. Once this was noticed adaptations were made, rebuilding to find ways in and out. Those around the table helpfully offered advice and architectural design. Trees became a key part of the scenes; everyone wanted to have foliage near their buildings to offer cool shady respite, and maybe a sturdy and protective sense of shelter.
>
> (Calais 26.05.2017)

Conclusion

For the people we encounter, what becomes salient is finding ways to survive. When nothing in life is stable and a person is living in a state of limbo, the materiality of the work may offer the idea of permanence, even though the objects built are transitory.

At the time of this writing (April 2024), some of the huge Calais boulders had been quietly shifted out of place, revealing small patches of ground with grass, weeds, and flowers reappearing from beneath the rocks. Structures can shift. Fleeting poetic acts carried out with miniature bricks can also somehow diminish the dehumanizing effect of the border. We have learned to trust that the materials we use, in this case the bricks, can offer creative, imaginative opportunities for people that are both humanizing and empowering. Reusable, environmentally responsible, and sustainable, our faith in the material is transmitted to the people who join the table, who in turn make use of its transformative potential.

References

Bachelard, G. (1994). *The poetics of space* (J. Solas, Trans.). Beacon Press (Original work published 1958).

Breeze, M. (2023). Temporary sheltering, empowering design, and the jungle. A case for architects. In G. Karunaratne (Ed.), *Informal settlements of the global south* (pp. 29–46). Routledge.

Carta, S., Usiskin, M., Lloyd, B., & Tabar, P. (2023). Digital and physical spaces in informal settlements. Migrants, refugee camps, and mapping. In G. Karunaratne (Ed.), *Informal settlements of the global south* (pp. 81–95). Routledge.

Cruickshank, D. (2015). The first cities. In W. Hall (Ed.), *Brick* (pp. 9–11). Phaidon Press.

Freeman, L., Nienass, B., & Daniell, R. (2015). Memory, materiality, sensuality. *Memory Studies, 9*(1), 3–12. https://doi.org/10.1177/1750698015613969

Human Rights Watch (2021, October 7). Enforced misery: The degrading treatment of migrant children and adults in Northern France. https://www.hrw.org/report/2021/10/07/enforced-misery/degrading-treatment-migrant-children-and-adults-northern-france

Kalmanowitz, D., & Lloyd, B. (2016). Art therapy at the border: Holding the line of the kite. *Journal of Applied Arts & Health, 7*(2), 143–58. https://doi.org/10.1386/jaah.7.2.143_1

Kapitan, L. (2015). Social action in practice: Shifting the ethnocentric lens in cross-cultural art therapy encounters. *Art Therapy, 32*(3), 104–111. https://doi.org/10.1080/07421656.2015.1060403

Latour, B. (2000). The Berlin key or how to do words with things. In P. Graves-Brown (Ed.), *Matter, materiality, and modern culture* (pp. 10–21). (L Davis, Trans) Routledge.

Lloyd, B., & Usiskin, M. (2020). Reimagining an emergency space: Practice innovation within a frontline art therapy project on the France-UK border at Calais. *International Journal of Art Therapy, 25*(3), 132–142. https://doi.org/10.1080/17454832.2020.1786417

Lloyd, B., Usiskin, M., & Press, N. (2018). The Calais winds took our plans away: Art therapy as shelter. *Journal of Applied Arts & Health, 9*(2), 171–184. https://doi.org/10.1386/jaah.9.2.171_1

Lloyd, B., & Usiskin, U. (2022). The community table: Developing art therapy studios on, in-between and across borders. In C. Brown & H. Ormond (Eds.), *Contemporary practice in studio art therapy* (pp. 102–116). Routledge.

Lusebrink, V. B. (2004). Art therapy and the brain: An attempt to understand the underlying processes of art expression in therapy. *Art Therapy, 21*(3), 125–135. https://doi.org/10.1080/07421656.2004.10129496

Moon, C. H. (Ed.). (2010). *Materials and media in art therapy: Critical understandings of diverse artistic vocabularies.* Routledge.

Papadopoulos, R. K. (2021). *Involuntary dislocation: Home, trauma, resilience and adversity-activated development.* Routledge.

Talwar, S. (2007). Accessing traumatic memory through art making: An art therapy trauma protocol (ATTP). *Arts in Psychotherapy, 34*, 22–35. https://doi.org/10.1016/j.aip.2006.09.001

Taylor, H. (2013). Refugees, the state and the concept of home. *Refugee Survey Quarterly, 32*(2), 130–152. https://doi.org/10.1093/rsq/hdt004

Tripp, T. (2007). A short term therapy approach to processing trauma: Art therapy and bilateral stimulation. *Art Therapy, 24*(4), 176–183. https://doi.org/10.1080/07421656.2007.10129476

Usiskin, M., & Lloyd, B. (2020). Lifeline, frontline, online: Adapting art therapy for social engagement across borders. *International Journal of Art Therapy, 25*(4), 183–191. https://doi.org/10.1080/17454832.2020.1845219

Usiskin, M., Lloyd, B., & Press, N. (2020). Temporary, portable, virtual: Making galleries on the France-UK border at Calais. In A. Coles & H. Jury (Eds.), *Art therapy, museums and galleries: Reframing practice* (pp. 265–288). Jessica Kingsley.

18

FESTIVAL PEDAGOGY
ACROSS AND BETWEEN

Pamela Whitaker

Festival opening: the art of gatherings

This chapter highlights the concept of placemaking in relation to festivals in Belfast, Northern Ireland, a city wounded by a history of sectarian conflict. Placemaking refers to strengthening the connection between people and the assets of their lived environments. In positioning its many festivals as sites of potential reconciliation and regeneration, the city of Belfast aims to bring people together for the purpose of cultural re-experiencing and the consideration of new ideas and approaches to life in Northern Ireland.

This chapter also introduces festival art therapy as a pedagogical method for employing art therapy as a public art and public health practice. Festivals are inclusive in the way they bring people together for the shared purpose of experiencing co-existence and the potential to influence new perspectives through public pedagogy and a citizenship of strangers (Biesta, 2012). The therapeutic alliance in this context is with people and places that are unexpected, and the therapeutic aim is contributing to creative health and well-being. Within this framework, the city becomes campus and art therapy pedagogy becomes a form of team teaching with cultural partners. The *walking studio* featured in this chapter is an example of a festival art event co-facilitated by the author in collaboration with

DOI: 10.4324/9781032720166-20

a trainee art therapist. It is a form of environmental art therapy within the midst of city life using the materiality of the urban landscape as a focus for personal and societal contemplation.

The materiality of festivals is about placemaking. It includes a series of venues, the physicality of participants experiencing and moving through events, and the meanings associated with festival locations and routes traversed. "Place creates individual and group identity through a number of interconnected constituents that include agency, behavior, and history" (Gheorghiu & Nash, 2013, p. 2) as well as territoriality. The attributes and materials of a place are associated with both contemporary and historical contexts that intertwine, so that the meaning of a shared space is dependent on a network of associations. Dean and Millar (2005) describe place as a process of interpenetrations and superimpositions generated from both historical and contemporary practices of habitation, which make and re-make the materiality of a place over time.

The festival venue is an overall *eventscape*, "a space that enables the construction and display of [individual and collective] identity and belonging and has the capacity to provide considerable change to the places that are part of its process" (Belboe, 2021, p. v). The *becoming* at a festival is occasion specific, an opportunity to be in the making with an event that is multifaceted and transformative. Festivals are educational, expressive, and challenging of preconceived ideas. They offer multiple occurrences and opportunities to be with people in curated events that are out of the ordinary.

Context

Belfast is a city with a 30-year history of political conflict between two communities in Northern Ireland—nationalists (seeking a united Ireland) and loyalists (seeking to maintain sovereignty with the United Kingdom). It can be considered a wounded city structured by a history of individual and social trauma that shapes expectations, opportunities for movement, and the use of space (Till, 2012). "Reactions to political violence are likely to limit the repertoire of flexible and creative responses by individuals and groups and to promote rigid and compulsive thinking and acting" (Papadopoulos, 2005, p. 37).

A festival composes a situation of affiliation and shared purpose, supporting discovery and change. Belfast City Council values the transformative capacity of the arts "in dealing with complex issues around legacy, conflict, and reconciliation" (Belfast City Council, 2024, para. 1). To this end, festivals are organized in the city as a form of mediation, positioning the city as a place for people to gather and co-create, re-making a once volatile city into one safe for accommodating differences of opinion. Belfast City Council (2023) considers placemaking to be a people-centered approach to both design and stewardship because it prioritizes inclusivity, safety, enjoyment, and opportunities for extended movement within the urban environment.

Festivals encourage new perceptions of self, others, and the urban landscape, with participants sculpting relations that extend beyond preconceived boundaries. A festival is a temporary community operating as a potential countermeasure for inhibition and binary thinking, encouraging instead unconventional, divergent, and varied perspectives (Whitaker, 2021b). Till (2012) proposes an ethos of place-based care that contradicts divisions between 'safe' and 'unsafe' territories. Within a wounded city, festivals provide symbolic regeneration through artistic interventions that attend to the recovery of both people and their localities.

Festivity as art therapy pedagogy

The aim of festival art therapy is to encourage health promotion through live arts within a culture of learning and connection. Festivity enhances expression, ideas, imagination, and cultural potential. As a formation of the public homeplace (Timm-Bottos, 2006, 2017), festival art therapy is a networking of identity across events that aim to challenge complacency, while also composing therapeutic ensembles of inquiry. A festival can encourage empathetic encounters with new people and places, evoking a sense of meeting life as it happens (Bell et al., 2018). Festival practitioners can 'perform' themselves within the materiality of these locations (Purrington, 2021), which act as scenes with props for experimentation.

Ideally, art therapy education is composed along a community-to-clinical continuum that incorporates public relations, including the contributions of lived experience experts, activists, change-makers, and social influencers. With a focus on "art therapy for active citizenship" (Whitaker & Riccardi, 2019, p. 105), art therapy students at the Belfast School of Art, Ulster University develop skills in social advocacy, co-production, event management, psychological first aid, open studio facilitation, and psychosocial support, all within the public sphere.

Educational benefits for festival participants can result from extending art therapy pedagogy into the thoroughfares of public life. Festivity is composed of multiple experiences, a series of *ands* that take participants to new places within themselves and their surroundings. Festivals can become a form of psychological first aid, encouraging agency, expression, empowerment, and communication through opportunities for engagement.

Art psychotherapy trainees in Belfast have contributed to disability activist festivals, mental health festivals, and arts festivals as the co-facilitators of artmaking workshops, exhibition openings, walking studios, and seminars. The chance to learn from the lived experiences of those most affected by social exclusion and discrimination has been a vital outcome of student participation. Festivals offer experiences of professional becoming within events that are transformative in their ability to generate thresholds of new cultural imaginings.

A festival offers a continuum of experiences across its varied events, which encourages psychological variation and capacity. "Art therapy in this context is not the making of an object, but the making of a range of experiences—the potential to move beyond limitations and to make more of one's life" (Whitaker, 2021b, p. 309). Festivals can be considered a social prescription that encourages creative health through cultural experiencing. They can promote the wellness factor of the arts for mutuality, regeneration, and togetherness (Whitaker, 2021b).

For art therapy trainees, festivals encourage site-specific creativity, contextual safeguarding (creating safety within public space), and the offering of psychosocial supports within a portable studio (Kalmanowitz & Lloyd, 2011). Art therapy studios within public events are informed by ethical standards, including an ethos of "trauma-informed practice which recognizes that trauma exposure can impact an individual's neurological, biological, psychological and social development" (Office of Health Improvement and Disparities, 2022, para. 4).

Festivals as public practice art therapy

The inspiration for the term *festival art therapy* has come from two sources: an article by McLachlan (2017) describing an art therapy sanctuary created for a community art festival in Edmonton, Alberta, and a chapter by Timm-Bottos (2012) referencing a co-produced community art exhibition for the Albuquerque Festival of the Arts in New Mexico. Both art therapists generated an interactive art experience that was a catalyst for public engagement and being "in relationship to another's way of seeing" (Timm-Bottos, 2012, p. 107).

McLachlan produced an art installation titled *The Listening Cave* for a family festival. It served as a retreat space from the busy thoroughfares of the festival, featuring a tent-like enclosure with a soft interior and ambient music. Afterwards, the cave became an inspiration for McLachlan's own art therapy studio located within a primary school.

> The listening cave was a surreal, different environment, a mini oasis that temporarily softened the noisiness outside, a place for families to snuggle in a big pile. Similarly, the therapy room is a small, very different place from the rest of the school, somewhat of a retreat for those children and families who are struggling in their everyday environments and their self-care.
>
> (McLachlan, 2017, p. 7)

Timm-Bottos co-created an art exhibition within a storefront space called *Art Street* where artists with differing social needs engaged in artmaking. Many of the participating artists did not have a home, but through artmaking within this public homeplace they found a place to be represented and acknowledged. As an act of intentional community making, each person's artistry was exposed to a wider audience and their life experiences were appreciated rather than interpreted or stigmatized (Timm-Bottos, 2012).

A festival can be an opportunity for activism in relation to social concerns. It transforms the way public space is inhabited by creating an unscripted or unexpected social experience. Deterritorialized art therapy pedagogy can encompass festivity as a form of learning that brings students to unexpected social "juxtapositions, realignments and confrontations between previously isolated groups, cultures and social forces" (Brandist et al., 2017, p. 850). A festival can be a transformative pedagogical event, producing new paradigms for knowledge, social innovation, and rites of passage.

French philosopher Gilles Deleuze characterized events as scenes that decodify space and invite a call to action, with reverberating effects. As a series of events, a festival is a rhizomatic production of space that temporarily reconfigures reality, "reshaping connectivity, relationships, and the material fabric of connectivity" (Beck & Gleyson, 2016, p. 329). Deleuze proposed the concept of nomadic space, which corresponds to festivity in the sense of occupying "a collective experience of a socially shared space and time" for emergent effects (Lorraine, 2006, p. 159). A festival has a place within art therapy pedagogy as it can teach students how to create a public art therapy experience with reverberating effects, one that extends participants' familiarity and comfort into encounters with formerly unknown places and stigmatized people.

Festivity as social sculpture

The artist Joseph Beuys championed cultural production within the immediate environments of people's lives as a representation of activist agency and artistry. As an expanded concept of art as social sculpture, this form of making was intended to elicit the public's collaboration in shaping new potentials within civic society.

> Beuys's concept of creativity and his statement that every human being is an artist does not chiefly mean that each individual should only develop [their] creative capacities, but that these capacities should be developed in the context of the wider field of social responsibility. How can people work together so that they can create a social sculpture in which every individual is represented and no one's substance and quality gets lost?
>
> (Zumdick, 2015)

Beuys expansion of art into lived environments was inspired by Fluxus, an international affiliation of artists dedicated to performance art, artistic endeavors influenced by chance encounters, and the alignment of artmaking with everyday life. The Fluxus philosophy encouraged alternative ways of experiencing social space and constructing its meaning.

In 1974, at the height of the political conflict in Northern Ireland, the Belfast School of Art was the site of a Joseph Beuys performative lecture. Beuys encouraged social activations as interventions for changing perceptions within contested urban territories. At the time of his lecture, Belfast city center was impacted by armed conflict, bombing, and civil unrest. Yet Beuys encouraged each person's artistic potential to extend beyond restriction into generative production. Beuys believed that *live art* is a form of recovery from the traumatized social body (Kuspit, 2023). "It loosens defense mechanisms through its play with meaning, identity, socialization [and] ambiguous space" (Whitaker, 2005, p. 29). The transgressive gestures of festivals, a form of live art, challenges predictability, enacting instead an *as if* formulation of life potential in the making (Whitaker, 2005).

Festivals bring to life the extraordinary, the uncomfortable, and the unexpected. They encourage new social rituals and choreograph bodies and minds into new actions, with activities that reinforce attachment and affiliation, and enhance a sense of belonging. They are a formulation of what is possible in the context of unscripted social encounters that encourage experimentation (Whitaker, 2021b).

Festivals as curriculum: the walking studio

Cultural practicums within the art psychotherapy training at the Belfast School of Art are short term, event-led projects that enhance service learning through community practice (Feen-Calligan et al., 2018; Nolan, 2019, 2023). Ulster University is committed to Belfast's development as a learning city, promoting lifelong learning for personal and social aims and an enhanced quality of life (Belfast Strategic Partnership, 2015). To this end, the art psychotherapy training contributes bespoke workshops to festivals with the aim of positioning the university as a public homeplace for both students and the public-at-large.

One of the features of festival participation by art psychotherapy students has been the facilitation of the walking studio—a curated walk through the arts quarter of Belfast co-produced by the author and art therapy students. The walk features street art, found poetry, art galleries, and historic alleyways. Walks have also included invited guests, such as an architect specializing in spatial design and a street artist sharing the stories behind the production of street art imagery. Within the arts district of Belfast, an annual street art festival invites artists to create works without a specific reference to the conflict in Northern Ireland. These artworks stand out against Belfast's political murals, which designate the boundaries of nationalist and loyalist neighbourhoods and typically include images of armed paramilitary figures. In contrast, street art ignites conversations, encouraging conviviality within unfamiliar places, and transforms neglected areas in need of regeneration. By subverting the expected order of urban spaces, street art prompts viewers to question their preconceptions and to think critically about the world around them (Street Buddha, 2023). As stopping points along the walking studio route, they serve as locations for extemporized artmaking and discussion.

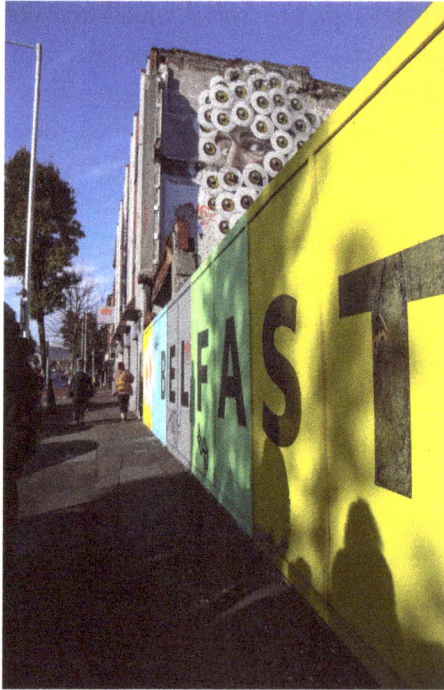

Figure 18.1 Photo Credit: Savannah Corbett (2023). The Walking Studio Street Art Tour [Personal Collection].

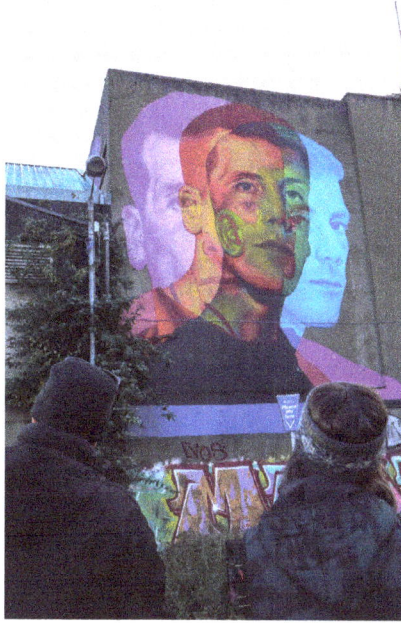

Figure 18.2 Photo Credit: Savannah Corbett (2023). The Walking Studio Street Art Tour [Personal Collection].

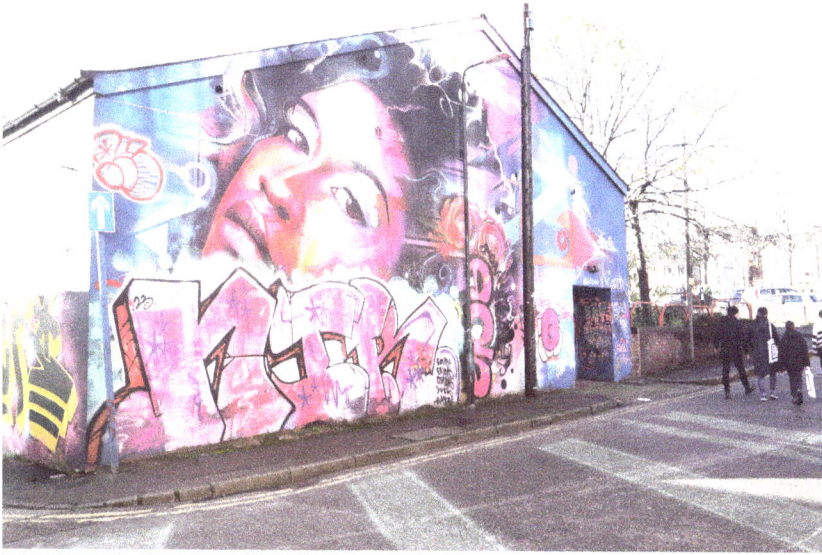

Figure 18.3 Photo Credit: Savannah Corbett (2023). The Walking Studio Street Art Tour [Personal Collection].

For art psychotherapy students, the guided walk is an opportunity to facilitate art viewing within public spaces at pre-determined stopping points that act as impromptu studios. Photography, spoken word poetry, mark making, and found materials influence participants' impressions of streetscapes and exhibitions. A performative activity is also included within the walk, which is typically each person sharing their walking poem (a collection of words found along the route) as they enact intentional movement through passageways between nearby streets.

A walking studio is a social sculpture, an aggregate of people walking together through civic spaces. "To walk is to study, reflect, connect with and understand your surroundings....Walking is a breathing in of the world; it is how we make sense of place" (Sullivan, 2015, p. 11). A walking route can also be considered a mapping of locations through psychogeography, a walking art practice pioneered by French philosopher Guy Debord in the 1950s (O'Rourke, 2013). It involves venturing into places one has never been before as an act of inquisitiveness, experimentation, and psychological versatility. To discover the extraordinary of an ordinary place is to suspend predictable patterns of behavior and responses.

> The scenes of walking…cannot be taken for granted, but must be realized as artistic material that coexists with embodiment and subjectivity out in the open. The walker is a researcher and an explorer. Walking is an extension of selfhood into a network of social implications.
>
> (Whitaker, 2021a, p. 50)

Encouraging multiple perspectives is a characteristic of the walking studio, leading to enhanced conversations about social contexts and varied environments. Participant-researchers walk the streets with a sense of inquiry rather than conclusion.

Walking in a wounded city involves situating oneself in zones that have been sites of conflict, violence, and trauma. Careri (2017) refers to these places as unexpressed parts of a city that evoke fear and loss of control. The walking studio provides opportunities to negotiate an assemblage of narratives about the meaning of various territories. "People live in the same city, even in the same part of a city, and yet perceive different worlds" (Tuan, 1974, p. 248). The navigation of these narratives is facilitated by art psychotherapy students who bring together the *ands* of people's different encounters with the places they find themselves in during the walking studio. Together, they create an art assemblage, a compilation of impressions put into both words and art.

The walking studio provides art therapy trainees an opportunity to practice community art therapy with its goals of inclusiveness, accessibility, and providing a place of belonging (Nolan, 2023). As a component of festival art therapy, it is not a treatment, but rather an artmaking experience within an event that brings people together. "People can engage with others who are different and then decenter their own experience, which opens them up to changing their perspectives while challenging their assumptions and biases" (Nolan, 2023, p. 19).

Closing ceremony: festival highlights

This chapter encourages integration of art therapy pedagogy into festival events. Public relations pedagogy embraces the city as campus and positions art therapy curriculums as public-facing events that enact civic responses to social concerns. A festival is immersive and generative. Through its events, it invites the challenging of defense mechanisms within a civic society that has experienced a history of conflict and sectarianism. Festivals can stage antidotes to fright and flight responses through somatic experiences that release tensions, physical sensations, and affects. Special events can mediate difference through the enactment of new cultural rites of passage geared toward peace building and conflict transformation.

Festivals offer new ways of perceiving a familiar context. They encourage fresh thinking patterns, expanded routes of travel, and flexibility in meeting new situations and people. Festivals are transitional, instilling urban environments with novel symbolic associations generated through connectivity, discussion, and knowledge making (Belfast Strategic Partnership, 2015). Challenging fixed thinking and trauma response patterns inspires the restaging of a wounded city's history. Given that metamorphosis and transition are hallmarks of festivals, these psychological qualities can help to shape a city's identity by rejuvenating culture, redressing conflict through cross-cultural experimentation, and creating unrestricted lifeways (St John, 2023). New routes of passage can be encouraged through the curation of public events that transport people to different places within themselves and within their community.

The walking studio is one example of a festival activity that positions the city as canvas and encourages the creative impulse within city wayfaring. Walking studio participants become street artists who produce both a walk's artefacts (found object assemblages, photography, writing, and mark making) and its performance of social sculpture (in the way the walking group occupies public spaces). The walking studio is a mobile workshop that choreographs encounters with landmarks, art, architecture, urban design, and conversation to "draw the spectator out of passivity" (Tunnacliffe, 2016, p. 11) and into active citizenship.

For art psychotherapy trainees, participating in festivals expands their learning in relation to activism, developing site-specific studios, collaborating with lived experience experts, and developing restorative arts practices in short-term locations. "Occupying an extraordinary eventscape of wonder and novelty, inhabitants are exposed to new knowledge, praxis, and skills that may be adopted in their post-event lives" (St John, 2023, p. 18). As a professional context, festivals provide a space for innovation and skill-building in response to citizens who are attempting to move beyond a history of sectarian conflict and engage in "one of the hardest things to do in the face of extreme events…to remain open" (Kalmanowitz & Lloyd, 2011, p. 109). Festival art therapy extends public practice art therapy into the realm of creative health and hopeful narratives. It is an expression of the extraordinary ability of people to move life into new directions.

Acknowledgments

Sincere gratitude is extended to Rebekah Wynn, Megan McLaughlin, and Maggie Mulhare for participating in festival-based cultural practicums during their art psychotherapy training and contributing their ideas to this chapter. Appreciation is also extended to Savannah Corbett who contributed her photographs of a walking studio within the arts district of Belfast.

References

Beck, C., & Gleyson, F. X. (2016). Deleuze and the event(s). *Journal for Cultural Research, 20*(4), 329–333. https://doi.org/10.1080/14797585.2016.1264770

Belboe, O. J. (2021). *Eventscape: A theoretical exploration of events as spatial processes* [Master's thesis, Norwegian University of Science and Technology]. https://ntnuopen. ntnu.no/ntnu-xmlui/handle/11250/2785207

Belfast City Council. (2023). *Placemaking and urban design.* https://www.belfastcity.gov. uk/documents/placemaking-and-urban-design

Belfast City Council. (2024). *Belfast 2024 Programme.* https://www.belfastcity.gov.uk/belfast2024/the-programme/the-art-of-reconciliation#:~:text=F%C3%A9ile%20an%20Phobail%2C%20in%20partnership,around%20legacy%2C%20conflict%20and%20reconciliation

Belfast Strategic Partnership. (2015). *Belfast a learning city: A learning charter for Belfast.* https://www.makinglifebettertogether.com/wpcontent/themes/makinglifebetter/resources/lifelonglearning/Belfast%20A%20Learning%20City%20A4%20WEB.pdf

Bell, S., Foley, R., Houghton, F., Maddrell, A., & Williams, A. (2018). From therapeutic landscapes to healthy spaces: Places and practices. *Social Science and Medicine, 196,* 123–130. https://doi.org/10.1016/j.socscimed.2017.11.035

Biesta, G. (2012). Becoming public: Public pedagogy, citizenship, and the public sphere. *Social and Cultural Geography, 13*(7), 683–697. https://doi.org/10.1080/14649365.2012.723736

Brandist, C., Gardiner, M. E., White, J., & Mika, C. (2017). Bakhtin in the fullness of time: Bakhtinian theory and the process of social education. *Educational Philosophy and Theory, 49*(9), 849–853. https://doi.org/10.1080/00131857.2016.1227208

Careri, F. (2017). *Walkscapes: Walking as aesthetic practice.* Culicidae Press.

Dean, T., & Millar, J. (2005). *Place.* Thames and Hudson.

Feen-Calligan, H., Moreno, J., & Buzzard, E. (2018). Art therapy, community building, activism, and outcomes. *Frontiers in Psychology, 9.* https://www.frontiersin.org/articles/10.3389/fpsyg.2018.01548/full

Gheorghiu, D., & Nash, G. (2013). Place, materiality, time, and ritual: Towards a relational archaeology. In D. Gheorghiu & G. Nash (Eds.), *Place as material culture: Objects, geographies and the construction of time* (pp. 1–13). Cambridge Scholars Publishing.

Kalmanowitz, D., & Lloyd, B. (2011). Inside-out, outside-in: Found objects and portable studio. In E. G. Levine & S. K. Levine (Eds.), *Art in action: Expressive arts therapy and social change* (pp. 104–127). Jessica Kingsley Publishers.

Kuspit, D. (2023, September 24). Joseph Beuys: The body of the artist. *Artforum.* https://www.artforum.com/features/joseph-beuys-the-body-of-the-artist-204066/

Lorraine, T. (2006). Ahab and becoming-whale: The nomadic subject in smooth space. In I. Buchanan & G. Lambert (Eds.), *Deleuze and space* (pp. 159–176). Edinburgh University Press.

McLachlan, C. (2017). Art therapy caves: Linking community art to a therapeutic space. *Canadian Art Therapy Association Journal, 30*(1), 4–10. https://doi.org/10.1080/08322473.2017.1303938

Nolan, E. (2019). Opening art therapy thresholds: Mechanisms that influence change in the community art therapy studio. *Art Therapy: Journal of the American Art Therapy Association, 36*(2), 7785. https://doi.org/10.1080/07421656.2019.1618177

Nolan, E. (2023). *Community art therapy: Theory and practice.* Routledge.

Office of Health Improvement and Disparities. (2022). *Working definition of trauma-informed practice.* https://www.gov.uk/government/publications/working-definition-of-trauma-informed-practice/working-definition-of-trauma-informed-practice#:~:text=Trauma%2Dinformed%20practice%20is%20an,biological%2C%20psychological%20and%20social%20development

O'Rourke, K. (2013). *Walking and mapping: Artists as cartographers*. MIT Press.

Papadopoulos, R. K. (2005). Political violence, trauma, and mental health interventions. In D. Kalmanowitz & B. Lloyd (Eds.), *Art therapy and political violence: With art, without illusion* (pp. 35–60). Routledge.

Purrington, B. (2021). Performance art therapy: Integrating performance art into expressive arts therapy [Master's thesis, Lesley University]. Digital Commons@Lesley. https://digitalcommons.lesley.edu/cgi/viewcontent.cgi?article=1421&context= expressive_theses

St John, G. (2023). Transfestive horizons: An introduction. *Journal of Festive Studies, 5*, 11–40. https://doi.org/10.33823/jfs.2023.5.1.187

Street Buddha. (2023). *Street art and the psychology of public spaces: Unravelling the urban mind*. https://thestreetbuddha.com/street-art-and-the-psychology-of-public-spaces-unraveling-the-urban-mind/

Sullivan, L. (2015). *Walking sculpture: 1967–2015*. Yale University Press.

Till, K. E. (2012). Wounded cities: Memory-work and a place-based ethics of care. *Political Geography, 31*, 3–14. https://doi.org/10.1016/j.polgeo.2011.10.008

Timm-Bottos, J. (2006). Constructing creative community. *Canadian Art Therapy Association Journal, 19*(2), 12–26. https://doi.org/10.1080/08322473.2006.11432285

Timm-Bottos, J. (2012). The "five and dime": Developing a community's access to art-based research. In H. Burt (Ed.), *Art therapy and postmodernism: Creative healing through a prism* (pp. 97–117). Jessica Kingsley Publishers.

Timm-Bottos, J. (2017). Public practice art therapy. *Canadian Art Therapy Association Journal, 30*(2), 94–99. https://doi.org/10.1080/08322473.2017.1385215

Tuan, Y. (1974). *Topophilia: A study of environmental perception, attitudes, and values*. Columbia University Press.

Tunnacliffe, C. M. (2016). The power of urban street art in re-naturing urban imaginations and experiences. *University College London*, DPU Working Paper No. 182. https://www.ucl.ac.uk/bartlett/development/sites/bartlett/files/migrated-files/ WP_182_Claire_Malaika_T_June_0.pdf

Whitaker, P. (2005). Moving art, moving worlds: Performing the body in visual arts and art therapy. *Canadian Art Therapy Association Journal, 18*(2), 27–34. https://doi.org/ 10.1080/08322473.2005.11432276

Whitaker, P. (2021a). The art of walking: Composing landmarks, performing territory. In D. Wong & R. P. M. H. Lay (Eds.), *Found objects in art therapy: Materials and process* (pp. 39–59). Jessica Kingsley Publishers.

Whitaker, P. (2021b). Full on – Festival art therapy. *European Journal of Psychotherapy and Counselling, 23*(3), 303–317. https://doi.org/10.1080/13642537.2021.1961835

Whitaker, P., & Riccardi, M. (2019). Public relations: Art therapy pedagogy out of bounds. *Canadian Art Therapy Association Journal, 32*(2), 104–114. https://doi.org/ 10.1080/08322473.2019.1667170

Zumdick, W. (2015). U-topos: Beuy's social sculpture as a real-utopia and its relation to social practice today. In M. J. Jacob & K. Zeller (Eds.), *A lived practice* (pp. 133–157). School of the Art Institute of Chicago.

INDEX

Abukhodair, N. 142

access needs and accommodations 59, 60; *see also* inclusive spaces

A'Court, B. 8

activism: and climate crisis 147–162; and community art studios 228; and festival events 285–286; and fostering social change 178–190; and video production 16; *see also* social action

Adam, H. 179

Adams, R. E. 75

Adamson, G. 71, 73

Aktaş, B. M. 43

Alamri, E. 5

Alders Pike, A. 7, 9, 58, 61, 63

Alter-Muri, S. 111

American Psychiatric Association 133

Anderson, L. 72, 75

Anderson, M. 5, 165

Ansloos, J. 11, 50

anthropocentrism 35–36, 40, 45

Anthropy, A. 213

Anzaldúa, G. 242

Archibald, J. 118, 119

Archibald, L. 7

Arslanbek, A. 51, 59

art and editing apps 14, 200, 205, 211, 221

art making alongside participants: in comics creation 202–204; with families and their transgender children 180–183; as Peer Art Therapists 132, 134, 140, 144; as shared ritual and feminist ethics of care 111–112; as temporary community with displaced people 267

art materials, media, and practices: familiarity with 56; history of 3–28; range, quality, quantity 56–57; *see also* ethics

artificial intelligence (AI) 14, 205

arts activism: and climate crisis 147–162; and community art studios 228, and festival events 285–286; and fostering a more just and compassionate; society 178–190; and video production 16

arts-based research 18

Asher, D. 255

Ausman, T. 240

Austin, B. 212, 221

avatars 212–213

Awais, Y. J. 55, 60

Bachelard, G. 222
Badr, S. 241, 242
Bahn, G. H. 222
Bailey, M. 97
Baldur's Gate 212
Balsara, C. 135
Barad, K. 39, 40, 44
Barnwell, G. 10
Baudrillard, J. 158
Bauman, W. A. 44
Baumann, D. 88
Baurick, T. 153
Bayne, H. B. 252
Bean, A. M. 212
Becerra, L. A. 18
Bechtel, A. 19, 62
Beck, B., 38
Beck, C., 286
Belboe, O. J. 282
Belfast City Council 283
Belfast Strategic Partnership 287, 291
Belkofer, C. M. 18
Bell, S. 283
Belluck, P. 182
belonging: and Black women 92, 119; and
    citizens of a wounded city 282, 287,
    291; and marginalized communities
    225–226, 231, 233; see also inclusive
    spaces and practices
Bennett, M. 203
Bhabha, H. K., 240, 241
Biesta, G. 281
Billard, T. J. 164
Black-centered practices: Black women
    87–102; Black communities 225–226
blackness as material 229–231
Boal, A. 88, 92, 96
Bodenbender, C. 214, 216
body-based art practices: body adornment
    51, 104, 106, 109–112; body as ground
    or material xxiii, 37–38, 96–97, 124–
    125, 219–220; virtual reality 213–218;
    walking 7–8, 287–291

book arts 6–7
Bonz, A. G. 59
Boon, L. 7
Borkar, N. 159
Botzakis, S. 194, 197
Braidotti, R., 40
Brammer, J. A. 240, 243
Brandist, C. 286
Brandoff, R. 50, 57
Brauen, M. 243
Breeze, M. 268
Brown, A. M. 233
Brown, J. K. 71
Brown, P. 182
brown, z. l. 91
Brunet, E. 205
Brushwood Rose, C. 104, 107, 108
Bryant, B. 158
Büch, M. 258, 259
burlesque and drag performance 109–110

Cabañas, K. M. xxiii
Camden-Pratt, C. E. 138
Cameron, L. 41
Careri, F. 290
Carl, E. 214
Carlton, N. R. 13, 16, 220
Carpendale, M. 57, 198, 199
Carpenter, J. 74
Carroll, L. 74
Carta, S. 268
Carter, T. 55
Center for Disease Control 120
challenges of therapeutic makerspaces
    234–235
Chan, K. C. 214, 217
Chansky, R. A. 73
Chapin Stephenson, R. 31, 60
Charmaz, K. 81
Chilton, G. 15
Chittister, J. 159
Choe, N. S. 14, 63
Choi, A. 181, 184

Choi, K. 156

Ciesemier, K. 163

Clare, E. 44

clay: challenging characterization as a regressive material 33, 135–136; history of use in art therapy 3; as natural material 7; *see also* miniature clay bricks

Cleveland, C. 91

climate crisis 7–10, 38, 147–160

climate justice 8–10

clothing as art material: altering transgender children's clothes 179–181; hospital gowns as symbols of structural injustice in maternal healthcare 185–188; sweat suits embroidered with testimonies of pregnant women deprived of medical treatment during ICE detentions; symbolism 179, 181; wedding dresses as symbols of reproductive injustice 181–185

Cole, S. 8

collage: images representing diverse identities and lifestyles 63; and its limited scope in art therapy 19; in research 18; in scanography 221; SoulCollage® 100

Collier, A. F. 73

Collins, P. H. 91

comics: art therapy applications 19, 194, 197–198, 202–204, 206–207; digital comics 14, 205; and the Expressive Therapies Continuum 202; as sequential narratives 199–200; for storytelling 200–201, 204–205

community-based practices: for asylum seekers and displaced people 266–279; for Black Women 87–102; for eco-art activism 147–162; for marginalized communities 225–236; for reconciliation and regeneration in urban settings 281–293; for social change 178–193; for transgender community care 163–175

The Community Table model 267, 270, 272, 277–278

complex identity systems: and integrating materials and media into therapy 134–142; and Lived Experience 131–134; and recommendations for therapists 142–144

contemporary art: and climate crisis 149–150, 157; and collage 19; and congruence with art therapy xxiii–xxiv, 42; and crafts 73; and improvisation 256–257; of Joseph Beuys 286–287; and new materialisms 42; and public art in Belfast 287–291; and scanography 218–219

Corkhill, B. 5

crafts/crafting: applications in art therapy 4–7; benefits 4–5, 79–80; as female empowerment 72–74; history 71–73; as self-care for women in helping professions 70–83

Crenshaw, K. 95, 104, 229

Crilley, M. 44

Critical Theory 36–39; applied to improv 258–259; as means to examine gaps in research and practice 19–20, 36–39

crocheting and knitting: benefits 5, historical perspective 71

Cross, G. 18

Cruickshank, D. 270

cultural appropriation: in art therapy 49–51; in art therapy research 18; defined 49–50; how to avoid it 52–55, 246–249; of Indigenous spiritual healing practices 121; of mindfulness and mandalas 238, 240–241, 244–249; responding to the harm it causes 51–52

cultural considerations: aims and significance of art materials and practices 11–12, 34–35, 58–59; cultural continuity in Indigenous creation practices 120–128; cultural humility 58; cultural safety 64; culturally responsive

practices for Black women; culturally
sanctioned art practices 80; 87–102;
gendered nature of materials 59; in
relation to the ExpressiveTherapies
Continuum 31–32; traditions and
prohibitions 11; *see also* economic
considerations
Curry, N. A.242, 246
Czerwiec, M. K. 194

Dachez, J. 198
Day, S. 180
Dead Pioneers 121
Dean, M. L. 6, 19, 37
Dean, T. 282
del Rey Cabero, E. 197, 198
de Vos, A. 153
Diggs, L. A. 13, 14
digital art tools and technologies:
advantages and challenges 13–14;
applications in art therapy 3, 13–17;
in comics creation 200–201, 205, 208;
design collaborations14; digital gaming
212–213; future developments 17;
integration into basket weaving 127–
128; music sampling 126–127; safety
considerations 63–64; scanography
218–222
Dillon, G. L. 119
disability: and ableism 60; and comics
194, 198;and disability justice 104, 106;
and disability studies literature 38–39;
and fashion 110; and fiber arts 5
displacement: and art materials used in
crisis contexts 268; and border politics
268–269; and cultural appropriation
244–245; and Indigenous peoples
123–124; and loss of home 272–273,
285; and nature of crisis contexts
267–269; and relationship with
ancestral homelands 117, 120–122;
and socio-political-environmental
antecedents 266

Dissanayake, E. 88
dissociative identity disorder *see* complex
identity systems
Divine Feminine 91–92
Divya 11
Do It Yourself (DIY) ethos 34, 73
doll making 6, 88, 97, 228
Donald, D. 42
Downing, J. 165
Drass, J. M. 133
drawing: in comics practice 199, 202–203;
of forbidden images 11; materials
168–169, 175; as research focus 18;
sand mandalas 151; as undertheorized
materials and practice 19, 37
Du, X. 14
Duran, E. 141

Eastwood, C. xxiv, 14, 133
eco-art 147–160
ecological approaches to art therapy: art
as environmental activism 147–160;
art as holding space for environmental
grief, pain, beauty, and empathy
147–160; challenges of outdoor
environments 8; environmentally
responsible use of materials 38–39,
57–58; Indigenous knowledges 7,
40–45; materials and settings 7–8,
62; overview of eco-art therapy 7–10;
relational accountability 117–128
economic considerations: crafts
and economic empowerment 4,
58; pathologization of economic
deprivation 60; socio-economic access
to materials 38–39, 59–60, 222, 259
Ehinger, J. 16
Ehinger, J. F. 220
Ehlert, R. 38
Elbrecht, C. 37
Elkin, L. xxiii
Elkis-Abuhoff, D. 18, 66, 246
Eliasson, O. 149

embroidery 5, 15, 72, 182–183

epistemic injustice 242

Erickson-Schroth, L.165

Eshuis, L. V. 214

ethics: of art materials, media, and practices 38–39, 49–69, 149–150, 270–271; of classical yoga principles and practices 239, 241; of culture-specific art forms 18, 246–248, 271; feminist ethic of care 107–108, 111–112; Indigenous, ecological, and new materialism's ethical relationality 9, 40–45, 117–118, 148–150; of therapist self-reflexivity xxiv, 105; *see also* cultural appropriation; cultural considerations; socio-economic considerations

Evans, J. S. B. T. 142

Evans, S. 212

Expressive Therapies Continuum 30–32, 168, 202

Fairbairn, M. 45

Fanon, F. 244

Feder, S. 165

Feen-Calligan, H. 287

femme identity 106–108

Fenner, P. 43, 136

Ferchaud, A. 213

Ferguson, D. 179

Fernandez, K. T. 194, 198

Ferranto, J. 5, 185

festival art therapy 281–294

fiber arts: history of use in art therapy xxiii, 3–6; as self-care for women in helping professions 70–83; in social practice 178–193; in textile comics 203–204

Figley, C. R. 75

figurines 139, 142–143

Fincher, S. 151, 242, 246

Finke, L. 165

Finlay, R. 194, 198

Fisher, J. 135, 138

Fishman, A. 194, 198

Flahavan, C. 5

Ford, E. 133

Forster, I. 257

found objects: in community care 228 practices; in eco-art 147–160; as economically just and environmentally responsible materials 59; history of use in art therapy 3, 6, 19; personal and socio-cultural significations 33–34; in scanography 218–219; as talismans 5

Fox, N. J. 39

Franco, G. E. 212

Franklin, M. 50, 247

Freeman, J. 13

Freeman, L. 273

Freire, P. 164

Fricker, M. 240, 242

Fridley, M. 252

Frost, S. 100

Frostig-Newton, K. 190

Fry, G. 182

Gallardo, L. 198, 205

Gantt, L. 10

Garcia, L. M. 187

Garlock, L. R. 5, 72, 73, 204

Gaspar da Silva, M. 5, 64

Gazit, I. 18

Geller, P. 229

gender-affirming care: and benefits of arts participation 166; centering hope and joy 164–165; as defined by transgender participants 173–174; and manicures 113; and materials/media considerations 168–169; with transgender children and their families 179–18

gender diversity and politics: association of crafts with women 71, 73, 79; avatars for gender exploration 17, 212–213; body as art material for transgressing gender norms 38; disrupting gendered nature of art materials 5–6, 59, 106, 110, 113, 179–181; legislative impact on gender-affirming care 165–167, 180, 181; misogyny in public greenspaces 8

Gerbeza, T. 218, 220, 221

Getahun, D. 188

Gheorghiu, D. 282

Gilligan, C. 148

Ginwright, S. 88

Gipson, L. xxiv, 38, 58, 87, 89, 92, 230, 242, 258

Giraldo, M. 260

Glinzak, L. 6

Golub, D. 184

Gómez Carlier, N. 12

González-Hidalgo, M. 10

Goodbrey, D. M. 200

Gopalakrishna, M. 58, 59

Goshen, I. 74

Grant, P. 199, 200

Graveline, F. J. 117

Graves-Alcorn, S. L. 31

Green, M. J. 194

Greenfield-Sanders, T. 90

Greenhalgh, P. 71

Grilo, D. 187

Gussak, D. 61

Gutierrez, A. 110

Hacmun, I. 17, 214, 216, 217

Hadley, S. 37

Haeyen, S. 17

Hagan, C. 241

Haines, S. 194, 197

Halpern, C. 255–257, 261

Hamilton, M. 218, 220, 221

Hamingson, Z. 252, 261

Han, B. 156

Hanania, A. 11

Harari, Y. 158

Haraway, D. J. 160

Hardy, L. J. 231, 232

Hardy, S. 181

Harper, N. J. 148

Harrigan-Farrelly, J. 188

Harvey, S. 256

Havard, J. 57

Havsteen-Franklin, D. 43, 198

Hellblade: Senua's Sacrifice 213

Henderson, P. 242, 246

Henderson, P. L. 4

Hendricks, M. L. 168

Hershler, A. 194, 197

Hetherington, R. 59, 61

Hickey-Moody, A. 39, 43, 44

Higginbotham, E. B. 97

Hinz, L. 19, 30–32, 199, 202, 204, 205

Hogan, S. 18, 188

Homer, E. S. 5, 204

Horovitz, E. G. 14, 61

Hoskin, R. A. 106–108

Houpt, K. 6, 252

Hu, J. 9

Huet, V. 133

Huizinga, J. 201

Human Rights Campaign 163

Human Rights Watch 271

Hunt, D. 64

Hurston, Z. N. 229

Husgafvel, V. 244

Huss, E. 59, 74

Huxtable, A. E. 194

Imarisha, W. 167

Immigration and Customs Enforcement (ICE) detentions 188–190

improv (theatrical improvisation): as art material and method 253, 255–257; defining characteristics 254–255; *yes, and* technique 253, 256–262

The Improvised Shakespeare Company 260

inclusive spaces and practices: challenging ethnocentric assumptions 58; contextualizing practice within a socio-cultural-political understanding

of history and current injustices 235, 266; 282–283; disrupting binaries of normativity 44; focusing on access for most marginalized to create access for all 229; welcoming people of diverse identities through space and materials 62–63, 267; *see also* access needs; belonging
Indigenous futurisms 119–120
Indigenous knowledges 40–45, 50, 118
Indigenous methodologies 117–118
Indigenous storywork 118–119, 122–128
Intentional Peer Support 134, 136
intersectionality: and cultural safety 64; and decolonized care 90–91, 106–107; and ethics 55; and Indigenous polyvocality 116–117; and New Materialism 44
Isaad, V. 96
Ishikawa, M. 240, 241, 243, 246, 247
Isis, P. 18, 242, 246

Jacobs, D. 194
Jacobson, L. 134
Jacobson-Levy, M. 6
Jagodowski, T. J. 254, 255
Jamerson, J. 201
James, S. E. 168
Janani, K. S. 108, 109
Jewell, M. 134, 136
Jhaveri, K. 51, 55, 246–248
Jin, H. 181
Johanson, R. 187
Johansson, J. 198
Johnson, J. L. 63, 64
Johnson, R. 38
Joseph, C. 166
joy: Black Woman joy 89, 101; trans joy 163–175
Judah, H. 149
Jung, C. G. 242
Jung, E. 148

Kabat-Zinn, J. 240, 242, 246
Kagin, S. L. 168
Kaimal, G. 4, 17, 18, 73, 74, 214–216, 244, 245
Kalmanowitz, D. 13, 61, 268, 284, 292
Kalwak, W. 10
Kanouse, S. 127
Kapitan, A. 50, 62
Kapitan, L. 6, 7, 12, 266
Karasawa, C. 256, 257
Katoshevski, M. 11
Katz, C. 150
Kaur, R. 186
Kausthub, S. 239
Kavitski, J. 16
Keaveny, R. 16
Kedar, I. 139
Kelly, B. T. 97
Keogh, K. 18
Kerr, C. 231
Khan, R. 198, 202, 204, 205
Ki, P. 36, 49, 55
Kichler, R. 163
Kikuchi, Y. 73
Kim, H. 149
Kim, H. K. 216
Kim, J. 13
Kindler, R. 252
Kinnaird, E. 141
kitchen as metaphor for art studios 225–227, 232–233
Knight, T. 154
Koch, S. C. 74
Kohut, M. 6
Kometiani, M. K. 13
Kopytin, A. 15
Kovach, M. 116–118
Krumer-Nevo, M. 74
Kuo, R. 53
Kuspit, D. 287

LaBar, L. 182
Lamar-Becker, S. L. 91

Lambert, B. 59
land art 9, 150
Latour, B. 273
Lazar, A. 14, 59
Lebaron, M. xxiii
Ledbetter, A. 187
Lee, J. 75
Lee, K. xxiii
Lee, L. C. B. 12
Leenerts, E. 73
Leone, L. 5, 185
Lepore, C. 165
Leung, W. 32
Levine, S. K. 9, 254–256
Lev-Wiesel 133
Li, L. 187
liberatory: climate justice 10;
    gender-affirming care 164–165;
    mindfulness centered in social
    justice 241; spaces 60, 227, 229–230,
    234–236
Lippard, L. R. 71
Liu, C. 220
Liu, Y. 214, 216
lived experience: of complex identity
    systems, autism, neurodiversity
    131–144; of disability 106, 111–112;
    of displacement 267; of loss, illness,
    trauma, and disability represented in
    comics 194, 197–198, 200–201; of
    people affected by social exclusion and
    discrimination 284; underrepresented
    in field's literature 19
Lloyd, B. 267, 268, 273, 284
Lloyd-Hazlett, J. 252
López-González, M. A. 254
Lorde, A. 150
Lorentzsen, K. 242, 246
Lorenzo de la Peña, S. 19
Lorraine, T. 286
Love, M. 258, 259
Lucas-Falk, K. 194
Lucie-Smith, E. 71
Lusebrink, V. B. 30, 168, 274

Mageary, J. 6
Mainardi, P. 72
Malchiodi, C. A. 133, 245, 246
Mallet, W. 218
mandala: in eco-art 147–160; cultural
    significance 158–159, 242–244; ethical
    guidelines for use in art therapy 246–
    249; in research 18; see also cultural
    appropriation
Manthe, L. 58, 150
Mardou Draws 198
Marin, D. 159
Martin, R. 14
Martinez, K. 167
Martínez-Vazquez, S. 187
Martinique, E. 156
Martyn, J. 59
Masotti, P. 117
maternal healthcare 181–190
Matott, D. L. 19
McAndrew, T. M. 255
McAvoy, J. 6
McCloud, S. 184, 200
McCreight, D. 194, 197, 198
McLachlan, C. 285
McNiff, S. 8, 18
Mead, S. 134, 136
Meade, N. A. 242, 244, 245
Medina, C. 167
Medina, J. 251
Mental Health Commission of
    Canada 88
Metzl, E. S. 63
Miller, G. 15, 17
Miller, J. J. 75
Miller, M. M. 228
Miller, S. M. 38
Millner, J. xxiii
Mims, R. 65
mindfulness: ethical guidelines for use
    in art therapy 246–249; historic roots
    239–240; problematic integration into
    Western therapy 240–242
Mingus, M. 60, 108, 166

miniature clay bricks 270–279
Miranda, D. A. 117
Misemer, L. 200, 201
Misluk-Gervase, E. 256
Monet, A. 92
Moon, B. L. 61, 62, 256
Moon, C. H. xxiv, 3, 4, 9, 12, 29, 33, 38, 43, 44, 58, 65, 74, 111, 133, 148–150, 233, 234, 248, 256, 271
Moore, V. T. Y. 252–254, 259, 260
Moretti, V. 194
Morris, J. 104, 108
Morrison, T. 93
Morton, L. 186
Mosinski, B. 64, 220, 221
Moxley, D. P. 5
Moyers, B. 92
Mulholland, M. J. 197, 198
Mullan, J. 106, 133, 141
Mulligan, M. 166
Mundt, K. xxiii, 51
mutual aid/care: as collective response to systemic injustice 228, 230; and disability justice principles 106; and DIY ethos 34; and relational safety 64–65; and social practice art therapy 58; and the transgender community 163

Naess, A. 150
nail polish 103–115
Napoli, M. 5, 7, 12, 50, 59
Nash, G. 7, 8, 62
Neal, L. xxiii, 9
Neville, B. 150
New Materialism: implications for art therapy 42–45; as informed by Indigenous knowledges 40–42; key concepts 39–40
Nixon, L. 119
Njoku, A. 188
Nolan, E. 287, 291
Nordenstam, A. 203, 204

Nordström, B. 6
Norris, M. 29

O'Connor, N. 7
Office of Health Improvement and Disparities 284
Oglesby, C. 226
O'Keefe, V. M. 120
O'Leary, M. E. 104
Omori 213
O'Neill Haaga, M.169
Open Brush 215
Orbach, N. 7, 57
O'Rourke, K. 290
Orr, P. 13
Ottiger, N. 15, 17

Pagano, C. J. 252
Page, C. 88
painting/paint: as applied with a wheelchair 60; cross-cultural significance 32; and digital painting apps 14, 200; and finger paint 135; history in art therapy 3, 19, 37; and improvisational principles 257; and nail polish 112–113; and paint pens 168
Papadopoulos, R. K. 272, 282
papermaking 18, 19, 58
Park, S. 11
Parker, R. 71, 72, 74
Parris, J. M. 246
Partridge, E. 59
Peahl, A. F. 186
pedagogy: 253, 281, 283–284, 286–292
Pedersen, H. 6
Peer Art Therapy (PATh) 131–144
Peled, E. 74
Pellow, D. 10
Pénzes, I. 17
performance art: and eco-art 159; examples in arts therapies literature 256; and maternal health disparities 185–188; and untapped therapeutic

potential 37–38, 110; and the walking
studio 290; *see also* Theatre of the
Oppressed
Peterson, B. C. 13
Phang, C. 194, 198
Phillips Sheesley, A. 252
photography: in art therapy history
3; and associated language 34; in
current art therapy practice 14–15;
and scanography 219–220; with
smartphones 17
Piepzna-Samarasinha, L. L. 104
Pinna-Perez, A. 256
place-based art forms (architecture,
installation art, built environment):
in border territories 268; in relation
to public events 285, 292; therapeutic
potential 20
placemaking 89, 101, 281–283
Pollanen, S. 73, 74
Portelli, G. M. 110
Potash, J. S. 32, 59
Prana, S. 241
Pruden, H. 117
psychoeducation and comics 197–198
public practice art therapy: festival
event in city wounded by sectarian
violence 281–283; makerspaces
in marginalized communities
232–234; Pride Festival to address
gender-affirming care 171–173; public
video screenings to address social
issues 16; traveling loom to reunite
neighborhoods 6
Purrington, B. 283
Putcha, R. S. 241, 243, 244, 249

Qian, J. 188
quilting 5–6, 182, 230–231

racism: within Immigration and Customs
Enforcement (ICE) detention
188–190; within maternal healthcare

185–188; and reproductive rights
181–185
Raffaelli, T. 18
Rambachan, A. 240
Ranganathan, S. 239–242, 245, 249
Rangarajan, S. 243, 244
Rankanen, M. 18
Reed, E. 163
Reer, F. 212
Reinholz, D. L. 60
relational aesthetic 8–9, 43–44;
65; 150
reproductive justice 181–190
research: on art and crafts materials,
media, and practices 3, 15, 17–20,
50–51; on crafts practices of women
in helping professions 70–80; on
gender-affirming care 163–177
Reynolds, F. 73
Rice, R. 212
Rifkind, C. 194
Riley, J. 73
Ringrose, J. 40
Ringstrom, P. 252
ritual: and culturally connected art forms
51, 58, 87, 92, 94–100, 247, 287; as
daily stabilizing practice 225, 227, 236;
in performance art 187; for personal
and collective healing 6, 15, 287; as
self-care 105, 109
Roberts, L. J. 4
Robertson, K. 179, 227
Roots & Roses 111, 133
Rootwork Gallery 89
Rosiek, J. L. 41, 42
Ross, C. 181
Roth, G.136
Royster, R. 6, 228
Rubin, J. A. 133
Rubin, R. 16
Rusch, D. C. 213
Rutan, S. J. 259
Ryu, S. 17

safer spaces and materials: cultural/ intersectional safety 64; physical safety 61–62; physiological safety 61, 168; psychological/emotional safety 62–64, 168–169; relational safety 64–65, 122, 134, 140–144

Sagan, O. 133

Said, E. W. 244

Sajnani, N. 246, 247

Salom, A. 11, 12

Sanger, M. 182

Sarris, G. 17

Saulnier, C. F. 74

Sawyer, S. 212

Sayre, D. 166

scapegoating and impotence *vs.* improvisational mindset 259–260

Scarborough, V. 56

Scavarda, A. 194, 198

Schorr, M. 61

Schwartz, A. 107

Schwenke, D. 252

sculpture: body sculpture 96–97; history in art therapy 3; social sculpture 286–287, 290, 292; as underexplored practice 19

Segalo, P. 5, 39

self-care: and commodification of culture specific practices 242–244; and manicures 105, 111; and marginalized communities affected by systemic injustice 228, 230; and women in helping professions 70–80

self-reflexivity xxiv, 18, 105–107, 266

Selvaraj, K. 50, 241, 242, 246, 249

Serano, J. 108

sewing: applications in art therapy 5, 98–99; for collective care and social change 182–185, 230–231; historical perspective 71

sex positivity 5, 63

Shah, A. 120

Shajarizadeh, A. 186

Shamri Zeevi, L. 16, 17, 214

Shange, N. 91

Sharman, Z. 165, 167

Shearer, M. 243

Sheikhai, S. 49, 55

Sherwood, P. 135

Shilling, R. D. 198

Shimoni, S. 76

Shimshak, C. 127

Shiner, L. 71

Sholette, G. 242

Shwed, A. 199

Siano, J. 58

Simpson, L. B. 119, 120, 122

Sins Invalid 106

Siossian, E. 154

Skaife, S. xxiii

Slaby, J. 32

Smith, B. 184

Smith, L. T. 118

Smolarski, K. 18

Snir, S. 18

Snyder, K. 201

Sochanik, J. 58

social action 10, 184, 233–234; *see also* activism

Social Constructivist Theory of Materiality 33–36

social media: in art therapy 15; helping participants navigate online exposure 63–64; as means for integrating cultural heritage and emerging facets of identity 11; as medium for voice and visibility of displaced people 269, 274

Song, J. E. 198

Sood, S. 242, 243

Soubosky, N. 110

spacemaking 87, 89–90, 92–96, 101

Spade, D. 233

Speigel, A. N. 194

Springham, N. 19

Staebler, C. 219

Starling, C. G. 245

StateoftheART Gallery 219
Steele, K. 135
Steinberg, J. 184
Stewart, N. 182
stickers 168, 175, 199
St John, G. 292
storytelling: in comics 194, 200–202, 204,
    208; as counternarrative 231–234; with
    digital media 13; for healing, agency,
    and community building 184–185, 190;
    as Indigenous cultural practice 118–
    119, 122–128; for transgender joy and
    authenticity 163
street art/artists 287–289, 292
Street Buddha 288
stress: among asylum seekers 269; among
    general public 178, 204, 240, 244, 246;
    among helping professionals 70–71,
    74–75, 77, 79; among postpartum
    patients 188; among transgender
    people in medical settings 168
Strom, D. 171
Strom, K. 40, 42
Sullivan, E. 189, 190
Sullivan, L. 290
Sundberg, J. 41
Suzuki, S. 178
Swanson, H. A. 150
Szuster, M. 255

Tachine, A. R. 119
Tajuddin, F. N. 179
TallBear, K. 41, 42, 44
Talwar, S. 4, 5, 59, 104, 111, 246–249,
    256, 258, 274
tattooing 37–38, 51, 109–111
Taylor, H. 272
Taylor-Johnson, H. 5
tele-art therapy 15, 61–62
Testa, R. J. 168
Thaller, S. 194, 197
Thayer, F. 63
Thayer-Cox, C. 133, 134
Theatre of the Oppressed 88, 92, 96

theory: color theories 141; critical race
    theory 229; feminist theory 74; nature
    of theory development 29; queer
    theory 106; social exchange theory 227;
    theory of mind 205, 216; theories of
    materiality and making 29–48; see also
    Critical Theory; Expressive Therapies
    Continuum; New Materialism; Social
    Constructivist Theory of Materiality
Thrall, J. 6
Till, K. E. 282
Timm-Bottos, J. 9, 57, 61, 167, 227,
    283, 285
Ting-Toomey, S. 228
TJ and Dave 258
Todd, S. 252
Todd, Z. 41
togetherness as material 227–228
Tordoff, D. M. 178
Torrealba, D. B. 188
transgender children 179–181
trauma: ableism trauma 60; art materials
    and practices for addressing trauma 5,
    73, 148, 197, 208, 212, 213; colonizing
    approach to trauma 141; COVID-19
    and collective trauma 181, 204;
    intergenerational trauma 54, 245,
    247–248; secondary trauma 74; sexual
    assault trauma 79, 104, 108, 109, 111;
    social trauma in city wounded by
    conflict 282, 284, 290–291
Tripp, T. 274
Tsing, A. L. 150
Tuan, Y. 291
Tubbs, C. 73, 74
Tunnacliffe, C. M. 292, 294
Tuval-Mashiach, R. 16

UNESCO 147
United States Department of
    Justice 120
Unpacking 213
U. S. Government 95
Usiskin, M. 15, 268, 269

Valldejuli, K. 12
Valoma, D. 121
Van Den Berg, Z. D. 59, 107
Van Der Kolk, B. 254
van Laar, C. 185
Van Leeuwen, T. M. 141
VanMeter, M. L. 31
Van Niel, F. 150
Vanzant, I. 95
van Zyl, J. 6
Varner, G. R. 51
Velasquez, M. 8
Vellodi, K. 36
Venba 213
video and animation: applications in art
    therapy 16; in digital comics 200–201,
    204; history in art therapy 3
virtual reality and avatars: aftercare 216;
    applications and challenges 16–17,
    212–215, 217–218, 221–222; in digital
    gaming 212–213; Open Brush digital
    game 215–216
Vivien, J. 12
Vuorinen, J. 221

Walker, A. 90, 92, 94
Walker, E. 198
walking art practice 281–282, 287–292
Waller, D. 136
Walley, B. 127
Walters, J. A. 15
Wardle, A. 8
Warson, E. 7
Watts, V. 42
Wazana Tompkins, K. 40
weaving, knotting, wrapping 5, 6,
    127–128
webcomics 200–201
Weinberg, T. 55

Weintraub, L. xxiii
Weiser, J. 14
West, C. 135
Whitaker, P. 8, 9, 62, 283, 284, 287, 290
Whitehead, A. L. 184
Whyte, M. K. 7, 11, 31, 32
Wiener, A. 156
Wiener, D. J. 252
Wierzbicka, A. 141
Wikler, A. 119
Wilkinson, R. A. 62
Wilson, S. 121
Winlaw, K. 136
Winnicott, D. W. 252
Wisenthal, P. 194
Wolk, N. 5, 185
womanist approach 87–90
Wong, D. 19
Wong, T. Y. W. 18
Woodford, A. E. 63
Woods, A. 133
World Health Organization 133
wounded city 281–283, 290–292
Wright, T. 148

Yalom, I. 259
Yam, R. 71, 73
Yi, C. S. 5, 38, 60, 110, 179, 256, 258
Yoon, I. H. 117
Youngson, B. 72

Zaken, S. B. 11
Zappa, A. 166
Zehavi, R. 71
Zigon, J. 228
Zittoun, T. 233
Zubala, A. 13
Zumdick, W. 286

For Product Safety Concerns and Information please contact our EU
representative GPSR@taylorandfrancis.com
Taylor & Francis Verlag GmbH, Kaufingerstraße 24, 80331 München, Germany

www.ingramcontent.com/pod-product-compliance
Lightning Source LLC
Chambersburg PA
CBHW070710280326
41926CB00089B/3447

9 781032 710181